Fundamentals of Anaesthesia and Acute Medicine

Anaesthes
Obstetrics and
Gynaecology

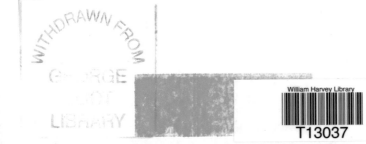

FUNDAMENTALS OF ANAESTHESIA AND ACUTE MEDICINE

Series editors

Ronald M Jones, Professor of Anaesthetics, St Mary's Hospital Medical School, London, UK

Alan R Aitkenhead, Professor of Anaesthesia, University of Nottingham, UK

Pierre Foëx, Nuffield Professor of Anaesthetics, University of Oxford, UK

Titles already available:

Cardiovascular Physiology (second edition)
Edited by Hans-Joachim Priebe and Karl Skarvan

Clinical Cardiovascular Medicine in Anaesthesia
Edited by Pierre Coriat

Intensive Care Medicine
Edited by Julian Bion

Management of Acute and Chronic Pain
Edited by Narinder Rawal

Neuro-Anaesthetic Practice
Edited by H Van Aken

Neuromuscular Transmission
Edited by Leo HDJ Booij

Paediatric Intensive Care
Edited by Alan Duncan

Forthcoming:

Pharmacology of the Critically Ill
Edited by Maire Shelly and Gilbert Park

Fundamentals of Anaesthesia and Acute Medicine

Anaesthesia for Obstetrics and Gynaecology

Edited by

Robin Russell

Consultant Anaesthetist and Honorary Senior Clinical Lecturer, Nuffield Department of Anaesthetics, John Radcliffe Hospital, Oxford

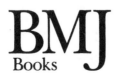

© BMJ Publishing Group 2000

First published in 2000
by the BMJ Publishing Group, BMA House, Tavistock Square,
London WC1H 9JR

www.bmjbooks.com

British Library Cataloguing in Publication Data

A catalogue record for this book is available from the British Library

ISBN 0-7279-1276-3

Typeset by Phoenix Photosetting, Chatham, Kent
Printed and bound by J W Arrowsmith Ltd, Bristol

Contents

Contributors

Michael Avidan
Clinical Lecturer, Department of Anaesthetics, King's College Hospital, London, UK

James Eldridge
Consultant Anaesthetist, Department of Anaesthetics, Queen Alexandra Hospital, Portsmouth, UK

Caroline Grange
Consultant Anaesthetist, Nuffield Department of Anaesthetics, John Radcliffe Hospital, Oxford, UK

Philippa Groves
Consultant Anaesthetist, Department of Anaesthetics, King's College Hospital, London, UK

Kym Osborn
Staff Specialist, Department of Women's Anaesthesia, Women's and Children's Hospital, Adelaide, South Australia

Michael Paech
Staff Specialist, Department of Anaesthesia, King Edward Memorial Hospital for Women, Perth, Western Australia

Jackie Porter
Consultant Anaesthetist, Department of Anaesthetics, St Thomas' Hospital, London, UK

Robin Russell
Consultant Anaesthetist and Honorary Senior Clinical Lecturer, Nuffield Department of Anaesthetics, John Radcliffe Hospital, Oxford, UK

Mark Scrutton
Consultant Anaesthetist, Department of Anaesthetics, St Michael's Hospital, Bristol, UK

Scott Simmons
Head of Department, Department of Women's Anaesthesia, Women's and Children's Hospital, Adelaide, South Australia

Richard Vanner
Consultant Anaesthetist, Department of Anaesthetics, Gloucestershire Royal Hospital, Gloucester, UK

Foreword

The Fundamentals of Anaesthesia and Acute Medicine series

The pace of change within the biological sciences continues to increase and nowhere is this more apparent than in the specialties of anaesthesia, acute medicine, and intensive care. Although many practitioners continue to rely on comprehensive but bulky texts for reference, the accelerating rate of biomedical advances makes this source of information increasingly likely to be dated, even if the latest edition is used. The series *Fundamentals of Anaesthesia and Acute Medicine* aims to bring to the reader up-to-date and authoritative reviews of the principal clinical topics which make up the specialties. Each volume will cover the fundamentals of the topic in a comprehensive manner but will also emphasise recent developments of controversial issues.

International differences in the practice of anaesthesia and intensive care are now much less than in the past and the editors of each volume have commissioned chapters from acknowledged authorities throughout the world to assemble contributions of the highest possible calibre. Three volumes will appear annually and, as the pace and extent of clinically significant advances vary among the individual topics, new editions will be commissioned to ensure that practitioners will be in a position to keep abreast of the important developments within the specialties.

Not only does the pace of advance in biomedical science serve to justify the appearance of an international series of this nature but the current awareness of the need for more formal continuing education also underlines the timeliness of its appearance. The editors would welcome feedback from readers about the series, which is aimed at both established practitioners and trainees preparing for degrees and diplomas in anaesthesia and intensive care.

RONALD M JONES
ALAN R AITKENHEAD
PIERRE FOËX

Preface

Obstetric anaesthesia continues to increase in popularity whilst advances in gynaecological surgery have implications for anaesthetic practice. This book is possibly the first text dedicated to both these aspects of women's anaesthesia.

Obstetric anaesthesia is rewarding in nature but appropriate training of correct technique can only increase the safety of both mother and baby during childbirth and is perhaps of greater significance. For those involved in the anaesthetic care of women undergoing gynaecological procedures there is now an increasing amount of laparoscopic work and an expansion in outpatient surgery. This book is aimed primarily at anaesthetists in training, with individual authors attempting to provide a thorough grounding of principles and practice of anaesthetic management based on current evidence. Due to its size the book is not a comprehensive review of all aspects of women's anaesthesia, but it should offer readers a helpful foundation on which to base their clinical practice.

ROBIN RUSSELL

1: Maternal changes in pregnancy

JAMES ELDRIDGE

During pregnancy a woman's physiology and anatomy change more rapidly than in any other stage of healthy adult life. What is normal in a non-pregnant woman may be abnormal during pregnancy and equally, what is abnormal when not pregnant may be normal in pregnancy. Optimal anaesthesia requires knowledge of how a woman's body adapts during pregnancy, labour, and delivery. This chapter reviews the changes of which the anaesthetist needs to be aware and examines the important issues when anaesthesia is to be provided for women who require non-obstetric surgery during pregnancy.

Physiological changes

Cardiovascular system

Haemodynamic studies in pregnancy are notoriously difficult to interpret. Many of the earlier studies reported that cardiac output and blood pressure fell in the third trimester but unfortunately, no precautions were taken to avoid aortocaval compression. Other investigations have used early post-partum values of cardiovascular variables as controls for pregnant values. These are unsuitable because some haemodynamic changes persist for several months into the postpartum period, especially in breastfeeding mothers. The most informative studies have followed mothers serially from before conception and then throughout pregnancy, avoiding the supine position during all assessments. Various techniques have been used to assess cardiac output during pregnancy, including the Fick method, thoracic impedance (which has proven unreliable), thermodilution (which requires invasive instrumentation), and echocardiography. Even though echocardiography is not as accurate as thermodilution, because it is not invasive, women find that serial measurements through pregnancy are acceptable.

Echocardiography has revealed that left ventricular mass increases during

1

pregnancy, just as it increases in athletes starting an exercise training programme. In this respect, pregnancy appears to be comparable to a prolonged period of moderate exercise. Cardiac output starts to increase early
in the first trimester, probably under a hormonal influence. By the eighth
gestational week, output has risen by over 20%[1] and it peaks at approximately 50% above the non-pregnant state by the end of the second
trimester. Cardiac output then changes little until term. The earliest rise in
cardiac output is a result of an elevated heart rate but by the end of the first
trimester, the increased stroke volume is the predominant cause. Although
in the third trimester, stroke volume may fall a little, cardiac output is maintained by the heart rate, which continues to increase slightly[2] (Fig 1.1).

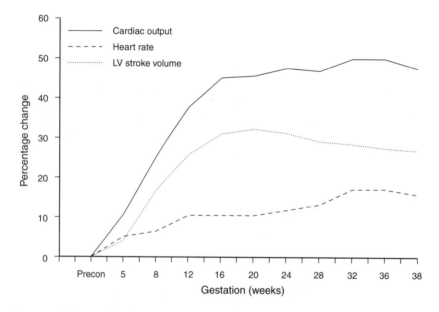

Fig 1.1   Changes in cardiac output, left ventricular stroke volume and heart rate
during pregnancy expressed as a percentage of the preconceptual value (from
Robson et al.[2] with permission)

Despite an elevated cardiac output, blood pressure falls in early pregnancy. Diastolic pressure reaches its nadir by midgestation, reflecting a
35% decline in the peripheral vascular resistance.[2] By term, the diastolic
pressure returns to pre-pregnant levels although the peripheral vascular
resistance remains 20% below its pre-pregnant value. The fall in peripheral
vascular resistance is predominantly due to the low resistance of the placental intervillous space, although progesterone, prostacyclin, and oestrogens also promote systemic vasodilation.

The aortic area increases by about 14% during a woman's first pregnancy
and this appears to be a permanent change. Aortic compliance also

increases, producing a marginal fall in systolic pressure during the second trimester but, in normal pregnancy, systolic pressure will have returned to pre-pregnant values by term.[2]

Pulmonary vascular resistance falls during pregnancy, so that pulmonary blood pressure does not change despite the increased cardiac output.[3] Pulmonary capillary wedge pressure is unchanged but as colloid oncotic pressure falls, the gradient in pulmonary transcapillary pressure is reduced. By term the transcapillary pressure has fallen by nearly 30%, suggesting a greater propensity for pulmonary oedema.[3]

Despite an increase in blood volume, central venous pressure is unaltered because of an increase in venous capacitance.

Cardiovascular changes in labour

Cardiovascular activity is increased further by labour. Women with cardiovascular disease are at particular risk during the peripartum period because of rapid changes in cardiac output, preload and afterload.

In labour, sympathetic activity increases, particularly in women who do not receive regional analgesia.[4] Between contractions, the heart rate may not alter but stroke volume, cardiac output, and blood pressure steadily rise. When the cervix has dilated to 8 cm, stroke volume is elevated by nearly 30%.[5]

With each contraction, direct compression of the intervillous space occurs and blood is forced out of the placental unit, producing an autotransfusion. The central venous pressure rises,[6] stroke volume is augmented, and cardiac output increases.[5,7] If the pain of labour is well controlled with a regional block, the heart rate may fall during a contraction but cardiac output still climbs by 10–15%.[7] Without regional analgesia, the increase in cardiac output is greater and the heart rate increases rather than falls.[8]

At delivery, the intervillous space is eliminated and there is an immediate reduction in venous capacity. The associated autotransfusion usually exceeds blood loss and so there is a rapid rise in central venous pressure and cardiac output to approximately 25% above prelabouring values.[5] Over the succeeding hours this declines slowly, returning to prelabouring values on the second postpartum day. Cardiac output remains above pre-pregnancy values for 12–24 weeks.

Aortocaval occlusion

Between 1932 and 1935, Ahltorp published three papers describing how pregnant women who were positioned supine became nauseated, hypotensive, and cyanotic and even lost consciousness. He found that the symptoms could be produced in some women even when they were prone if the uterus was lifted and pushed posteriorly. He correctly hypothesised that the symptoms might be due to inferior vena cava compression.[9] These symptoms are now referred to as the supine hypotensive syndrome. All pregnant women are at risk of developing the supine hypotensive syndrome because the posterior aspect of the enlarging uterus is in close proximity to the great vessels of the abdomen. Angiography reveals that inferior vena caval compression is commonplace.[10] If venous return to the right atrium is significantly impaired, cardiac output falls and this may be followed by hypotension. However, in many women the collateral circulation through the epidural and azygous veins is sufficient to maintain an adequate cardiac output. Even so, vena caval occlusion can still be detected by a rise in femoral venous pressures.

Elevated femoral venous pressures have been demonstrated in the supine position as early as the 16th week of gestation,[11] but it is very unusual for women to develop supine hypotension before 20 weeks. If a woman at term is placed in a supine position, femoral venous pressures rise to twice their normal value[11] and complete occlusion of the inferior vena cava occurs in over 90% of individuals.[10] Only 60% of women, however, become symptomatic when supine because collateral venous circulation and compensatory systemic vasoconstriction are sufficient to maintain blood pressure. Even at term, less than 10% of women actually develop overt supine hypotensive syndrome.[12] If symptoms do occur, they usually become apparent within 3–10 minutes of adopting a supine position, although occasionally symptoms may take up to 30 minutes to appear.

Inferior vena caval occlusion not only causes femoral venous pressures to rise but also causes elevated pressures in uterine veins which may compromise placental perfusion. This is less likely if the placenta has implanted in the fundus of the uterus because ovarian veins, which usually drain into the inferior vena cava above the site of compression, commonly provide sufficient collateral circulation to prevent engorgement of the placental bed.[13]

Placental blood flow may also be compromised by aortic compression. Complete occlusion is rare but partial occlusion is common at term. The site of compression is usually at the pelvic brim and occurs most frequently during contractions in early labour. Partial occlusion of the aorta may not affect brachial artery blood pressure but systemic vascular resistance rises and cardiac output may fall. Pressure in the femoral arteries falls and, more importantly, the pressure in the uterine arteries is reduced because the origin of the uterine vessels is usually below the site of aortic compression. This, in combination with elevated venous pressure, compromises placental perfusion and hence fetal oxygenation. Kauppila and colleagues found that intervillous blood flow was reduced by 20% when pregnant women were turned from a left lateral to a supine position.[14] During labour, as the fetal head descends into the pelvis, the severity of aortic occlusion is reduced.[15]

Various maternal positions have been suggested to reduce the incidence of aortocaval occlusion. Techniques such as adopting a semirecumbent position or flexion of the hips have been suggested but these are not as effective as tilting the mother laterally.[15] To reduce the pressure of the uterus on the inferior vena cava, the left lateral wedge is most commonly employed. Over 90% of women find that a left wedge alleviates symptoms more effectively than a right wedge. Classically, a 15° tilt is recommended, although partial vena caval occlusion may be present even in the full lateral position. It is only in the prone position, with the uterus hanging freely, that caval compression does not occur. Aortic compression is also known to be present even with a tilt of over 30° and is only relieved in the full lateral position.[15] If a 15° tilt does not relieve symptoms of supine hypotension, then the tilt should be increased until symptoms abate.

Respiratory system

As the pregnant uterus enlarges into the abdominal cavity, the diaphragm becomes elevated and the transverse diameter of the thoracic cage increases. By term the thoracic cage is nearly fully expanded and inspiration is almost exclusively produced by diaphragmatic descent. Although total lung capacity is slightly reduced during pregnancy, vital capacity hardly changes.[16,17] Tidal volume increases and by term reaches 30% greater than pre-pregnant values with half of the increase occurring in the first trimester.[18] Early in pregnancy the increase in tidal volume is accommodated by a reduced inspiratory reserve volume. In the third trimester, it is the expiratory reserve volume that is reduced, while the inspiratory reserve volume actually increases. By term, expiratory reserve volume has fallen by 25% and residual volume is also reduced by 15%. The combination of these changes produces a 20% fall in functional residual capacity (FRC) (Fig 1.2).[16] The reduction in FRC occurs predominantly in the third trimester and, not surprisingly, is dependent on maternal posture with a much greater reduction in FRC occurring when women are supine. Even though the closing volume is unchanged by pregnancy,[17] the fall in FRC causes airway closure in 50% of supine women at term, making them vulnerable to hypoxia.[19]

The reduced FRC and increased oxygen demand make pregnant women prone to desaturate more rapidly than non-pregnant women during periods of apnoea. Archer and Marx found that after intubation and ventilation with 97% oxygen for four minutes followed by 60 seconds of apnoea, arterial oxygen tension fell by 7.8 kPa in non-pregnant women, while in pregnant women the fall was 21 kPa.[20] This reinforces the importance of preoxygenation before induction of anaesthesia in pregnant women.

Gas flow through the airways is little changed by pregnancy. Although the hypocapnia of pregnancy would tend to cause bronchconstriction, the large airways dilate (probably under the influence of progesterone), maintaining the conductance of the airways. Flow volume loops, forced

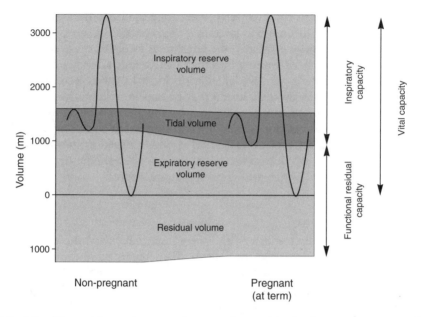

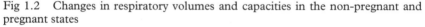

Fig 1.2   Changes in respiratory volumes and capacities in the non-pregnant and pregnant states

expiratory volume in one second (FEV_1) and the ratio of FEV_1 to forced vital capacity (FEV_1/FVC) are all unchanged.[17]

Oxygen consumption increases by nearly 60% during pregnancy.[18] The increased demand is predominantly due to fetal requirements but maternal cardiac, respiratory, renal, and uterine consumption also contribute. Carbon dioxide production mirrors this increase.[18] The respiratory rate is only marginally increased by pregnancy but the combination of an increased tidal volume and a reduction in physiological dead space[21] nearly doubles the alveolar ventilation. The reduced physiological dead space is probably caused by improved perfusion of ventilated alveoli. The change in alveolar ventilation is under hormonal control as the supply of oxygen and the excretion of carbon dioxide are in excess of requirements.[22] The controlling agent is, once again, most likely to be progesterone as the arterial partial pressure of carbon dioxide is inversely related to the progesterone concentration.[23] Progesterone increases the sensitivity of the respiratory centre to carbon dioxide and acts as a direct respiratory stimulant.[24]

The hyperventilation of pregnancy decreases arterial carbon dioxide partial pressure to approximately 4.0 kPa. This fall occurs by the end of the first trimester and is maintained thereafter.[18] The gradient between endtidal and arterial carbon dioxide partial pressure is also reduced during pregnancy. In non-pregnant women this gradient is usually 0.5–0.8 kPa. At the end of the first trimester the gradient is often negligible and by term the gradient occasionally reverses. Therefore in pregnant women, the endtidal carbon dioxide partial pressure can usually be assumed to correlate closely with the arterial carbon dioxide partial pressure.

Arterial oxygen partial pressure increases marginally during pregnancy provided the supine position is avoided. This increase is most marked in the first trimester and declines towards pre-pregnant values by term.[25] The fall in physiological dead space contributes to improved oxygenation, as does a change in arteriovenous oxygen difference. The arteriovenous oxygen difference is reduced in pregnancy, because oxygen supply is increased more than oxygen demand.

Renal compensation for respiratory alkalosis occurs with serum bicarbonate falling from 24 to 20 mmol/l, although arterial pH remains slightly raised.[26] Despite maternal alkalosis, the P_{50} of the oxyhaemoglobin dissociation curve increases steadily throughout pregnancy,[27] most probably because of an elevated 2,3 diphosphoglycerate concentration (although not all studies have found raised 2,3 diphosphoglycerate levels). Elevation of the P_{50} increases the delivery of oxygen from maternal haemoglobin to fetal haemoglobin as well as to maternal tissues.

During labour, painful contractions cause further hyperventilation and arterial pH values in excess of 7.50 are not uncommon. This reduces respiratory drive and may cause periods of apnoea and maternal hypoxia between contractions, particularly if systemic opiates are given for pain relief. Indeed, Deckardt found that primiparous women in labour who received epidural analgesia with local anaesthetics alone had a mean oxyhaemoglobin saturation of 94.3% while those given systemic opiate had a mean saturation of 88.8%.[28] However, epidural opiates may also cause hypoxic episodes. Porter and colleagues found that women given epidural analgesia with an infusion of 0.0625% bupivacaine plus 2.5 µg/ml fentanyl have significantly more periods of desaturation below 95% than women receiving an epidural infusion of plain 0.125% bupivacaine.[29]

Gastrointestinal system

Over 70% of pregnant women suffer from heartburn.[30] Anatomical changes and hormonal effects on smooth muscle tone promote reflux of gastric contents into the oesophagus. During pregnancy, the stomach is shifted cephalad and the intra-abdominal portion of the oesophagus is often displaced into the thoracic cavity[30] which reduces the efficiency of the lower oesophageal sphincter. (The lower oesophageal sphincter is sometimes referred to as the lower oesophageal high pressure zone, as no true anatomical sphincter exists in the lower oesophagus.) Moreover, the pressure which the lower oesophageal sphincter can exert is reduced in pregnancy by the smooth muscle relaxant action of progesterone. While the competence of the lower oesophageal sphincter is reduced, the intragastric pressure rises because the enlarging uterus compresses the intra-abdominal contents. The barrier pressure is the difference between the intragastric pressure and the lower oesophageal sphincter pressure. Reduction in barrier pressure is associated with heartburn in women in their first trimester,[31] although at what stage in gestation an asymptomatic woman is at increased risk of regurgitation remains a matter of debate. The hormonal influence on lower oesophageal tone starts in early pregnancy but compression of intra-abdominal structures by the uterus is insignificant before the 20th week of pregnancy. Vanner studied 100 women undergoing termination of pregnancy, 50 during the first trimester and 50 in the second.[32] He found that the incidence of gastro-oesophageal reflux into the lower oesophagus was not significantly different between groups. Potentially more serious was that reflux into the upper oesophagus occurred in two women, one in each trimester. However, this was no more frequent than would be expected in the non-pregnant population.

Should regurgitation occur, the consequences are determined, at least in part, by the volume and acidity of the intragastric contents. Serial studies of acid production throughout pregnancy have proved difficult to perform because women are understandably reluctant to swallow nasogastric tubes repeatedly. Gastrin has been used as a surrogate marker for gastric secretion. It is a polypeptide hormone secreted by the antrum of the stomach and induces copious gastric secretions. Maternal plasma gastrin concentration rises steadily through the second and third trimesters of pregnancy.[33] However, to conclude that this indicates a steadily rising level of gastric secretion may be wrong, as direct measurements of gastric volume in cohorts of women in each trimester of pregnancy suggest that both the basal and histamine-augmented gastric secretion and acidity are unchanged in the first and third trimesters and are actually marginally reduced in the second.[34]

Gastric emptying also affects the residual volume in the stomach. Over the years, various methods have been used to assess gastric emptying, including gastric aspiration, realtime ultrasound, epigastric impedance, applied potential tomography, X-ray studies and radioisotope techniques. Most studies, however, have used the paracetamol absorption technique because of its simplicity and ready acceptance by pregnant women. The technique correlates closely to the rate of clearance of liquid from the stomach. The majority of recent studies suggest that there is little change in gastric emptying times between non-pregnant controls and women in the first, second or third trimesters.[34] Even in early labour gastric emptying is rarely prolonged[35] but some delay does occur in women near to delivery.[36] Gastric emptying is dramatically slowed if systemic opiates are given for pain relief in labour.[35,37] In contrast, pain relief with an epidural infusion of local anaesthetic and fentanyl at up to 20 μg/h does not alter gastric emptying,[38] although large boluses of epidural opiates may have some effect.

8

The risk of regurgitation in the postpartum period decreases rapidly. Reduction in intra-abdominal pressure occurs immediately on delivery and, 20 hours postdelivery, the acidity and volume of gastric contents are the same as in non-pregnant controls. Lower oesophageal sphincter tone may take longer to return to pre-pregnant strength. In a study of 25 conscious women between 24 and 80 hours postpartum who were placed in four positions including lithotomy, five regurgitated. However, this was a lower proportion than in non-pregnant controls and considerably lower than the 17 of 25 in whom reflux was observed before delivery.[39] In the same study, reflux did not occur in any woman more than 48 hours post delivery. These data suggest that by 48 hours postpartum, women do not routinely require intubation providing there are no other specific indications.[40]

Haematology

Both red cell mass and plasma volume increase during pregnancy. However, the increase in plasma volume is proportionally greater and this results in the well-known physiological anaemia of pregnancy. Plasma volume starts to increase in the first trimester and expands rapidly in the second, with a small further increment in the third trimester. Early studies suggested that plasma volume actually decreased in the third trimester but this was probably the result of women being placed supine when measurements were made. By term plasma volume has expanded by nearly 50% (1500 ml).[41,42] This expansion is under hormonal control.[43] Progesterone increases aldosterone production and oestrogens increase renin activity, promoting salt and water retention. The increase in total body water varies markedly between women but is about 6000 ml by the later part of the third trimester.

The haematocrit falls during pregnancy by nearly 15%,[42] although the red cell mass actually increases. Studies on the red cell mass before the 12th week of gestation are contradictory but from the end of the first trimester, it is clear that the red cell mass increases steadily, reaching 30% above the pre-pregnant level by term.[42,44] The increase in red cell mass parallels, and is probably caused by, an increase in erythropoietin. The source of erythropoietin is not established but is likely to be predominantly renal, although some placental or fetal production may contribute.[45]

The physiological anaemia of pregnancy may be important in preventing placental infarcts. Koller noted that haemoglobin concentrations above the norm for any particular stage of gestation were associated with intrauterine growth retardation and placental infarcts while anaemia in pregnancy led to placental enlargement.[46] He hypothesised that the higher viscosity produced by increased haemoglobin concentration was a causative factor for placental infarcts.

Platelet count is unaltered between the second and third trimesters but platelet turnover changes. Platelet distribution width is an indicator of thrombocytopoietic activity in the bone marrow. During pregnancy, distribution width increases, implying an increased production of platelets. As the platelet count is unaltered, platelet consumption must also be increased. Several studies have suggested that platelet half-life is reduced in pregnancy, although this is only marked in pre-eclamptic women.[47] Not only is platelet activity increased but platelet function is also changed, as bleeding time is reduced during pregnancy. In the peripartum period platelet activation is, not surprisingly, increased further. Platelet factor 4 and β-thromboglobulin are indicators of platelet activation and both are increased during labour, peaking during delivery itself.[48]

Reduced prothrombin and partial thromboplastin times in addition to changes in thromboelastography all indicate that a hypercoagulable state exists during pregnancy. Although partly caused by the change in platelet function, the clotting cascade and fibrinolytic system are also modified. Most, but not all of the clotting factors are increased. Plasma concentrations of factors I, VII, VIII, IX, X, and XII are all elevated, while those of factors II and V are unaltered.[49,50] Furthermore, the concentration of antithrombin III, an inhibitor of the clotting cascade, is reduced by term. The fibrinolytic system is activated during pregnancy. Fibrin degradation products are significantly elevated at term, implying a state of accelerated coagulation and fibrinolysis.[51] Although fibrinolytic activity is depressed during labour itself, it rises within 15 minutes of delivery and within one hour fibrin degradation products are increased. Plasma fibrinogen decreases rapidly with placental separation.[50]

Blood loss at delivery varies widely. Following vaginal delivery, average blood loss is approximately 600 ml, while at caesarean section it may be up to 1000 ml.[52] During the first five postpartum days, the haematocrit continues to fall. The haematocrit on the second postpartum day correlates most closely with the haematocrit six weeks postpartum.[53] Blood volume decreases over the first seven days, returning to near pre-pregnant levels by nine weeks postdelivery.

Hepatic function

The gross anatomy of the liver is little changed by pregnancy although it is displaced laterally and cephalad in the third trimester. The elevated cardiac output of pregnancy is not reflected by any change in liver blood flow. However, physiological function of the liver is altered. A proliferation of smooth endoplasmic reticulum occurs, with a steady increase in hepatic microsomal activity. Progesterone in particular induces this increased hepatic activity. At the same time progesterone also competitively inhibits oxidative reactions. In contrast, conjugative reactions are unaffected.

Total body albumin is increased in pregnancy, although serum albumin concentration falls by 25%. The ratio of albumin to globulin is also reduced.[54] Serum concentrations of some specific carrier proteins, such as thyroid-binding globulin, may rise during pregnancy.[55]

Many liver enzymes are increased to the upper limits of their normal range including aspartate transaminase, alanine transferase, lactate dehydrogenase, and γ-glutamyl transpeptidase.[54] Although alkaline phosphatase increases by up to 400%, this is predominantly caused by placental production of the enzyme.

Certain signs of liver disease, including palmar erythema and spider naevi, are common during pregnancy but are rarely indicators of significant pathology. However, pregnant women are more prone to gallstone production. Bravermann demonstrated that, following a test meal, gallbladder emptying is prolonged in early pregnancy and is both prolonged and incomplete during the third trimester.[56]

Renal function

During pregnancy the kidneys increase in length by about 1 cm[57] and both the ureters and the pelvicalyceal system dilate. Ureteric dilation is produced by increased smooth muscle mass during the first trimester. This is enhanced in the second trimester by the enlarging uterus compressing the ureters at the pelvic brim, producing partial ureteric obstruction.[58] Both the ureters and the pelvicalyceal systems return to pre-pregnant dimensions by 12 weeks postpartum.

Renal blood flow increases early in the first trimester, reaching about 75% above pre-pregnant levels by term.[59] The increase in renal blood flow is associated with a 50% rise in glomerular filtration rate (GFR). Early studies demonstrated a fall in both renal blood flow and GFR in the third trimester but this only occurs when estimates are made with women in a supine position.

Although production of urea and creatinine is little altered during pregnancy, the increase in GFR reduces the plasma concentrations of both. These reach a nadir by the end of the first trimester and are maintained near this level until term. During pregnancy estimates of renal function should always be compared with values that have been established as being "normal" for the particular gestation. Such is the case for uric acid, the concentration of which has become one of the standard markers of renal function in pre-eclampsia. Normal renal handling of serum uric acid is complex, involving free filtration by the glomeruli, then almost complete reabsorption in the proximal tubule with a small proportion being resecreted back into the tubular lumen before a further phase of reabsorption. Altogether, only 10% of the filtered load is excreted. During pregnancy, although there is little change in purine metabolism, uric acid levels fall in the first trimester but then gradually increase to near pre-pregnancy levels at the time of delivery.[60]

The increase in GFR presents more glucose to the distal tubules. As pregnant women do not increase their tubular reabsorption of glucose in parallel with the increase in GFR, glucosuria is not uncommon. During pregnancy glucosuria does not necessarily indicate either renal disease or diabetes mellitus and usually resolves within a week of delivery.

Osmoregulation is also altered by pregnancy with a fall of approximately 10 mOsm/kg during gestation. This is not compensated by an increased water excretion, indicating a change in antidiuretic hormone secretion. However, total body sodium does increase by 500–900 mmol.[58] Although progesterone promotes sodium excretion, its effects are more than counterbalanced by the elevated levels of aldosterone, renin, angiotensin, and oestrogens, all of which promote sodium reabsorption.

Renal compensation for the respiratory alkalosis of pregnancy occurs (see above), with the serum bicarbonate falling from 24 to 20 mmol/l. However, capacity for renal bicarbonate reabsorption remains unaltered during pregnancy.

Immune function

Pregnancy produces a unique immunological state in which the host tolerates the presence of foreign tissue. The survival of the human species is dependent on this tolerance but the precise mechanism by which it occurs remains to be determined.

The immune system can be divided into two distinct components: cell-mediated immunity and humoral immunity. These interact to protect the host from both pathogenic and neoplastic invasion. Cell-mediated immunity is produced by phagocytes, which activate a non-specific response, and by T-lymphocytes which confer specific immunity. Between 50% and 70% of phagocytes are neutrophils. Natural killer cells form a subpopulation of phagocytes, making up 5–10% of monocytes, and provide resistance to viral infections and suppression of neoplastic cells. Humoral immunity is composed of the antibody and the complement systems. Antibodies are produced by modified B-lymphocytes called plasma cells and the complement system is made up of a series of proteins, which, when activated, culminate in the formation of a membrane attack complex.

Even in the non-pregnant individual, immune activity varies with time, which complicates comparative studies between the pregnant and non-pregnant state because the control level of activity is difficult to assess. However, although studies are contradictory, most indicate that pregnancy is associated with only minor changes in overall function of the immune system.[61] While T-cell activity and quantity appear to be unaltered,[62] the effectiveness of the natural killer cells is diminished although their number is maintained.[63] The leucocyte count increases only marginally through pregnancy but in labour it rises rapidly to approximately 11 000 mm^{-3} and peaks on the first postpartum day at 15 000 mm[-3]. This rise is predominantly due to increased numbers of neutrophils. The leucocyte count returns to normal by the sixth postpartum week.

The concentrations of immunoglobulins A, G, and M and *in vitro* antibody function are unchanged by pregnancy,[55] although specific humoral antibody titres may alter. In the immediate postpartum period the B-lymphocyte population may decrease, although it is constant during pregnancy itself. The concentration of complement proteins and their activity are either maintained or increased during pregnancy.[64]

Most epidemiological studies of infections during pregnancy also suggest an immune system that is functioning normally,[61] although some infections are more common. In particular, viral infections with polio, hepatitis A and B, and cytomegalovirus are more prevalent and pathological. Protozoal infections with malaria, toxoplasmosis, amoebiasis, giardiasis, and trypanosomiasis are also more common. Autoimmune diseases, however, may improve during pregnancy.

Despite apparently normal function, the immune system adapts in ways not fully understood, allowing a pregnant woman to carry her fetus. Whilst the exact mechanism remains to be determined, some factors have been established.[61] On a cell surface, the human leucocyte antigen (HLA) determinants are one of the major sites for assessing antigenicity. HLA determinants are usually polymorphic structures but on trophoblast cells they are monomorphic and other antigenic markers appear to be missing. This low density of immunogens may limit a pregnant woman's ability to respond to trophoblast cells. In addition, although the T-lymphocyte's response to a systemic challenge of fetal cells is normal, local response at the placental site appears suppressed. Even when cytotoxic T-lymphocytes are present, they appear unable to kill trophoblast cells.[65] This is probably due to a local release of immunosuppressive agents from placental tissues.

Central nervous system

There is little evidence of major change in central nervous system (CNS) activity during pregnancy but minor changes in pain threshold, susceptibility to general and local anaesthetics, and alterations in sympathetic activity all occur.

In animal experiments, pain threshold during pregnancy has been found to increase. The mechanism is probably mediated through opiate receptors, as intrathecal or systemic opiate antagonists reverse the change in pain threshold.[66] These receptors may be stimulated by an increased concentration of endorphins. In human pregnancy, the plasma concentration of β-endorphin has been variously reported as either unchanged or elevated but during labour the concentration increases significantly.[67] The source of the endorphins is not clear. The placenta may contribute and the fetal unit may also produce endorphins, as the umbilical arterial concentration of endorphins is higher than the umbilical venous concentration. However, endorphins do not readily cross the blood–brain barrier and in humans the concentration of β-endorphin is not increased in cerebrospinal fluid, even in labour,[67] so the exact site of analgesic action of β-endorphin remains to be determined.

As pregnancy progresses, there is a steady rise in the activity of the sympathetic nervous system. In particular, sympathetic tone of venous capacitance beds in the legs is increased,[68] suggesting a susceptibility to sympatholytic events such as epidural anaesthesia.

The pharmacodynamic responses to general and local anaesthetics are altered by pregnancy. The minimum alveolar concentration (MAC) of halogenated inhalational agents in ewes is reduced by 25–40%.[69] This is probably caused by the increased progesterone concentration, although changes in serotonin[70] and endorphin levels may also have a role.

In pregnancy the rise in progesterone concentration also reduces the amount of local anaesthetic required to block nerve conduction. Interestingly, acute exposure to progesterone does not alter the sensitivity of nerves to local anaesthetic agents,[71] but prolonged exposure does.[72] This suggests that progesterone induces a mediator that actually produces the alteration in neuronal function. During pregnancy a given dose of either intrathecal or epidural local anaesthetic blocks more dermatomes than in non-pregnant controls, the effect starting in the first trimester. This may be due to increased susceptibility of the nerve fibres to the local anaesthetic but the anatomical changes in the epidural space that occur during pregnancy also contribute.

Anatomical changes

The vertebral canal

During pregnancy the lumbar lordosis of the vertebral column is often more prominent. This alters the relationship of the iliac crest to the lumbar spine. At term, the line between the crests is at the height of the L3–4 interspace while in non-pregnant women, it is more commonly at the L4–5 interspace.

Location of the epidural space may be more exacting for several reasons. Subcutaneous deposition of adipose tissue and interstial oedema may make palpation of the vertebral spines difficult whilst the lumbar lordosis reduces the distance between adjacent lumbar spines. In addition, the presence of a gravid uterus at term may prevent a women from adequately flexing her back. The ligaments are softened by the change in the hormonal milieu during pregnancy and this alters the feel of the ligamentum flavum. Finally, the epidural veins become engorged, especially during uterine contractions, and so are more likely to be punctured during insertion of an epidural

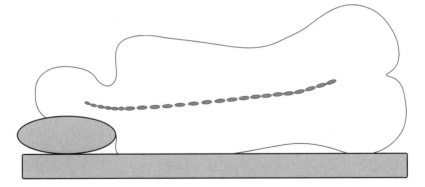

Fig 1.3　When lying laterally, a pregnant woman's hips are usually broader than her shoulders. The spinal canal is therefore tilted head down and this may increase the cephalad spread of hyperbaric intrathecal solutions

catheter. Distension of epidural veins may increase the spread of local anaesthetic within the spinal canal. Rostral movement of intrathecal local anaesthetic is also increased in pregnancy as engorged epidural veins compress the dural sac. This is enhanced in a lateral position because, at term, maternal hips are usually significantly wider than shoulders and therefore the vertebral column is tilted slightly head down (Fig 1.3).

Airway changes

The increase in interstitial fluid that occurs in pregnancy, combined with capillary engorgement, results in mucosal oedema and hyperaemia. This often causes nasal stuffiness and nose bleeds are common.[73] The false cords and arytenoids may be swollen and occasionally vocal cord oedema can cause life-threatening airway obstruction.[74] Airway management may also be hindered by enlargement of breast tissue, making insertion of a laryngoscope into the mouth awkward. Below the vocal cords the bronchi are usually slightly dilated during pregnancy and although the physiological dead space is reduced, the anatomical dead space is unchanged. The upward displacement of the diaphragm causes a widening of the bronchial angle and the lateral diameter of the chest is increased.[73]

Pharmacological changes

Pharmacokinetics

Maternal pharmacokinetics are altered by the physiological changes of pregnancy. Uptake, distribution, metabolism, and elimination of drugs are all affected and the overall effect on free plasma concentration of agents may be unpredictable.

15

Although gastric emptying during pregnancy is little changed, the reduced intestinal motility alters uptake of oral drugs. Drugs that are slowly absorbed in the small bowel, such as digoxin, may have increased bioavailability.[75] More dramatically, if systemic opiates are given during labour and gastric emptying arrested, any subsequent orally administered drug has little effect unless it is absorbed in the stomach. In the immediate postpartum period, when gastric emptying returns to normal, the reverse is true. A large dose of drug may be presented to the small bowel and this may result in an excessive plasma concentration. Oral uptake may be affected by iron supplements and antacids which are commonly prescribed in pregnancy. These agents may chelate other pharmacological agents, preventing their absorption.[75]

Uptake of inhalational agents is affected by respiratory and cardiovascular changes of pregnancy. Both gestational hyperventilation and reduction in functional residual capacity produce a more rapid equilibration of inhaled, alveolar and hence arterial partial pressure of agents. This effect is counteracted by the increased cardiac output of pregnancy but respiratory effects predominate.

The volume of distribution of most agents is increased. This particularly affects polar water-soluble drugs, which are predominantly dispersed across the extracellular space. This increases by as much as 5 l during pregnancy. Lipid-soluble drugs also have an increased volume of distribution but the proportional increase is rather smaller. The activity of these drugs is usually more affected by changes in protein binding.

Albumin concentration falls by about 25% at term.[55] Acidic drugs, such as salicylates and most anti-epileptic agents, and some neutral drugs, such as warfarin, are primarily bound to albumin. The fall in albumin concentration increases the free drug fraction of these agents. This effect is enhanced by the increase in the fatty acid concentration that occurs in pregnancy as fatty acids competitively reduce the number of binding sites on each albumin molecule. With fewer binding sites available, free drug fraction of an agent increases. The increase in free drug fraction counteracts the fall in total drug concentration produced by expansion of the volume of distribution so that, despite an apparent decrease in total drug concentration, free drug concentration may actually rise.[76]

Basic drugs such as local anaesthetics are bound to α_1-acid glycoprotein, the concentration of which changes little during pregnancy. However, α_1-acid glycoprotein is an acute-phase protein and serum concentration may increase by 50% in the peripartum period.[77] The clinical significance of this increase has not been addressed. The concentration of some binding proteins such as thyroxine-binding globulin, caeruloplasmin, and transferrin also increases during pregnancy.[55]

Most drugs are eliminated either through the renal system or by hepatic metabolism or both. Renal excretion predominates for many water-soluble agents. The increase in renal blood flow, glomerular filtration rate, and creatinine clearance that occurs during pregnancy is accompanied by an increase in excretion of water-soluble drugs such as pancuronium. Lipid-soluble agents are more commonly metabolised in the liver before excretion.

Drugs with a high first-pass hepatic extraction, such as lignocaine, are relatively unaffected by changes in liver enzyme activity. Although they would be affected by changes in liver blood flow, this actually alters little during pregnancy and so metabolism of these agents is not significantly changed. In contrast, drugs with a low first-pass metabolism are relatively immune to changes in liver blood flow but are affected by changes in enzyme activity. Progesterone is a potent inducer of hepatic enzymes and this results in an increase in hepatic extraction of drugs such as phenytoin, paracetamol, and some β-blockers.[75]

Plasma cholinesterase concentration falls by about 25% by term and in the immediate postpartum period it falls by a further 35%.[78] Agents that are eliminated by plasma cholinesterase, such as suxamethonium, mivacurium, and remifentanil, might be expected to have a prolonged duration of action. The effect of reduced plasma cholinesterase concentration on suxamethonium, however, is offset by an increase in volume of distribution and consequently the duration of action of suxamethonium is actually unchanged at term. In contrast, in the immediate postpartum period, as volume of distribution falls rapidly, the duration of action of suxamethonium is prolonged by about three minutes.[79]

In general, during pregnancy the half-life of polar drugs is reduced whereas, for more lipid-soluble agents, it is increased. However, it is not always possible to predict the changes that actually occur because of the multiple factors that influence the pharmacokinetic properties of an agent.

Anaesthesia for non-obstetric surgery during pregnancy

Between 0.75% and 2.2% of pregnant women undergo non-obstetric operations during their pregnancy.[80,81] A wide variety of surgical procedures are performed. Of 5405 non-obstetric operations carried out on pregnant women in Sweden between 1973 and 1981, 25% were classified as abdominal surgery, 19% genitourinary and gynaecological, and an additional 10% were classified as laparoscopic surgery. Almost all the laparoscopic surgery was performed in the first trimester.[80]

Although some diagnostic or surgical procedures have the potential to harm the fetus, important treatments should not be denied to pregnant women as the fetus is inescapably dependent on maternal health for continued survival. However, where possible, elective surgery should be postponed until after delivery.

When surgery is required, anaesthetists need to consider the effect of pregnancy on the mother and how anaesthetic technique can affect a developing fetus. The association between non-obstetric surgery and fetal outcome has been the focus of several investigations. Shnider found an 8.8% spontaneous abortion rate when he reviewed 147 women who underwent surgery during pregnancy.[82] Similarly, Brodsky found a fetal loss of 8.0% when surgery was performed in the first trimester and 6.9% in the second trimester compared to control rates of 5.1% and 1.4% respectively.[81] In the largest series reported so far, Mazze reviewed 720 000 births in Sweden.[80] He identified 5405 operations performed for non-obstetric reasons. In the group of women who underwent surgery, the incidence of premature delivery increased to 7.47% compared with a control rate of 5.13% (a 46% increase), with an associated increase in the number of neonates with very low birth weight. The predominant reason for fetal loss and premature delivery is probably the underlying medical condition rather than exposure to anaesthetic agents.

However, anaesthetic mishaps producing maternal hypoxia and hypotension are a threat to the fetus and even relatively small changes in maternal physiology may significantly compromise fetal health. To prevent fetal asphyxia, uterine blood flow and maternal oxygenation must be maintained. Studies in the pregnant ewe demonstrate that when uterine blood flow is reduced by 65%, fetal arterial oxygen tension falls by over 1 kPa and fetal acidosis follows within 10 minutes.[83] As uterine blood flow is not autoregulated, arterial hypotension or elevated venous pressure results in reduced uterine blood flow. Aortocaval compression must be avoided as it causes both. Furthermore, anaesthesia may be associated with hypocapnia, alkalosis or catecholamine release, all of which may lead to uterine arterial vasoconstriction.

In premature neonates, high fetal oxygen tensions may cause retrolental fibroplasia and promote closure of the ductus arteriosus. *In utero*, however, the fetus is protected from these potentially harmful effects because placental oxygen consumption and inequalities in distribution of placental blood flow prevent the fetus from achieving an arterial oxygen tension much above 9 kPa even when maternal arterial partial pressure of oxygen is above 85 kPa.[84] Thus, while maternal inspired oxygen concentrations above 50% have little benefit for the fetus, they cause it no harm and so higher maternal inspired oxygen concentrations can be safely used if required.

Teratogenicity may be defined as any significant postnatal change in form or function in an offspring after prenatal treatment. The risk of exposing a fetus to a teratogen varies with the gestational age of the fetus. Within two weeks of conception, teratogenic changes are unlikely as fetal loss is the more probable outcome for an affected fetus. Fetal abnormalities are more likely if exposure to a teratogen occurs between the fourth and 11th gestational week as this is the period of organogenesis. Some organs continue to develop after this period and so exposure to teratogens may still be harmful but changes are more likely to be minor morphological or functional changes. Causes of teratogenicity are diverse and include infection, pyrexia, hypoxia, and acidosis as well as the more well-recognised hazard of ionising radiation.

The association of drugs with teratogenicity is an emotive issue. Whilst evidence is often contradictory, few drugs are actually proven teratogens and none of these is routinely used in anaesthesia. Many drugs have, however, been implicated as possible teratogens. Most of the evidence giving rise to this concern has come from either epidemiological studies or animal experiments. As effects are usually rare, epidemiological studies must assess very large numbers of patients to establish a causative effect. Few prospective studies have been performed and none of them are large, but retrospective studies have been reported. Between 1963 and 1989 seven epidemiological studies were published that reviewed fetal deformities in women who had received an anaesthetic during pregnancy. A total of over 9100 patients were analysed. In all seven of these studies, the incidence of fetal deformities was no different from the matched control rate in women who did not undergo surgery. Unfortunately, these reports included a mixture of anaesthetic and surgical techniques and not all series specified in which trimester surgery took place.[80,85] By including patients who had a low risk of teratogenicity, such as those in the second or third trimester, a change in fetal deformity rate may have been masked. The group thought to be at greatest risk are those who undergo general anaesthesia in the first trimester. Of 2252 women identified by Mazze and Kallen who had surgery in the first trimester, more than 60% received general anaesthesia and a further 25% were given an unknown anaesthetic. Even in this high-risk group, the number of neonates with congenital abnormalities was almost identical to the expected number (44 vs 42.6) with the observed/expected ratio of 1.0 (confidence intervals of 0.8–1.4).[80] This would suggest that the risk of anaesthesia causing teratogenic changes is very small.

Despite reassuring information from these studies, there is still concern over particular agents, often because of information derived from animal studies. Extrapolation from animal studies to humans, however, must be treated cautiously especially as the duration and dosage of exposure to agents during the animal experiments often do not match those used clinically.

Premedication

Although several epidemiological studies suggested a link between chronic exposure to diazepam in the first trimester and subsequent cleft lip formation, this has not been supported by more recent studies.[86] No study has suggested that a single dose, as might be used for premedication, is associated with teratogenicity. Long-term administration may lead to neonatal withdrawal symptoms following delivery and exposure just before delivery may cause neonatal drowsiness and hypotonia.

Ranitidine and cimetidine are not known to be harmful but caution is advised with chronic exposure to cimetidine because of known androgenic effects in adults.

Induction agents

Thiopentone has been used for many years and does not appear to be associated with fetal abnormalities although formal studies have not been conducted. Chronic exposure to barbiturates may be associated with fetal anomalies although evidence is contradictory.

Reproductive studies in animals have suggested that propofol may lead to delayed or abnormal ossification. However, the effect of administering propofol to humans during early pregnancy has not been investigated and its use is therefore controversial. Studies using propofol during caesarean section at term suggest it is a safe agent to use in the third trimester although neonatal depression has been reported.

Animal studies of etomidate suggest that this agent is not teratogenic. Nevertheless, it is a potent inhibitor of cortisol synthesis and neonates have lower cortisol concentrations when women are given etomidate for induction of anaesthesia for caesarean section.[87]

Ketamine in early pregnancy increases intrauterine pressure, which may cause fetal asphyxia even though blood pressure is maintained. In the third trimester this increase in intrauterine pressure does not occur.

Inhalational agents

Halothane and isoflurane have been extensively used during pregnancy, suggesting that these are safe agents. Some animal data, however, give cause for concern. Several investigators have reported increased fetal loss and teratogenicity in animals following gestational exposure to halothane but these findings have not been reproduced by others.[88,89,90] One animal study suggested that isoflurane in high concentration might be toxic to the fetus, but this was not confirmed when lower doses were used.[91]

In humans the use of twice the minimum alveolar concentrations of halogenated vapours causes a significant reduction in maternal blood pressure and cardiac output with an associated fall in uterine blood flow, despite uterine vasodilation. Such high concentrations should therefore be avoided. Lower concentrations may also cause a fall in blood pressure but this appears to be compensated by uterine vasodilation. The halogenated vapours also cause uterine relaxation, which may be beneficial for surgery during pregnancy as premature labour may be prevented.

Nitrous oxide has been extensively investigated. It oxidises the cobalt in vitamin B_{12} from cob(I)alamin to cob(II)alamin. This inactivates the action of vitamin B_{12} as a coenzyme for methionine synthetase. Methionine syn-

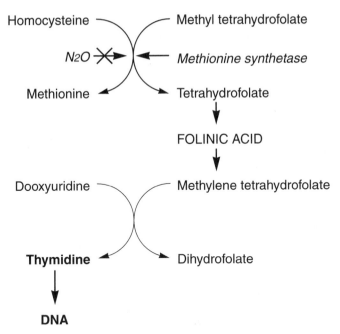

Fig 1.4 Nitrous oxide inhibits methionine synthetase, blocking the production of methionine and ultimately thymidine and DNA

thetase is required for the formation of methionine as well as thymidine, one of the subunits of DNA (Fig 1.4). The consequences of its inhibition are complex. Interference with DNA synthesis obviously gives rise to concern for teratogenic effects and animal studies have lent some support to this. Nitrous oxide has consistently been found to have teratogenic effects on Sprague-Dawley rats, although these effects only appear when the animals are exposed to 50–75% nitrous oxide for 24 hours on days 8 or 9 of their gestation, which is the period of greatest vulnerability. Confusingly, although folinic acid restores the ability to synthesise DNA, it does not prevent the teratogenic effects of nitrous oxide whilst simultaneous exposure to halothane does prevent these effects,[91] suggesting that the teratogenic mechanism may not simply involve methionine synthetase inhibition.

In humans, several epidemiological studies of occupational exposure to nitrous oxide during pregnancy have suggested an association between exposure and an increased incidence of teratogenicity and spontaneous abortion. Tannenbaum and Goldberg, however, reviewed 14 studies and concluded that despite the consistently positive results, the number of methodological errors was such that they could not accept the conclusion that occupational exposure to nitrous oxide caused adverse effects.[92] The American Society of Anesthesiology commissioned a similar report, which also failed to demonstrate any significant increase in congenital abnormalities or spontaneous abortion with occupational exposure to nitrous oxide.[93]

Muscle relaxants

Because muscle relaxants only cross the placenta in very small quantities, fetal exposure to these agents is limited. Animal data using doses of pancuronium, vecuronium, atracurium, and tubocurare nearly 300 times higher than the concentration of normal fetal exposure suggested that morphological changes may occur.[94] However, there are no data associating the commonly used depolarising or non-depolarising muscle relaxants with teratogenicity in concentrations comparable with those that a fetus is likely to be exposed to during clinical practice.

Anticholinesterase inhibitors

These agents are highly ionised and so, like muscle relaxants, do not readily cross the placenta. There is no evidence to suggest teratogenicity, although pyridostigmine, when used chronically to treat myasthenia gravis, may cause premature labour.

Analgesics

Although the opiates readily cross the placenta, brief exposure is safe. Long-term exposure will cause symptoms of withdrawal when the fetus is delivered. Animal studies have not demonstrated any teratogenic changes associated with exposure to morphine, fentanyl or alfentanil, providing the side-effects of hypoventilation and impaired feeding are eliminated. Use of any opiate near the time of delivery may cause neonatal depression.

Non-steroidal anti-inflammatory agents act through the inhibition of prostaglandin synthesis and their use in early pregnancy may cause bleeding and fetal loss. Case reports have also suggested that chronic exposure in the third trimester may cause premature closure of the ductus arteriosus and persistent pulmonary hypertension of the newborn.

Bupivacaine and lignocaine have a very good safety record. However, at nearly 10 times the maximum dose recommended for use in humans, bupivacaine has embryocidal effects in rats. When used at delivery, bupivacaine has no significant neonatal neurobehavioural effects, while lignocaine may have a mild effect.[95] Cocaine abuse during pregnancy may increase the incidence of fetal abnormalities in the genitourinary and gastrointestinal tracts.

Anaesthesia during the first trimester

When a pregnant woman is anaesthetised, the fetus is exposed to the anaesthetic agents. However, as already discussed, the direct risks from this are low. Of greater importance are the indirect effects on the fetus that may occur when anaesthesia alters maternal physiology. Periods of maternal hypoxia, hypotension, hyper- or hypocarbia must be avoided and uterine perfusion needs to be optimised. Haemorrhage causing significant maternal anaemia may also cause fetal hypoxia. Every effort must be made to maintain maternal physiological parameters in the range appropriate for gestational age throughout the perioperative period. Although each trimester has slightly different anaesthetic implications, these general principles should be observed at every stage of gestation.

The most common surgical procedure in the first trimester is laparoscopy but cervical cerclage is also common in the latter part of the first and early in the second trimester. Even when the initial expectation is that fetal loss is inevitable, anaesthesia should be performed with the assumption that the fetus will survive. To reduce the risks of teratogenicity and fetal loss, semi-urgent surgery should be delayed from the first to the second trimester whenever possible.

There are insufficient data to conclude whether regional or general anaesthesia is the safer option for either mother or fetus. However, many obstetric anaesthetists would argue that, when possible, regional anaesthesia should be used. In part, this is because drug exposure is minimal, especially when intrathecal local anaesthetics are used, and in part because regional anaesthesia allows the mother to continue to protect her own airway. Airway management in the first and early second trimester is a controversial subject. Within the first few weeks of pregnancy, the lower oesophageal barrier pressure falls. Because of this, some anaesthetists would recommend a rapid-sequence induction whenever general anaesthesia is administered to pregnant women, no matter what gestation. However, gastric emptying time is little changed by pregnancy.[34] Vanner and colleagues demonstrated that significant reflux is not increased in asymptomatic women during the first trimester.[32] Although aspiration is an important cause of maternal mortality, when Atrash reviewed maternal mortality in the United States between 1979 and 1986, none of the 21 deaths that were due to aspiration were attributed to surgery associated with medical abortion or hydatidiform mole.[96] These were the two procedures that were most likely to be performed without intubation. Furthermore, rapid-sequence induction is not completely devoid of risk. It is associated with a higher incidence of failed intubation,[97] which may promote loss of airway control. Suxamethonium, the most commonly used muscle relaxant for a rapid-sequence induction, is associated with potentially fatal side-effects. Anaphylactic reactions occur in between one in 5000 and one in 20 000 administrations and bradycardias, hyperkalaemia, and malignant hyperpyrexia may also occur with its use.

The overall balance of risk between intubation and mask anaesthesia for asymptomatic women during the first and early second trimester remains difficult to assess. While the issue remains unresolved, the majority of anaesthetists are happy not to intubate the trachea of otherwise uncomplicated pregnant women at 12 weeks gestation, while most would intubate pregnant women undergoing surgery after 20 weeks gestation.

Anaesthesia during the second trimester

From midgestation, some pregnant women become vulnerable to aortocaval occlusion. Although collateral circulation may be sufficient to prevent overt supine hypotension, uterine perfusion may still be compromised. Therefore all women after 20 weeks gestation should be tilted or wedged to the left during surgery.

During this trimester perioperative fetal monitoring becomes possible. From the 16th week of gestation the fetal heart can be detected with Doppler techniques and from around the 20th week, baseline variability of the fetal heart rate becomes apparent. At this point information about fetal well-being can be derived. This is only advantageous if the monitoring does not interfere with the surgery and if a useful intervention can be made to correct a detected abnormality. The value of fetal monitoring remains to be demonstrated but case reports of modification of anaesthetic technique and suppression of premature labour suggest that there are benefits to the fetus.[98] It should be realised, however, that interpretation of fetal heart rate during anaesthesia may be difficult. Loss of variability is to be expected with exposure to anaesthetic agents and mild fetal bradycardia is also common, especially if maternal hypothermia occurs. While a normal fetal heart rate is reassuring, abnormal fetal heart rates by themselves do not necessarily indicate fetal distress. Nevertheless, an advantage of monitoring is that if an abnormal fetal heart rate is detected, the anaesthetic technique can be reviewed to confirm that optimal conditions are being maintained.

Monitoring uterine activity postoperatively may offer the greatest benefit, as premature labour is a significant risk after surgery. Once the uterus has reached the umbilicus, an external pressure transducer can detect uterine contractions. If regular uterine contractions occur either pre- or postoperatively, appropriate tocolytic therapy can be instituted. Routine fetal and uterine monitoring of all pregnant women undergoing surgery has been recommended.[98]

Anaesthesia during the third trimester

In the third trimester the anaesthetic considerations are very similar to those of caesarean section at term except that uterine relaxation is advantageous and fetal depression is to be expected. As the fetus is viable, detection of fetal compromise becomes increasingly important because the baby may be delivered if necessary. While general anaesthesia is required for many surgical procedures, most obstetric anaesthetists would recommend regional anaesthesia whenever possible because at term regional anaesthesia has a 16-fold lower mortality rate than general anaesthesia.[99]

During the third trimester women become particularly vulnerable to hypoxia because of the combination of increased oxygen consumption and the reduced FRC, especially in the supine position. Adequate preoxygenation and denitrogenation are crucial. A rapid-sequence induction should always be used and, as in the second trimester, pregnant women must always be tilted or wedged to the left. Although excessive doses of volatile agents should be avoided, adequate doses must be maintained to avoid awareness. MAC is reduced during pregnancy but inadequate anaesthesia is associated with increased catecholamine release, which reduces placental blood flow. For the same reason postoperative analgesia must be effective. Although opiates can be used, they may result in maternal hypercarbia; regional analgesia with local anaesthetic agents may be advantageous.

In the third trimester every effort should be made to monitor the fetal heart rate and uterine activity as far as possible both during and after surgery. If severe fetal distress is detected and cannot be rapidly corrected, the baby should be delivered.

Surgical procedures during pregnancy

Intracranial haemorrhage causes almost 5% of maternal deaths.[100,101] Because intracranial pathology is relatively common during pregnancy, neurosurgery is actually performed surprisingly frequently. In Mazze's study of surgery during pregnancy, over 6% of operations were neurosurgical.[80]

Neuroanaesthetists often use mild hyperventilation to control intracranial pressure. Because a pregnant woman is already hypocapnic, arterial carbon dioxide partial pressure has to be reduced further to reduce intracranial pressure. Such hyperventilation impairs uterine blood flow, shifts the oxyhaemoglobin dissociation curve to the left and reduces fetal oxygenation. While the benefits of hypocapnia must be assessed carefully before use, in practice the fetus can usually tolerate a period of hypocapnia. Some centres also use deliberate mild hypothermia for neurosurgery, which the baby usually tolerates although fetal heart rate variability is lost and mild bradycardia is common. Osmotic diuretics (mannitol) are sometimes requested during neurosurgery but these can cause fetal dehydration and should be avoided if possible. Deliberate hypotension should only be employed if absolutely necessary as a sustained fall in blood pressure causes fetal hypoxia and acidaemia.

The incidence of cardiac surgery during pregnancy is probably rising. Pregnancy does not seem to increase the maternal mortality associated with the surgery, but fetal loss as high as 25% is to be expected with such operations. If cardiopulmonary bypass is required, the fetus appears to tolerate mild hypothermia well, although fetal heart rate patterns may become very abnormal. Whenever possible, blood pressure should be maintained above 60 mmHg, even during bypass. Fetal heart rate monitoring should be used and if the trace is unexpectedly abnormal, a remedial cause should be sought. Careful consideration should be given to the effect on the uterine circulation of the vasoactive drugs used. When possible, α-agonists should be avoided. However, maternal well-being should remain paramount.

References

1 Capeless EL, Clapp J. Cardiovascular changes in early phase of pregnancy. *Am J Obstet Gynecol* 1989;**161**:1449–53.

2 Robson SC, Hunter S, Boys R, Dunlop W. Serial factors influencing changes in cardiac output during human pregnancy. *Am J Physiol* 1989;**256**:H1060–H1065.

3 Clark S, Cotton DB, Lee W, *et al*. Central hemodynamic assessment of normal term pregnancy. *Am J Obstet Gynecol* 1989;**161**:1439–42.

4 Jouppila R, Puolakka J, Kauppila A, Vuori J. Maternal and umbilical cord plasma noradrenaline concentrations during labour with and without segmental extradural analgesia, and during caesarean section. *Br J Anaesth* 1984;**56**:251–255.

5 Robson SC, Dunlop W, Boys R, Hunter S. Cardiac output during labour. *BMJ* 1987;**295**:1169–72.

6 Hendricks CH. The hemodynamics of a uterine contraction. *Am J Obstet Gynecol* 1958;**76**:969–82.

7 Lee W, Rokey R, Miller J, Cotton DB. Maternal hemodynamic effects of uterine contractions by M-mode and pulsed-Doppler echocardiography. *Am J Obstet Gynecol* 1989;**161**:974–6.

8 Robson SC, Dunlop W, Boys R, Hunter S. Cardiac output in labour. *Br J Anaesth* 1987;**295**:1169–72.

9 Ahltorp G. Uber Ruckenlagebeschwerden bei Graviden [On problems in the supine position in pregnant women]. *Acta Obstet Gynecol Scand* 1935;**15**:295–341.

10 Kerr MG, Scott DB, Samuel E. Studies of the inferior vena cava in late pregnancy. *BMJ* 1964;**1**:532–3.

11 McLennan CE. Antecubital and femoral venous pressure in normal and toxemic pregnancy. *Am J Obstet Gynecol* 1943;**45**:568–91.

12 Kinsella SM, Lohmann G. Supine hypotensive syndrome. *Obstet Gynecol* 1994;**83**:774–87.

13 Bieniarz J, Yoshida T, Romero-Salinas G, *et al*. Aortocaval compression by the uterus in late human pregnancy. IV. Circulatory homeostasis by preferential perfusion of the placenta. *Am J Obstet Gynecol* 1969;**103**:19–31.

14 Kauppila A, Kokinen M, Puolakka J, Tuimala R, Kuikka J. Decreased intervillous and unchanged myometrial blood flow in supine recumbency. *Obstet Gynecol* 1980;**55**:203–5.

15 Kinsella SM, Whitwam JG, Spencer JAD. Aortic compression by the uterus: identification with the Finapres digital arterial pressure instrument. *Br J Obstet Gynaecol* 1990;**97**:700–5.

16 Alaily AB, Carrol K. Pulmonary ventilation in pregnancy. *Br J Obstet Gynaecol* 1978;**85**:518–24.

17 Baldwin GR, Moorthi DS. New lung functions and pregnancy. *Am J Obstet Gynecol* 1977;**127**:235–9.

18 Spatling L, Fallenstein F, Huch A, Huch R, Rooth G. The variability of cardiopulmonary adaptation to pregnancy at rest and during exercise. *Br J Obstet Gynaecol* 1992;**99**:1–40.

19 Russell IF, Chambers WA. Closing volume in normal pregnancy. *Br J Anaesth* 1981;**53**:1043–7.

20 Archer GW, Marx GF. Arterial oxygen tension during apnoea in parturient women. *Br J Anaesth* 1974;**46**:358.

21 Shankar KB, Moseley H, Vemula V, Kumar Y. Physiological dead space during general anaesthesia for Caesarean section. *Can J Anaesth* 1987;**34**:373–6.

22 Clapp J, Seaward BL, Sleamaker R, Hiser J. Maternal physiologic adaptations to early human pregnancy. *Am J Obstet Gynecol* 1988;**159**:1456–60.

23 Machida H. Influence of progesterone on arterial blood and CSF acid-base balance in women. *J Appl Physiol* 1981;**51**:1433–6.

24 Skatrud JB, Dempsey JA, Kaiser DG. Ventilatory response to medroxyprogesterone acetate in normal subjects: time course and mechanism. *J Appl Physiol* 1978;**44**:939–44.

25 Templeton A, Kelman GR. Maternal blood-gases, (PAO2 – PaO2), physiological shunt and VD/VT in normal pregnancy. *Br J Anaesth* 1976;**48**:1001–4.

26 Blechner JN, Cotter JR, Stenger VG, Hinkley CM, Prystowsky H. Oxygen, carbon dioxide, and hydrogen ion concentrations in arterial blood during pregnancy. *Am J Obstet Gynecol* 1968;**100**:1–6.

27 Kambam JR, Handte RE, Brown WU, Smith BE. Effect of normal and preeclamptic pregnancies on the oxyhemoglobin dissociation curve. *Anesthesiology* 1986;**65**:426–7.

28 Deckardt R, Fembacher PM, Schneider KTM, Graeff H. Maternal arterial oxygen saturation during labor and delivery: pain-dependent alterations and effects on the newborn. *Obstet Gynecol* 1987;**70**:21–5.

29 Porter JS, Bonello E, Reynolds F. The effect of epidural opioids on maternal oxygenation during labour and delivery. *Anaesthesia* 1996;**51**:899–903.

30 Bassey OO. Pregnancy heartburn in Nigerians and Caucasians with theories about aetiology based on manometric recordings from the oesophagus and stomach. *Br J Obstet Gynaecol* 1977;**84**:439–43.

31 Brock-Utne JG, Dow GB, Dimopoulos GE, Welman S, Downing JW, Moshal MG. Gastric and lower oesophageal sphincter (LOS) pressures in early pregnancy. *Br J Anaesth* 1981;**53**:381.

32 Vanner RG. Gastro-oesophageal reflux and regurgitation during general anaesthesia for termination of pregnancy. *Int J Obstet Anesth* 1992;**1**:123–8.

33 Attia RR, Ebeid A, Fischer JE, Goudsouzian NG. Maternal, fetal and placental gastrin concentrations. *Anaesthesia* 1982;**37**:18–21.

34 O'Sullivan G. The stomach – fact and fantasy: eating and drinking during labor. *Int Anesthesiol Clin* 1994;**32**:31–44.

35 Nimmo WS, Wilson J, Prescott LF. Narcotic analgesics and delayed gastric emptying during labour. *Lancet* 1975;**i**:890–3.

36 Nimmo WS, Wilson J, Prescott LF. Further studies of gastric emptying in labour. *Anaesthesia* 1977;**32**:100–101.

37 La Salvia LA, Steffen EA. Delayed gastric emptying time in labor. *Am J Obstet Gynecol* 1950;**59**:1075–81.

38 Kelly MC, Carabine UA, Hill DA, Mirakhur RK. A comparison of the effect of intrathecal and extradural fentanyl on gastric emptying in laboring women. *Anesth Analg* 1997;**85**:834–8.

39 Vanner RG, Goodman NW. Gastro-oesophageal reflux in pregnancy at term and after delivery. *Anaesthesia* 1989;**44**:808–11.

40 Bogod DG. The postpartum stomach – when is it safe? *Anaesthesia* 1994;**49**:1–2.

41 Hytten FE, Paintin DB. Increase in plasma volume during normal pregnancy. *J Obstet Gynaecol Br Commonwealth* 1963;**70**:402–7.

42 Taylor DJ, Lind T. Red cell mass during and after normal pregnancy. *Br J Obstet Gynaecol* 1979;**86**:364–70.

43 Longo LD. Maternal blood volume and cardiac output during pregnancy. *Am J Physiol* 1983;**245**:R720–R729.

44 Lund CJ, Donovan JC. Blood volume during pregnancy: significance of plasma and red cell volumes. *Am J Obstet Gynecol* 1967;**98**:393–403.

45 Cotes PM, Canning CE, Lind T. Changes in serum immunoreactive erythropoietin during the menstrual cycle and normal pregnancy. *Br J Obstet Gynaecol* 1983;**90**:304–11.

46 Koller O. The clinical significance of hemodilution during pregnancy. *Obstet Gynecol Surv* 1982;**37**:649–52.

47 Tygart SC, McRoyan DK, Spinnato JA, *et al.* Longitudinal study of platelet indices during normal pregnancy. *Am J Obstet Gynecol* 1986;**154**:883–7.

48 Gerbasi FR, Bottoms S, Farag A, Mammen EF. Changes in hemostasis activity during delivery and the immediate postpartum period. *Am J Obstet Gynecol* 1990;**162**:1158–63.

49 Talbert LM, Langdell RD. Normal values of certain blood factors in the blood clotting mechanism in pregnancy. *Am J Obstet Gynecol* 1964;**90**:44–50.

50 Bonnar J, McNicol GP, Douglas AS. Coagulation and fibrinolytic mechanism during and after normal childbirth. *BMJ* 1970;**2**:200–3.

51 Gerbasi FR, Bottoms S, Farag A, Mammen EF. Increased intravascular coagulation associated with pregnancy. *Obstet Gynecol* 1990;**75**:385–9.

52 Ueland K. Maternal cardiovascular dynamics. VII. Intrapartum blood volume changes. *Am J Obstet Gynecol* 1976;**126**:671–7.

53 Taylor DJ, Lind T. Puerperal haematological indices. *Br J Obstet Gynaecol* 1981;**88**:601–6.

54 McNair RD, Jaynes RV. Alterations in liver function during normal pregnancy. *Am J Obstet Gynecol* 1960;**80**:500–5.

55 Mendenhal HW. Serum protein concentrations in pregnancy. I. Concentrations in maternal serum. *Am J Obstet Gynecol* 1970;**106**:388–99.

56 Braverman DZ, Johnson ML, Kern FJ. Effects of pregnancy and contraceptive steroids on gallbladder function. *N Engl J Med* 1980;**302**:362–4.

57 Bailey RR, Rolleston GL. Kidney length and ureteric dilation in the puerperium. *J Obstet Gynaecol Br Commonwealth* 1971;**78**:55–61.

58 Lindheimer MD, Katz AI. Renal changes during pregnancy: their relevance to volume homeostasis. *Clin Obstet Gynecol* 1975;**2**:345–64.

59 Dunlop W. Serial changes in renal hemodynamics in normal human pregnancy. *Br J Obstet Gynaecol* 1981;**88**:1–9.

60 Lind T, Godfrey KA, Otun H. Changes in serum uric acid concentrations during normal pregnancy. *Br J Obstet Gynaecol* 1984;**91**:128–32.

61 Feinberg BB, Gonik B. General precepts of the immunology of pregnancy. *Clin Obstet Gynecol* 1991;**34**:3–16.

62 Gehrz R, Christianson WR, Linner KM, Conroy MM, McCue SA, Balfour HH. A longitudinal analysis of lymphocyte proliferation responses to mitogens and antigens during pregnancy. *Am J Obstet Gynecol* 1981;**140**:665–70.

63 Toder V, Nebel L, Gleicher N. Studies of natural killer cells in pregnancy. I. Analysis at the single cell level. *J Clin Lab Immunol* 1984;**14**:123–7.

64 Kovar IZ, Riches P. C3 and C4 complement components and acute phase proteins in late pregnancy and parturition. *J Clin Pathol* 1988;**41**:650.

65 Head JR. Can trophoblast be killed by cytotoxic cells? In vitro evidence and in vivo possibilities. *Am J Reprod Immunol* 1998;**20**:100–5.

66 Gintzler AR. Endorphin-mediated increases in pain threshold during pregnancy. *Science* 1980;**210**:190.

67 Steinbrook RA, Carr DB, Datta S, Naulty JS, Lee C, Fisher J. Dissociation of plasma and cerebrospinal fluid beta-endorphin-like immunoactivity during pregnancy and parturition. *Anesth Analg* 1982;**61**:893.

68 Edouard D, Pannier B, London G, Safar M. Differential influence of pregnancy on limb venous tone in humans. *Anesthesiology* 1990;**73**:A955.

69 Palahniuk RJ, Shnider SM, Eger EI. Pregnancy decreases the requirement for inhaled anesthetic agents. *Anesthesiology* 1974;**41**:82–3.

70 Spielman FJ, Mueller RA, Corke BC. Cerebrospinal fluid concentration of 5-hydroxyindoleactic acid in pregnancy. *Anesthesiology* 1985;**62**:193.

71 Bader AM, Datta S, Moller RA, Covino BG. Acute progesterone treatment has no effect on bupivacaine-induced conduction blockade in the isolated rabbit vagus nerve. *Anesth Analg* 1990;**71**:545–8.

72 Flanagan HL, Datta S, Moller RA, Covino BG. Effect of exogenously administered progesterone on susceptibility of rabbit vagus nerves to bupivacaine. *Anesthesiology* 1988;**69**:A676.

73 Leontic EA. Respiratory disease in pregnancy. *Med Clin North Am* 1977;**61**:111–28.

74 Brock-Utne JG, Downing JW, Seedat F. Laryngeal oedema associated with pre-eclamptic toxaemia. *Anaesthesia* 1977;**32**:556–8.

75 Reynolds F, Knott C. Pharmacokinetics in pregnancy and placental drug transfer. *Oxford Rev Reprod Biol* 1989;**11**:389–449.

76 Dean M, Stock B, Patterson RJ, Levy G. Serum protein binding of drugs during and after pregnancy in humans. *Clin Pharmacol Therapeut* 1980;**28**:253–61.

77 Flynn RJ, Moore J, Dwyer R, Duly E, Dundee JW. Changes in alpha 1 acid glycoprotein during labor. *Anesth Analg* 1988;**67**:s61.
78 Whittaker M, Crawford J, Lewis M. Some observations of levels of plasma cholinesterase activity within an obstetric population. *Anaesthesia* 1988;**43**:42–5.
79 Leighton BL, Cheek T, Gross JB, et al. Succinylcholine pharmacodynamics in peripartum patients. *Anesthesiology* 1986;**64**:202–5.
80 Mazze RI, Kallen B. Reproductive outcome after anesthesia and operation during pregnancy: a registry study of 5405 cases. *Am J Obstet Gynecol* 1989;**161**:1178–85.
81 Brodsky J, Cohen EN, Brown BW, Wu M, Whitcher C. Surgery during pregnancy and fetal outcome. *Am J Obstet Gynecol* 1980;**138**:1165–67.
82 Shnider SM, Webster GM. Maternal and fetal hazards of surgery during pregnancy. *Am J Obstet Gynecol* 1965;**92**:891–900.
83 Skillman CA, Plessinger MA, Woods JR, Clark K. Effect of graded reductions in uteroplacental blood flow on the fetal lamb. *Am J Physiol* 1985;**149**:1098–105.
84 Levinson G, Shnider SM. Anesthesia for surgery during pregnancy. In: Shnider S, Levinson G, eds. *Anesthesia for obstetrics*. Baltimore: Williams and Williams, 1993:259–80.
85 Duncan PG, Pope WDB, Cohen MM, Greer N. Fetal risk of anesthesia and surgery during pregnancy. *Anesthesiology* 1986;**64**:790–4.
86 Shiono PH, Mills JL. Oral clefts and diazepam use during pregnancy. *N Engl J Med* 1984;**311**:919–920.
87 Reddy BK, Pizer B, Bull PT. Neonatal serum cortisol suppression by etomidate compared with thiopentone, for elective caesarean section. *Eur J Anaesthesiol* 1988;**5**:171.
88 Basford A, Fink BR. Teratogenicity of halothane in the rat. *Anesthesiology* 1968;**29**:1167–73.
89 Pope WDB, Halsey MJ, Lansdown ABG, *et al.* Fetotoxicity in rats following chronic exposure to halothane, nitrous oxide or methoxyflurane. *Anesthesiology* 1978;**48**:11–16.
90 Wharton RS, Wilson AI, Mazze RI, Baden JM, Rice S. Fetal morphology in mice exposed to halothane. *Anesthesiology* 1979;**51**:532–7.
91 Mazze RI, Fujinaga M, Rice S, *et al.* Reproductive and teratogenic effects of nitrous oxide, halothane, isoflurane and enflurane in Sprague-Dawley rats. *Anesthesiology* 1986;**64**:339–44.
92 Tannenbaum TN, Goldberg RJ. Exposure to anaesthetic gases and reproductive outcome. A review of epidemiologic literature. *J Occup Med* 1985;**27**:659–68.
93 Burrings JE, Hennekens CH, Mayrent SL, Rosner B, Greenberg ER, Colton T. Health experiences of operating room personnel. *Anesthesiology* 1985;**62**:325–30.
94 Fujinaga M, Baden JM, Mazze RI. Developmental toxicity of nondepolarising muscle relaxants in cultured rat embryos. *Anesthesiology* 1992;**76**:999–1003.
95 Abboud TK, Khoo SS, Miller F, Doan T, Henriksen EH. Maternal, fetal, and neonatal responses after epidural anesthesia with bupivacaine, 2-chloroprocaine, or lidocaine. *Anesth Analg* 1982;**61**:638.
96 Atrash HK, Koonin MN, Lawson HW, Franks AL, Smith JC. Maternal mortality in the United States, 1979–1986. *Obstet Gynecol* 1990;**76**:1055–60.
97 Samsoon GLT, Young RB. Difficult tracheal intubation: a retrospective study. *Anaesthesia* 1987;**42**:487–90.
98 Liu PL, Warren TM, Ostheimer GW, Weiss JB, Liu LMP. Foetal monitoring in parturients undergoing surgery unrelated to pregnancy. *Can Anaesth Soc J* 1985;**32**:525–32.
99 Hawkins JL, Koonin LM, Palmer SK, Gibbs C. Anesthesia-related deaths during obstetric delivery in the United States,1979–1990. *Anesthesiology* 1997;**86**:277–84.
100 Berg C, Atrash HK, Koonin LM, Tucker M. Pregnancy-related mortality in the United States, 1987–1990. *Obstet Gynecol* 1996;**88**:161–7.
101 *Report on confidential enquiries into maternal deaths in the UK. 1991–1993*. Department of Health London: HMSO, 1996.

2: The effects of anaesthesia and analgesia on the baby

JACKIE PORTER

Drugs given to a parturient during pregnancy or labour may affect the fetus and newborn either by a direct pharmacological effect following placental drug transfer or indirectly because they affect maternal physiology, placental perfusion, maternal acid-base balance or the progress of labour.

Placenta

Anatomy

Following fertilisation of the ovum, the dividing cells develop into two parts: the trophoblast, which forms the placenta, and the blastocyst, which develops into the fetus. Eleven to 13 days after conception the trophoblast sends out processes into the decidual layer of the endometrium, invading thin-walled maternal blood vessels. Blood spills from the spiral arterioles, creating a lake of maternal blood in which placental villi float (Fig 2.1). The fetal loops in each villus are in close contact with maternal blood although the two circulations remain separated by a thin placental layer of trophoblast, fetal capillary endothelium, and connective tissue, the "placental barrier'. The fetal capillaries in each villus are supplied by two umbilical arteries carrying deoxygenated blood, while oxygenated blood returns to the fetus through one umbilical vein. Oxygen and nutrients pass to the fetus while carbon dioxide and fetal waste products pass into deoxygenated maternal blood in endometrial basal veins.

Drug transfer

There is no absolute barrier to the passage of drugs across the placenta. Passage of a drug from mother to fetus is governed by its physicochemical properties and the dynamics of the two circulations. The rate and extent to which free drug crosses the placenta depend on several factors.

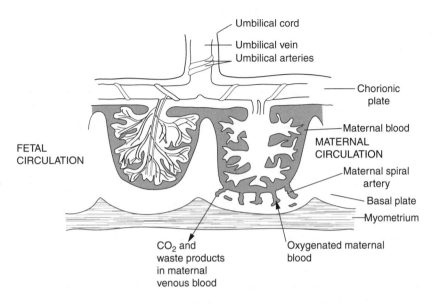

Fig 2.1   Anatomy of the uteroplacental circulation

- Lipid solubility of the drug
- Placental permeability
- Concentration gradient for the unbound diffusible drug, which in turn depends on:
  - pH gradient across the placenta
  - blood flow on either side of the placenta
  - plasma protein binding

Lipid solubility
The cells of the placental barrier form a continuous lipid membrane across which drugs may pass. Most drugs cross by simple diffusion in their unionised form and the more lipid soluble the drug, the more freely it may cross.

Placental permeability
Polar drugs cross more slowly than unionised molecules, the rate being dependent on the permeability of the placenta for that drug. This depends on the area and thickness of the placenta and on the molecular weight or size of the drug molecule. Whilst drugs with a molecular weight less than 600 Da cross the placenta freely, for those with a higher molecular weight

31

placental permeability limits the rate of transfer. These drugs are said to undergo "permeability-dependent transfer".

Concentration gradient

pH gradient

Lipid-soluble drugs diffuse down a concentration gradient. Since only unionised drug diffuses in significant quantity, the degree of ionisation will in part determine this gradient. The degree of ionisation of a drug depends on the pH gradient across the placenta and on the pKa value of the drug. The more acid the environment, the more ionised weak bases become. The healthy fetus is slightly more acid than the mother by about 0.1 pH unit. When the unionised portion of a weak base passes across the placenta from mother to fetus a greater proportion of the drug becomes ionised and therefore "trapped" in the fetus. This maintains a concentration gradient for unionised drug across the placenta favouring maternal to fetal transfer. In a compromised fetus the pH becomes more acid and the fetal load of weakly basic drug is increased. Conversely, weakly acidic drugs are more ionised in the mother and so less drug will cross. The ratio of drug concentration in the fetus to that in the mother, the fetal/maternal (F/M) ratio, is generally higher for weak bases than for weak acids and often exceeds unity. Opioids and local anaesthetics are examples of weak bases, while thiopentone is a weak acid.

Placental blood flow

For highly lipid-soluble drugs that equilibrate within one circulation through the placenta, the rate of transfer across the placenta depends on how quickly the drug can be delivered to, and removed from, the placenta, thus determining the concentration gradient. The blood flow on the maternal side depends on maternal blood pressure and on blood vessel diameter. More important in maintaining the concentration gradient for these drugs, however, is the rate at which the drug is removed on the fetal side which depends, therefore, on the umbilical venous blood flow. These drugs are said to exhibit "flow-limited transfer" and include lignocaine and pethidine. A reduction in perfusion on either side of the placenta will slow transfer of these drugs.

Plasma protein binding

Most drugs are bound to plasma proteins; the more lipophilic the drug, the greater the degree of binding and it is only the unbound, free fraction that can cross the placenta. Albumin tends to bind acidic drugs such as thiopentone although a few neutral or weakly basic drugs, such as fentanyl and diazepam, are also predominantly albumin bound. An acute-phase protein, α_1-acid glycoprotein, binds basic drugs including local anaesthetics and opioids. The extent to which a drug is bound in both maternal and fetal circulations and the transplacental concentration gradients for each protein determine F/M ratios. At term the concentration of albumin is greater in the fetus than in the mother so at equilibrium drugs bound extensively to albumin will, in theory, be in higher concentration in the fetus than in the mother and the F/M ratio will be high. In practice, however, binding is often weak so drug dissociates from albumin and crosses the placenta freely. For drugs that are less than 90% bound, this factor is of little clinical relevance. Conversely, the concentration of α_1-acid glycoprotein is greater in the mother than the fetus so drugs that are extensively bound to this will have a F/M ratio well below one. Drugs in this category include bupivacaine, ropivacaine, and some of the fentanyls.

Fetal/maternal ratios

The fetal/maternal (F/M) ratio is used to calculate the proportions of a substance on either side of the placenta. It is often calculated using umbilical venous (UV) blood concentrations. However, UV blood reflects only equilibration of a drug locally across the placenta and when considering the effects of a drug on the baby, the concentration of drug in fetal tissues is more relevant. In order to reflect this more accurately, many authors quote F/M values using umbilical arterial (UA) or capillary blood concentrations. Even drugs that exhibit flow-limited placental transfer and equilibrate between maternal and umbilical venous blood within one passage through the placenta take time to penetrate deeper into fetal tissues. The concentration in fetal tissues continues to rise over time, until fetal tissue, UV, and maternal plasma concentrations are in equilibrium. The F/M ratio at this time depends on the pKa of the drug, the pH gradient across the placenta, and the extent of plasma protein binding. Although net maternal-to-fetal transfer occurs during this period, by the time equilibrium is reached both the maternal and UV plasma concentrations have fallen well below peak maternal plasma concentration. Thus unlike the mother, the baby never experiences the full extent of drug effect. However, with repeated doses or infusions, fetal tissue concentrations of many drugs approximate to maternal plasma concentrations and any drug effects are similar to those in the mother. Furthermore, accumulation of the drug in the mother and baby occurs if the interval between doses is less than the elimination half-life ($T_{1/2\beta}$) of the drug, as is the case with most analgesic drugs.

Neonatal drug elimination

After birth the baby has to metabolise and/or excrete the drug. Hepatic and renal mechanisms are poorly developed in the newborn so many drugs that pass to the fetus before delivery have a more prolonged elimination half-life than in the adult and drug effects persist for longer.

Assessment of the baby

Assessment during labour

Fetal heart rate

Continuous or intermittent electronic fetal heart rate monitoring is widely used during labour to detect fetal hypoxia. Changes associated with fetal distress occur when fetal oxygenation becomes inadequate and include loss of beat-to-beat variability, late and variable decelerations, and prolonged fetal bradycardia. Whilst these changes are often associated with hypoxia, acidosis, and low Apgar scores, they are not specific. Even in the presence of severe heart rate changes, approximately 50% of fetuses will have a normal pH (see below) suggesting absence of fetal hypoxia. Furthermore, episodes of fetal sleep and some maternal drugs may reduce fetal heart rate variability. Systemic and intrathecal opioids have been shown to reduce the variability. Neuraxial blockade may reduce maternal blood pressure and uterine blood flow and precipitate cardiotocographic changes suggestive of fetal distress. Even in the absence of maternal hypotension, bolus doses of epidural bupivacaine have been associated with decelerations in fetal heart rate.[1] Lignocaine and 2-chloroprocaine have also been associated with these changes although the incidence is lower than for bupivacaine.[1] Several well-conducted controlled trials have shown deficiencies in the use of electronic fetal heart monitoring to predict fetal hypoxia and adverse outcomes. Whether the monitor itself is insufficiently sensitive or whether the fault lies in interpretation of the trace is unclear, but until the predictive value of fetal heart rate monitoring improves, the significance of the changes induced by maternal analgesia remains elusive. So far the changes associated with systemic opioids and epidural local anaesthetics, in the absence of hypotension, have not been shown to be associated with adverse fetal outcome.

Fetal scalp blood analysis

pH measurements

In the presence of severe fetal heart rate changes, scalp blood analysis may be performed to confirm or refute a diagnosis of hypoxia. The most commonly used method is intermittent blood sampling from the fetal scalp in labour, performed through the cervix. A low pH provides an indirect measure of hypoxia. Continuous readings have been obtained using a pH electrode applied to the subcutaneous tissues of the fetal scalp. Whilst this provides trend data and perhaps an earlier warning of fetal hypoxia than intermittent sampling, the correlation between pH values following intermittent sampling and the pH electrode remains in question. Confirmation of its value in predicting neonatal outcome requires large studies.

Respiratory gas measurements

Intermittent values for fetal oxygen and carbon dioxide tensions may be obtained at the same time as intermittent pH readings but the procedure is invasive. Transcutaneous measurements provide a non-invasive measure of fetal respiratory gas status. Continuous readings of transcutaneous arterial oxygen saturation (SpO_2) can be measured using a transvaginal pulse oximeter. Transcutaneous gas tensions for oxygen ($tcPO_2$) and carbon dioxide ($tcPCO_2$) require a transvaginal electrode applied to the fetal scalp by suction. The data collected correlate well with umbilical arterial values. However, technical problems preclude its routine use. Maintaining sensor contact is often difficult. Interference is a problem, particularly in the second stage of labour, as are maternal movement, fetal hair, and scalp oedema. Even if reliable recordings are made, there is no evidence that a fall in fetal SpO_2 results in an adverse outcome.

Doppler studies

Doppler ultrasonography is a non-invasive means of assessing uteroplacental blood flow through measurement of vascular resistance. Measures of blood flow velocity waveform in the umbilical artery (Fig 2.2) and cross-sectional area in uterine, umbilical or major fetal blood vessels enable blood flow to be estimated. The ratio of systolic to end-diastolic flow velocity (S/D ratio) in the uterine artery is often used (Fig 2.2a) since a higher ratio warns of fetal acidosis (Fig 2.2b), while absent flow to the fetus in diastole or flow away from the fetus, "reverse flow" (Fig 2.2c), are serious indicators of inadequate uteroplacental flow.

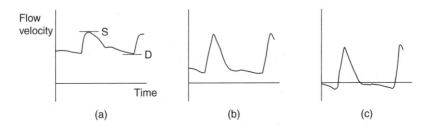

(a)   (b)   (c)

Fig 2.2   Diagrammatic representation of flow velocity in the uterine artery as measured by Doppler ultrasonography. (a) Normal pattern in third trimester with good flow in diastole. (b) Abnormal trace in which end-diastolic flow velocity is reduced and S/D ratio is increased. (c) Critical trace with reverse end-diastolic flow. S: peak systolic flow velocity; D: end-diastolic flow velocity

After delivery

Apgar scores

The Apgar score, described by Virginia Apgar in 1953,[2] is a simple and widely used measure of the condition of the neonate at birth. Pulse, respiration, colour, tone, and reflex irritability are scored at one, five, and 10 minutes after birth, with a maximum possible score of 10 at each testing. An Apgar score of less than seven one minute after delivery is generally taken to indicate neonatal depression. However, it is strongly influenced by the *in utero* environment and it is performed only during the first 10 minutes of life, a highly stimulating time for the newborn, so subtle degrees of neonatal depression are unlikely to be detected. Following maternal sedation in labour, Brazelton[3] reported neonates with "excellent Apgar scores" who later slipped into a state of unresponsiveness lasting a few hours to one day.

Neonatal umbilical gas and acid-base status

Umbilical venous (UV) and arterial (UA) gas and acid-base measurements taken at birth are commonly used as an indication of neonatal welfare.[4] However, they reflect *in utero* status and give no indication of a baby's ability to sustain adequate respiration and circulation or of neurological status. UV values reflect maternal arterial status while UA values reflect more accurately gas and acid-base status of neonatal tissues.

Neurobehavioural scores

Neonatal neurobehavioural tests assess well-being further into the neonatal period. They examine behavioural responses of the newborn and are used to detect neonatal depression caused by asphyxia or maternal drug administration. The Brazelton Neonatal Behavioural Assessment Scale (BNBAS)[5] was originally designed to be used clinically and examines primary reflexes, habituation to stimuli, irritability or consolability, and motor tone. However, it is rarely used now except as a research tool by developmental psychologists since it requires considerable training and the 49 individual items take 35–40 minutes to perform.

Scanlon's Early Neonatal Neurobehavioural Scale (ENNS)[6] was designed specifically to investigate the neurobehavioural effects of anaesthetic drugs during the first eight hours of life and concentrates on neonatal muscle tone, primary reflexes, state of alertness, and responses to stimulation. Habituation tests examine the ability of the newborn to cease responding to a repetitive test such as a noise or light stimulus. A failure to habituate may occur following exposure to systemic opioids in labour or from neonatal asphyxia. Although it is quicker to perform than the BNBAS, taking only 5–10 minutes, the ENNS still requires significant training to achieve reliable results.

The Neurologic and Adaptive Capacity Score (NACS) was proposed by Amiel-Tison *et al.* in 1982.[7] It aims to differentiate between the depressant effects of drugs used in labour from those effects secondary to birth trauma and perinatal asphyxia, by including an examination of tone differences in the extensor and flexor muscles of the neck. When performed at two and 24 hours of life, a low initial score resulting from maternal medication should improve in the later examination. It is easier to learn than the ENNS and takes less than five minutes to perform the 20 criteria. It is the test currently favoured by obstetric anaesthetists examining the effects of maternal medication on the newborn.

Neonatal respiration

Although an assessment of respiratory status is included in the Apgar score subtle degrees of respiratory depression, such as might result from small maternal doses of an opioid used systemically or neuraxially, are unlikely to be detected. Various methods have been used to evaluate neonatal respiration. Time to first breath and time to sustained respiration are used immediately after delivery but do not assess respiration over a prolonged period of time. Respiratory rate and tidal volume are not particularly sensitive measures of respiratory depression while spirometry, pneumotachography, and plethysmography are cumbersome. Minute ventilation has been measured[8,9] and alveolar ventilation has been derived from measures of carbon dioxide (CO_2) excretion and either endtidal CO_2 concentration or blood carbon dioxide tension (PCO_2).[10] The ventilatory response to CO_2 is the most sensitive measure of opioid-induced ventilatory depression. Blood gases give a good indication of neonatal respiratory status. Arterial sampling may be considered the gold standard, via either an indwelling arterial line or repeated arterial stab, while heel prick capillary samples have also been used but all these methods are invasive. Transcutaneous gas measurements[4,11] and pulse oximetry[12,13] provide non-invasive and continuous monitoring of respiratory gas status.

Effects of maternal anaesthesia and analgesia

Inhalational analgesia

Nitrous oxide

The passage of nitrous oxide across the placenta is rapid but so too is its excretion through the lungs after birth. Its use in labour has no known clinically significant side-effects for the fetus or newborn.

Nitrous oxide interferes with methionine synthase activity by inactivating its cofactor vitamin B_{12}. This enzyme is required for the synthesis of deoxythymidine, an essential base in deoxyribonucleic acid, so the subsequent effects on metabolism are potentially far reaching. Prolonged use of nitrous oxide in adults has resulted in bone marrow depression, megaloblastic anaemia, and a demyelinating condition resembling subacute combined degeneration of the cord usually seen in patients with vitamin B_{12} deficiency. The doses received during labour or general anaesthesia for delivery are much less and there is no evidence to suggest that either parturients or neonates are at risk from these effects.

37

Nitrous oxide may increase the incidence of maternal hypoxia in labour although the relevance of this to fetal and neonatal welfare is unclear. Episodes of hypoxaemia occur during painful labour.[14] Painful uterine contractions stimulate the mother to hyperventilate and the arterial carbon dioxide tension ($PaCO_2$) can fall markedly. This reduces ventilatory drive and subsequent hypoventilation or apnoea[15] between contractions may result in maternal oxygen desaturation, a situation potentially harmful to the fetus. A reduction in maternal oxygen tension has been associated with a reduction in fetal oxygenation and, in some cases, fetal heart rate decelerations.[15] Oxygen delivery to the fetus may be reduced further by maternal alkalosis, causing a left shift of the oxygen dissociation curve, reducing the release of oxygen to the fetus. Furthermore, maternal hyperventilation and hypocarbia cause generalised vasoconstriction including the uteroplacental and umbilical vessels, reducing uterine blood flow and so reducing fetal oxygenation and pH. Whilst these changes are unlikely to affect the healthy term fetus, any concurrent reduction in placental oxygen transfer may be exacerbated, resulting in fetal distress.

Entonox combined with systemic pethidine has been found to exacerbate the episodes of maternal hypoxaemia.[12,14] However, neither Deckardt et al.[12] nor Griffin and Reynolds[14] examined the effect of Entonox without systemic narcotics and therefore it cannot be stated conclusively that Entonox alone exacerbates maternal hypoxaemia over and above that seen in normal, painful labour. In the absence of epidural or opioid analgesia, no increase in maternal hypoxaemia has been reported with Entonox.[16] However Wilkins et al.,[17] using healthy volunteers, demonstrated significantly greater falls in SpO_2 with Entonox when compared with either nitrogen 50% or 79% in oxygen during periods of hyperventilation. They concluded that Entonox may exert this effect by altering respiratory drive or the ventilatory response to hypoxia or by diffusion hypoxia. Even though maternal hypoxaemic episodes occur, they have rarely been shown to be harmful to the baby as indicated by either fetal heart rate monitoring, Apgar scores, Neurologic and Adaptive Capacity Scores or cord blood acid-base and gas status.[12,14,15,18]

Jacobson et al.[19] suggested that babies born to mothers treated with opioids and Entonox in labour have an increased risk of developing drug addiction in later life and an imprinting method was suggested. However, this study has been heavily criticised, being retrospective with poorly matched controls, so further studies are needed in order to confirm or refute these claims.

Trichloroethylene and methoxyflurane

Although popular in the past, neither trichloroethylene nor methoxyflurane is in current use. Both cross the placenta freely and cause neonatal depression. Their blood-gas solubility coefficients are higher than nitrous oxide (Table 2.1) so elimination from the baby is slower and the babies born to

Table 2.1   Blood/gas solubility coefficients at 37°C of inhalational agents

Inhalational agent	Blood/gas solubility coefficient
Nitrous oxide	0.47
Trichloroethylene	9.0
Methoxyflurane	13.0
Enflurane	1.9
Isoflurane	1.4
Desflurane	0.42

mothers who had received either trichloroethylene or methoxyflurane were sleepy and unresponsive following delivery. Methoxyflurane is metabolised to free fluoride ions in the liver to a greater extent than the other fluorinated ethers and in high concentration these ions are toxic to the kidney. After the use of methoxyflurane, serum inorganic fluoride ion concentrations are raised in the newborn although the concentrations reached were well below those at which clinical nephrotoxicity would be expected.

Enflurane, Isoflurane, and Desflurane

Like all volatile anaesthetic agents, enflurane, isoflurane, and desflurane are highly lipid soluble, unionised, and non-protein bound and therefore cross the placenta freely in a flow-limited manner. Blood-gas partition coefficients for enflurane and isoflurane lie between that of nitrous oxide and those of trichloroethylene and methoxyflurane (Table 2.1) and speed of elimination from the baby is similar. Neither enflurane nor isoflurane has been shown to have a depressant effect on the newborn following use during labour and delivery as demonstrated using Apgar scores, neurobehavioural scores, and umbilical acid-base status. These agents are usually mixed with oxygen rather than air, which may be beneficial to the compromised fetus. Desflurane has a blood-gas partition coefficient even lower than that of nitrous oxide (Table 2.1) so elimination from both mother and baby is rapid. Apgar scores, neurobehavioural scores, and cord acid-base status are similar following either desflurane 1.0–4.5% in oxygen or nitrous oxide 30–60% in oxygen during the second stage of labour.[20] However, the 23% incidence of amnesia in the mother[20] and the high cost of this agent preclude its widespread use in labour.

Systemic opioids

Pethidine

Placental transfer

Like most opioids, pethidine has a low molecular weight and high lipid solubility (Table 2.2), crosses the placenta freely, and exhibits "flow-dependent placental transfer". Following maternal intravenous injection of

Table 2.2   Physicochemical and pharmacokinetic properties of opioids. A: adult; N: neonate; $T_{1/2\beta}$: elimination half-life; F/M ratio: ratio between drug concentration in umbilical and maternal plasma; lipid solubility: octanol/water partition coefficient at 37°C and pH 7.4

| | Protein binding (%) | | $T_{1/2\beta}$ (hours) | | pKa | | Lipid | % unionised |
	A	N	A	N	(25°C)	F/M ratio	solubility	at pH 7.4
Pethidine	40–70	85	3.3–4.0	11–22	8.6	0.3–1.5	39	7.4
Norpethidine	–	–	17–25	62	–	–	–	–
Fentanyl	80–89	63	3.1–3.7	1.2–7.3	8.4	0.3–1.1	813	9.1
Alfentanil	84–92	67	1.2–1.6	2.8	6.5	0.3	128	88
Sufentanil	92	80	2.7–4.6	5–19	8.0	0.4–0.8	1778	19.7
Diamorphine	40–63	–	0.5	–	7.8	–	280	29
Morphine	30–40	–	1.7–3.0	5.2–28	7.9	–	1.4	24

pethidine, the drug appears in fetal blood within two minutes and equilibrium occurs between maternal and fetal plasma levels after six minutes. In contrast, morphine is more polar than other opioids and transfer is partially limited by placental permeability.

Opioids are basic drugs and most are bound predominantly to (x_1-acid glycoprotein. The higher concentration of α_1-acid glycoprotein in the mother compared with the fetus should, in theory at least, limit placental transfer. However, pethidine is only 40–70% plasma protein bound in the mother (Table 2.2) and binding is weak, so free drug passes across the placenta readily. Following maternal administration there is net transfer of unbound pethidine to the fetus (Fig 2.3a) with rapid equilibration between concentrations in maternal arterial (MA) and umbilical venous (UV) blood. UV concentrations of free drug therefore mirror maternal plasma concentrations and start to fall within one hour of administration. However, the concentration in fetal tissues, represented by umbilical arterial

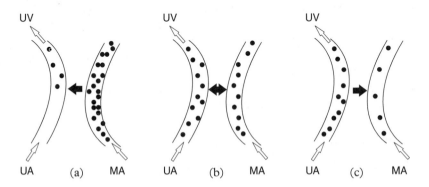

Fig 2.3   Pethidine transfer across the placenta. UA: umbilical artery; UV: umbilical vein; MA: maternal arterial blood; • unbound pethidine molecule. Filled arrows represent direction of net pethidine transfer. Unfilled arrows represent direction of blood flow. See text for explanation

(UA) or fetal capillary concentrations, continues to rise, reaching a peak 2–3 hours after administration.[21] The ratio between total pethidine concentration in UA and in maternal blood increases with time. The longer the dose-to-delivery interval, the higher the ratio and often unity is reached after 2–4 hours (Fig. 2.3b). Belfrage et al.[21] demonstrated unity for the UA/UV ratio 120 minutes after intramuscular pethidine and greater than one thereafter. After this time, if no more pethidine is administered, there is net transfer of pethidine back to the mother (Fig. 2.3c). The concentration in the UA exceeds that in the UV and the fetal/maternal ratio may exceed unity. Several investigators have reported mean UV/MV ratios for pethidine of 0.8–1.31 at delivery.

Pethidine is a weak base with a pKa of 8.72 (Table 2.2). Because the healthy fetus has a pH slightly below that in the mother, a higher proportion of the opioid will be ionised in the fetus compared with in the mother. This maintains a concentration gradient down which unionised free drug may pass. In the presence of hypoxia the fetus becomes more acid, more opioid passes from mother to fetus, ion trapping occurs, and the fetal concentration of the drugs rises.

Metabolism

The primary metabolic pathway for pethidine is hepatic N-demethylation to norpethidine in both mother and baby. Norpethidine and a small proportion of pethidine are hydrolysed to pethidinic and norpethidinic acid respectively and, following partial conjugation, are excreted in the urine. A small amount of pethidine is excreted unchanged in the urine.

Direct effects on the baby

In utero Intravenous or intramuscular opioids given to mothers in labour may decrease fetal heart rate variability within minutes of injection, lasting for up to 30 minutes.[22,23] Following maternal pethidine administration, a reduction in fetal movements and fetal scalp oxygen tension may occur. Modification of fetal EEG activity has also been shown, these changes lasting for at least four days. The significance of these changes is not clear but knowledge of these effects is important since loss of beat-to-beat variability on the cardiotocograph may be interpreted as a sign of fetal distress, resulting in unnecessary intervention.

Postdelivery Large doses of pethidine administered systemically to the parturient depress all aspects of the Apgar score.[10,24] However, it is not a particularly sensitive test and frequently Apgar scores have been reported as normal.

Neurobehavioural scores have shown babies exposed to pethidine *in utero* to be more sleepy, less vigorous, and less able to develop sucking skills. Such babies are therefore slower to establish breastfeeding and spend less time crying than babies whose mothers received no medication. The effects may last for up to 72 hours after delivery. Kuhnert et al.[25] found reduced neurobehavioural scores using the BNBAS for up to three days after delivery following intravenous administration of pethidine during labour. Brackbill et al.[26] found that babies exposed to pethidine as well as epidural analgesia took twice as long to habituate to a sound stimulus compared with controls whose mothers received epidural analgesia alone. Total scores using the BNBAS were reduced and there was a significant correlation between pethidine dose and overall score. Apgar scores were normal, however, demonstrating the low sensitivity of this test to subtle aspects of neonatal functioning. Using the BNBAS, Belsey et al.[27] showed a correlation between higher cord blood levels of pethidine and an increased tendency towards respiratory difficulties, drowsiness, and unresponsiveness at delivery, with poor scores for some of the tests continuing over the first six weeks of life. However, the changes were subtle and there was no significant difference in BNBAS scores when compared with an unmedicated control group.

The use of systemic pethidine for pain relief in labour has been associated with depression in all aspects of neonatal respiration.[10,21,24] Roberts et al.[8] demonstrated a reduced minute ventilation during the first few hours of life in babies exposed to pethidine in utero compared with control babies whose mothers did not receive opioids. Hamza et al.[13] compared babies born to mothers receiving pethidine by intravenous infusion with those whose mothers received no opioids. During active but not quiet sleep, babies exposed to opioid during labour demonstrated greater degrees of oxygen desaturation below SpO_2 90% and more frequent apnoeic episodes. Neonatal CO_2 retention, respiratory acidosis, and reduced CO_2 excretion persisting for up to 24 hours have all been reported following the administration of pethidine in labour compared with unmedicated controls.[10]

The depressant effects of pethidine on the newborn have been shown to be maximal when delivery occurs 1–3 hours after administration.[21,24] Shnider and Moya[24] found no significant depressant effects, using time to sustained respiration and Apgar scores, in babies whose mothers had received pethidine 50–100 mg within one hour of delivery compared with an unmedicated control group. If delivery occurred 2–3 hours after pethidine, the incidence of depressed babies was significantly increased. Belfrage et al.[21] examined babies for opioid-induced respiratory depression using time to sustained respiration and respiratory rate, before and after naloxone administration to the newborn. They reported a prolonged time to sustained respiration and an increase in respiratory rate after naloxone in babies born more than one hour after maternal pethidine administration compared with those born within one hour. Rooth et al.[4] demonstrated higher $PaCO_2$ values in babies whose mothers received pethidine at least one hour before delivery compared with those receiving pethidine within one hour of delivery or with unmedicated controls. Opioid-induced respiratory depression persists for several hours after delivery.[8]

If delivery occurs 1–3 hours after a single dose of pethidine, the extent of neonatal depression depends on the amount of pethidine that has crossed the placenta. If the dose-to-delivery interval is greater than three hours there is net transfer of pethidine back to the mother and total fetal pethidine concentrations fall. However, both mother and fetus convert pethidine to norpethidine, although the fetal liver does so at a slower rate.

Norpethidine can be measured in maternal plasma within one hour of an intramuscular injection of pethidine and concentrations continue to rise over several hours.[21] Like pethidine, it crosses the placenta freely but while net pethidine transfer to the fetus occurs only over the first 2–3 hours, norpethidine continues to cross several hours after maternal pethidine injection. Thus the fetal tissue concentration of norpethidine at delivery increases with dose-to-delivery interval.[21] Norpethidine is less analgesic and sedative than pethidine but has a greater respiratory depressant effect and is also proconvulsant. Furthermore, these effects are present for longer since the elimination half-life of norpethidine is prolonged compared with pethidine (Table 2.2). This is particularly marked in the newborn because of slower hepatic metabolism and a low glomerular filtration rate, although the enzyme activity in the neonatal liver increases rapidly over the first 72 hours of life. Kuhnert et al.[25] demonstrated less optimal BNBAS performance with longer dose-to-delivery interval and suggested this was due to norpethidine. The prolonged elimination half-life of norpethidine in the baby explains why the depressant effects on neonatal neurobehaviour last up to three days after delivery despite very low pethidine concentrations.[25] Repeat doses of pethidine increase the load of both pethidine and norpethidine to the fetus and so enhance the subsequent depression.[21]

Respiratory support with a bag and mask may be required initially for severe neonatal respiratory depression following the use of pethidine during labour. The neonatal depressant effects of opioids can be reversed using naloxone, the pure opioid antagonist.[10,28] Naloxone 40 μg, given via the umbilical vein at birth, has been shown to reverse the effects of maternal pethidine on the baby's respiration and behaviour.[28] However, the effect lasts only 30 minutes. In part, this is because the elimination half-life of naloxone in the newborn is only three hours compared with up to 22 hours for pethidine. Furthermore, whilst pethidine is readily antagonised by naloxone, the effects of norpethidine are less easily reversed.[29] In a study by Wiener et al.,[28] the effects of 200 μg naloxone given intramuscularly persisted for 48 hours and in clinical practice, naloxone is usually given in relatively large doses intramuscularly (100 μg/kg) to prolong its duration of action.

Other effects Jacobson et al.[19] suggested that babies exposed to opioids in utero during labour have an increased risk of developing drug addiction in later life although the studies on which this was based have been heavily criticised (see above).

Indirect effects on the baby

The use of systemic opioids exacerbates maternal oxygen desaturation seen during painful labour (see above). Pethidine provides poor analgesia and so has little, if any, effect on reducing hyperventilation during contractions. However, it potentiates hypoventilation between contractions by a direct depressant effect on the respiratory centre and women receiving pethidine have been shown to desaturate more compared with women receiving no analgesia.[14] Despite these findings, evidence that this is harmful to the healthy fetus is scarce. Deckardt et al.[12] demonstrated lower umbilical arterial pH in babies born to mothers using pethidine and nitrous oxide analgesia in labour compared with babies whose mothers had received epidural analgesia. Interestingly, amongst the mothers who received pethidine and nitrous oxide the incidence of haemoglobin oxygen desaturation was much greater. Fetal heart rate was unaffected, probably because it is a relatively insensitive guide to fetal oxygenation. An acute reduction in fetal oxygen tension must be substantial in the uncompromised fetus to produce late decelerations. However, in a compromised fetus with a basal oxygen saturation already reduced, a further reduction in maternal oxygenation may reduce fetal oxygenation to a critical level.

Morphine and diamorphine

Morphine has a low molecular weight but, unlike other opioids, has two polar hydroxyl groups so lipophilicity is reduced (Table 2.2) and placental transfer is slower. Early studies on the effects of morphine suggested that the fetus may be more susceptible to its opioid effects. Although this has not been substantiated by other investigators, morphine has no significant advantages over pethidine and is therefore little used in obstetric practice. Morphine is conjugated in the liver to morphine-3-glucuronide, which has negligible affinity for the μ-receptor, and to the active metabolite morphine-6-glucuronide, before excretion in the urine.

Diamorphine is chemically similar to morphine but two acetyl groups replace two hydroxyl groups, conferring greater lipophilicity (Table 2.2). It is metabolised to morphine and its metabolites. Systemic diamorphine is used in only 4% of labours, mainly in Scotland.[30] There is little available literature regarding its use in labour but in the National Birthday Trust Survey[30] there was an association between low Apgar scores and diamorphine use which was more marked than after pethidine.

The fentanyls

The fentanyls (fentanyl, alfentanil, and sufentanil) are more lipid soluble than pethidine (Table 2.2) so unbound drug crosses the placenta more rapidly. Fentanyl has been detected in fetal blood within one minute of maternal intravenous injection. In animal studies maternal fentanyl concentrations after intravenous bolus administration declined rapidly due to rapid redistribution and uptake into maternal tissues. UV plasma concentrations mirror these changes because of rapid equilibration across the placenta. All are more protein bound than pethidine or the morphines (Table 2.2) due to their higher lipophilicity. Fentanyl is 80–89% plasma protein bound in parturients but unlike most opioids, it is bound significantly to both albumin and $(x_1$-acid glycoprotein as well as several other proteins. Since the concentration of albumin is greater in the neonate than the mother, binding is similar in both mother and fetus and the net fentanyl load to the fetus is likely to be even greater than for pethidine. After fentanyl administration in labour F/M ratios are usually greater than 0.7 and frequently around one for total drug and slightly higher for free drug (Table 2.2).[31,32] Fentanyl undergoes hepatic metabolism but, unlike morphine and pethidine, it has no active metabolites.

There have been several reports on the use of systemic fentanyl in labour, either by intermittent intravenous injection or by patient-controlled analgesia.[23,33,34] It may offer some advantages over pethidine since it has a more rapid onset of action, no active metabolites, and fewer maternal side-effects. However, since the elimination half-life of fentanyl in the newborn is up to 440 minutes (Table 2.2) it has the potential for prolonged neonatal depression. Furthermore, like pethidine, doses of intravenous fentanyl currently used frequently do not achieve adequate analgesia, particularly in late labour.[34] Maternal sedation and respiratory depression may occur so the potential for maternal hypoxaemia and its subsequent adverse effects on the baby exists.

Rayburn et al.[23] randomised women to receive intravenously either fentanyl 50–100 µg/h or pethidine 25–50 mg two to three hourly. Pain relief was similar in the two groups but the incidence of neonatal side-effects was greater and naloxone was used more frequently (13% vs 2%) in the pethidine group. However, NACS did not differ significantly between the two groups. In an earlier, unrandomised study comparing intravenous fentanyl with no analgesia the incidence of naloxone use in the fentanyl group was only 0.7% despite doses of up to 600 µg.[22] Kleiman et al.[33] reported the use of fentanyl by patient-controlled analgesia in a parturient for 3.5 hours, using a total dose of 400 µg. A period of reduced fetal heart rate variability, which responded to maternal oxygen administration and the left lateral position, occurred 30 minutes after starting analgesia. Apgar scores were nine at one and five minutes after delivery and the respiratory rate of the baby was within normal limits for six hours after delivery. Although no indices of maternal respiration or gas status were measured the authors suggested that the availability of pulse oximetry and naloxone would be prudent in these women. Morley-Forster and Weberpals[34] reported the use of patient-controlled intravenous fentanyl in women in whom epidural analgesia was contraindicated. Forty four percent of neonates were "depressed" with one-minute Apgar scores of six or less, with 21% requiring naloxone for respiratory depression, an incidence of 9% overall. Mothers of narcotised neonates had received a higher total dose of fentanyl compared with mothers of non-narcotised babies.

Sufentanil and alfentanil are synthetic analogues of fentanyl. Both are more lipid soluble (Table 2.2) and therefore faster acting. Although both fentanyl and sufentanil have been shown to cross the placenta rapidly *in vitro*, sufentanil crosses the placenta more readily than fentanyl, probably because of its higher lipophilicity. Both alfentanil and sufentanil are more extensively bound to plasma proteins than fentanyl, being approximately 88% and 90% bound respectively in parturients (Table 2.2). Binding is mainly to α_1-acid glycoprotein and thus the ratio of α_1-acid glycoprotein on either side of the placenta is an important determinant of the concentration gradients for both alfentanil and sufentanil. Because plasma α_1-acid glycoprotein levels are lower in the fetus than in the mother, sufentanil and alfentanil are only 80% and 67% bound respectively in the baby. Thus total concentrations in the neonate are lower than in the mother, with UV/MV ratios of approximately 0.3 for alfentanil and 0.4 for sufentanil being commonly reported (Table 2.2). Despite the low total fetal concentrations, however, free concentrations are similar to those in the mother, demonstrating rapid transfer and equilibration across the placenta. The proportion of alfentanil or sufentanil as free drug in the fetus is therefore greater than in the mother. This has the potential to lead to respiratory depression and other opioid effects, even though the total drug concentration is relatively low. Sufentanil has a higher affinity for the μ-opioid receptor than fentanyl but duration of action and values for elimination half-life tend to be similar (Table 2.2).

Remifentanil is the newest synthetic opioid to be used for pain relief in labour. It is very short acting due to rapid metabolism by plasma and tissue esterases, with an elimination half-life of 8–12 minutes. It therefore has to be administered by continuous intravenous infusion or by intravenous patient-controlled analgesia. Its pharmacokinetic and pharmacodynamic profiles may well be altered by the physiological changes of pregnancy. There have been few reports on the use of remifentanil in obstetric patients and it is not yet licensed for use in pregnancy. Hughes *et al.*[35] used remifentanil to supplement epidural anaesthesia for caesarean section. At delivery, the mean UV/MA ratio was 0.82, suggesting it crosses the placenta rapidly. NACS at 60 minutes after delivery were significantly lower in the remifentanil group compared with control babies who received no opioid, but this difference was not apparent at 30 minutes. Its effects on maternal blood pressure, uterine blood flow, and contractility and its pharmacokinetic profile in the newborn have not yet been reported.

Partial agonist/antagonists

Several partial agonist/antagonist opioids have been used for pain relief in labour in the hopes that side-effects would be fewer but this has not been found to be the case.

Meptazinol in labour has been shown to produce equivalent analgesia to equal doses of pethidine but less neonatal depression.[36] However, this was not the case in a study by Morrison et al.[37] who compared intramuscular meptazinol and pethidine in doses of 100–150 mg. Pain relief was similar but so too was neonatal outcome and mothers vomited more with meptazinol. Furthermore, de Boer et al.[36] showed no less respiratory depression in the newborn at 60 minutes of age following meptazinol despite its shorter elimination half-life in the baby. Pentazocine is another mixed x-receptor agonist/antagonist claimed to have fewer maternal and neonatal depressant effects. However, it has never become popular because of dysphoria, tachyphylaxis, and the need for frequent administration. Nalbuphine 20 mg has been compared with pethidine 100 mg, both by intramuscular injection.[38] Analgesia was equivalent but neurobehavioural scores were worse in the nalbuphine group. Although it is claimed to have a ceiling effect for respiratory depression, in a comparison of patient-controlled intravenous nalbuphine 3 mg or pethidine 15 mg, the former provided better analgesia but equal maternal and neonatal side-effects.[39] Its use has also been associated with a sinusoidal fetal heart rate pattern, the significance of which remains unclear.

Regional analgesia

Regional analgesia for pain relief in labour may affect the fetus either by direct drug transfer across the placenta or indirectly through a change in maternal physiology. The drugs most commonly used to provide regional analgesia in obstetrics are local anaesthetics and opioids.

Local anaesthetics

Pharmacokinetics

Lignocaine and bupivacaine　The dose of local anaesthetic crossing the placenta is dependent mainly on the maternal plasma concentration and this in turn is determined by absorption from the epidural space, which is rapid. Lignocaine has been detected in the maternal circulation within three minutes of epidural injection, with peak concentrations occurring at approximately 20 minutes. Peak plasma concentrations of bupivacaine occur approximately 15–30 minutes after bolus injection.

Once in the maternal bloodstream, unbound local anaesthetic crosses the placenta readily since these drugs are all highly lipophilic (Table 2.3). Bupivacaine appears in the fetal circulation within 10 minutes of epidural injection and equilibrium between maternal and fetal plasma concentrations

47

Table 2.3   Physicochemical and pharmacokinetic properties of local anaesthetics. A: adult; N: neonate; MW: molecular weight; F/M ratio: ratio between drug concentration in umbilical and maternal plasma; $T_{1/2\beta}$: elimination half-life; lipid solubility: n-heptane/buffer partition coefficient at pH 7.4

| | Protein binding (%) | | | pKa | % ionised | F/M | $T_{1/2\beta}$ (hours) | | Lipid |
	A	N	MW	(25°C)	at pH 7.4	ratio	A	N	solubility
Lignocaine	56–75	14–24	234	7.9	75	0.5–0.7	1–2	1.6–3	2.9
Bupivacaine	88–95	50–66	288	8.1	83	0.2–0.4	1.2–5.0	4.5–18	27.5
Ropivacaine	92–95	82	274	8.1	83	0.2–0.3	2–7	11	6.1
Etidocaine	95	<95	276	7.7	67	0.3	2.6	6.4	141
Mepivacaine	65–77	–	246	7.9	61	0.6–0.7	1.9	9	0.8

occurs after 30 minutes. Although bupivacaine is more lipid soluble than lignocaine (Table 2.3), F/M ratios at equilibrium are lower than for lignocaine. F/M ratios for lignocaine following continuous epidural analgesia in labour are in the order of 0.5–0.7,[40–42] whilst for bupivacaine ratios are 0.23–0.44.[32, 40–42]

There are several reasons for this difference in F/M ratios between lignocaine and bupivacaine. The first relates to the difference in protein binding of the two local anaesthetics. Whilst all local anaesthetics are weakly basic drugs and highly bound to α_1-acid glycoprotein (Table 2.3), bupivacaine is more protein bound in the maternal circulation than lignocaine and therefore less drug is free to cross the placenta. This property confers a slower passage across the placenta for bupivacaine than lignocaine. Furthermore, the fetal glycoprotein content is lower than that in the mother, so only 50–66% is bound to fetal protein compared with 88–95% in the mother. Values for lignocaine are approximately 24% and 56% respectively. The second reason for the low F/M ratio for bupivacaine is its longer duration of action. Repeat doses of epidural bupivacaine are required less frequently and, in contrast to lignocaine, there is little or no accumulation. The same is not true for lignocaine as tachyphylaxis is observed. Lignocaine also accumulates in the mother and toxic concentrations of greater than 10 µg/ml may be reached in the fetus. A third reason relates to the potential for placental binding. Highly lipid-soluble and protein-bound drugs, such as local anaesthetics, bind to the placenta. The extent of binding depends on lipid solubility so bupivacaine binds more than lignocaine, further limiting transfer from mother to fetus. Thus, bupivacaine is preferable to lignocaine for maintaining epidural analgesia in labour. Following continuous epidural analgesia in labour, maternal plasma concentrations of bupivacaine have been shown to be well below the plasma level of 1.5 µg/ml above which mild symptoms of systemic toxicity may occur.

2-Chloroprocaine   2-Chloroprocaine is an ester-linked local anaesthetic used in the USA but unavailable in the UK. It undergoes rapid hydrolysis in the plasma and has an elimination half-life of approximately 40 seconds. Even with large bolus doses administered rapidly, placental transfer is small and maternal toxicity unlikely. However, despite its extreme safety for mother and baby, extensive motor block precludes a wider use in obstetrics.

Ropivacaine Ropivacaine is a new amide local anaesthetic, structurally related to bupivacaine and mepivacaine. Whilst bupivacaine is a racemic mixture of S- and R-enantiomers, ropivacaine is a single S-enantiomer. The pharmacokinetics of ropivacaine are shown in Table 2.3. Its pKa is identical to that of bupivacaine so equal proportions of the drugs are ionised at a given pH. Both bupivacaine and ropivacaine are predominantly bound to α_1-acid glycoprotein although ropivacaine is slightly less lipid soluble and therefore slightly less bound than bupivacaine. The lower lipophilicity of ropivacaine confers a smaller volume of distribution and a shorter half-life.[43] This suggests that bupivacaine may accumulate in tissues to a greater extent. Ropivacaine is slightly less potent than bupivacaine. Following bolus doses of bupivacaine and ropivacaine 0.5% for caesarean section, Ala-Kokko et al.[43] found the mean UV/MV ratio for total ropivacaine concentration to be similar to that for bupivacaine at 0.28. Mean total plasma concentrations of each drug were similar, whether in maternal or umbilical blood, but concentrations of unbound ropivacaine were approximately twice those of bupivacaine in both mother and baby. In part, this may be explained by the slightly lower plasma protein binding. Bader et al.[32] also suggested that bupivacaine may accumulate in lipid-rich fetal tissues, thus lowering free fetal plasma concentrations. However, continuous epidural infusion of bupivacaine in animals has not demonstrated a significant increase in brain concentration and bupivacaine has not been shown to accumulate in the human fetus beyond 40 minutes of administration.

Like opioids, local anaesthetics are weak bases so more drug is ionised in the fetus than in the mother. This maintains a concentration gradient for unionised drug, encouraging more to pass from mother to fetus. The situation is exacerbated in the presence of fetal distress when the pH in the fetus falls.

Direct effects on the baby

In utero effects Local anaesthetics have been shown to have a direct effect on the fetal heart with decelerations occurring within 30 minutes of epidural injection.[1] Whilst bupivacaine, particularly when used in high concentrations, is the most likely agent to affect the fetus, changes in fetal heart rate have also been reported following lignocaine and 2-chloroprocaine.[1] This is surprising in view of the low F/M ratio of bupivacaine compared with lignocaine (Table 2.3) or chloroprocaine. Abboud et al.[1] suggested that the mechanism may be bupivacaine uptake into the fetal heart. Epidural local anaesthetic may also have an indirect action, causing fetal bradycardia secondary to episodes of maternal hypotension and uterine hypoperfusion.

Neurobehaviour Subtle behavioural effects have been associated with the use of epidural local anaesthetics in labour.[6,44,45] Neonatal depression has been demonstrated more readily following the use of lignocaine and mepivacaine for labour and delivery since they cross the placenta more extensively than bupivacaine or chloroprocaine. Scanlon *et al.*[6] demonstrated significantly reduced muscle tone in babies born to mothers who received either epidural lignocaine or mepivacaine during labour compared with babies born to mothers who did not receive epidural analgesia, although their responses to habituation tests were normal. They described babies as "floppy but alert". This study was, however, unrandomised, poorly controlled and did not differentiate between babies exposed to lignocaine or mepivacaine. However, in another unrandomised study, Tronick *et al.*[45] also claimed poor muscle tone following either epidural lignocaine or mepivacaine compared with an unmedicated control group. Kuhnert *et al.*[46] compared neonatal neurobehaviour following either lignocaine or chloroprocaine for vaginal or caesarean delivery. Babies were more depressed following lignocaine and they suggested this was probably due to the different pharmacology of the drugs. Some of the tests of neurobehaviour demonstrated better scores in the chloroprocaine group for up to three days after delivery. Higher cord concentrations of lignocaine correlated with lower BNBAS scores. However, the changes detected were very subtle and the authors commented that type of delivery affected the scores more than the type of local anaesthetic used, with worse scores following vaginal delivery compared with caesarean section.

Since F/M ratios for bupivacaine are well below unity the effects of epidural bupivacaine on neonatal neurobehaviour are more subtle than lignocaine or mepivacaine and require very sensitive tests to detect them. The BNBAS is more sensitive to these effects than some of the other scoring systems and lower total scores, and correlations of cord concentrations of drug with performance, have been demonstrated following both epidural lignocaine and bupivacaine. Rosenblatt *et al.*[44] examined neonatal behaviour using BNBAS for six weeks after delivery of babies born to mothers receiving epidural bupivacaine 0.375% by intermittent injection. Infants with greater exposure to bupivacaine were less alert at delivery and achieved lower scores on some of the Brazelton assessment items. Although these effects were maximal on day 1, some persisted for the first six weeks of life. It must be remembered that this was an uncontrolled study and comparison with a group of historical unmedicated controls demonstrated no detectable differences in behaviour. Kuhnert *et al.*[47] compared bupivacaine with chloroprocaine, also using the more sensitive BNBAS, and related the effects to cord concentrations. Neonates in the bupivacaine group performed better than those in the chloroprocaine group. No adverse effects on muscle tone were attributed to bupivacaine and there was no correlation between UV bupivacaine concentration and neurobehavioural performance. There was, however, no unmedicated control group.

No studies using Scanlon's ENNS or Amiel-Tisson's NACS have demonstrated adverse effects following the use of epidural bupivacaine, while the only effect demonstrated by Kileff et al.[48] was poor sucking at 24 hours. Corke[49] examined babies using a modified form of ENNS and found no adverse effects following exposure to epidural bupivacaine compared with unmedicated controls. McGuinness et al.[50] compared epidural bupivacaine with spinal tetracaine and found no neurobehavioural differences with ENNS despite the use of much higher doses of bupivacaine. Scanlon et al.[41] also reported no detrimental neurobehavioural effects in babies born to mothers receiving epidural bupivacaine in labour, using their previous study as historical controls.[6] Abboud et al.[40] compared babies exposed to epidural bupivacaine, chloroprocaine, and lignocaine and, in contrast to Scanlon's findings,[6,41] found Apgar scores, neonatal acid-base status, and NACS to be equally good in all three groups. Writer et al.[51] compared epidural bupivacaine with ropivacaine for pain relief in labour and reported fewer babies with low NACS at 24 hours, but not at two hours, in the ropivacaine group. However, other studies comparing these two drugs given epidurally for caesarean section have shown no difference in either ENNS or NACS. From these findings it appears that the neurobehavioural changes associated with local anaesthetics are slight at most, requiring sophisticated tests to detect them, and thus are unlikely to be clinically meaningful.

How may local anaesthetics affect neurobehaviour? As plasma concentrations of local anaesthetics rise, they first cause central nervous system stimulation by inhibition of inhibitory pathways, followed by central nervous system depression at higher concentrations. This effect is probably mediated through an effect on transmission at the neuromuscular junction. They also depress spinal reflexes. Although mild toxic effects may occur at concentrations of bupivacaine greater than 1.5 µg/ml the subtle effects observed by Rosenblatt et al.[44] occurred at the much lower mean UA and UV plasma concentrations of 80 ng/ml, well within the range normally achieved during continuous epidural for labour analgesia. They postulated that this increased sensitivity was associated with a more permeable blood–brain barrier in the newborn. Similar concentrations were measured by Scanlon et al.[41] (100 ng/ml) but no effects were detected using the ENNS, demonstrating the lower sensitivity of this assessment scale.

Indirect effects on the baby

The indirect effects of regional local anaesthetic blockade can be either advantageous or detrimental to the fetus.

Maternal blood pressure and uteroplacental flow   Uterine and placental blood flow is determined by maternal blood pressure and the degree of vasoconstriction in the uteroplacental blood vessels. Any fall in maternal systolic blood pressure results in a reduction in uteroplacental and intervillous blood flow (Fig 2.4).

Sympathetic preganglionic fibres leave the spinal cord through the first to 12th thoracic nerve roots. Depending on the height of the block, local anaesthetics administered epidurally or spinally block these fibres, causing vasodilation that may result in hypotension. The reduction in uteroplacental blood flow, and therefore intervillous flow, may cause fetal hypoxaemia and acidosis. Since a block to T5 is required for caesarean section, hypotension is more likely to occur and to be more profound than following epidural analgesia in labour.

In the supine parturient, vena caval compression impairs venous return to the heart and may cause a reduction in maternal cardiac output. If insufficient blood bypasses the vena cava through the vertebral venous plexuses, venous return remains inadequate and blood pressure is maintained by reflex sympathetic stimulation producing vasoconstriction and tachycardia. In the presence of sympathetic blockade following epidural or spinal analgesia, reflex vasoconstriction is obtunded and hypotension is more pronounced, particularly after the extensive block required for caesarean section. Even if maternal blood pressure is maintained in the supine position, uteroplacental flow and intervillous perfusion may be reduced by compression of the aorta by the gravid uterus.

A fluid preload is commonly given before regional blocks are sited to prevent or attenuate maternal hypotension. Up to 500 ml of Hartmann's solution/Ringer's lactate or normal saline are usually given before labour analgesia and larger volumes before anaesthesia for caesarean section, to

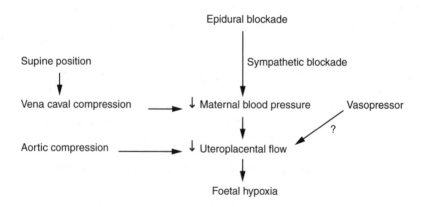

Fig 2.4   Interrelation between maternal causes of hypotension under epidural analgesia and fetal hypoxia

increase blood volume and cardiac output. Dextrose is not used because it has been associated with increased fetal acidosis. Left uterine displacement is also vital to avoid aortocaval compression. However, these measures may be insufficient to prevent hypotension and vasopressors may be employed to prevent or treat it. Since a sensory block to T10 is all that is required for labour analgesia, vasopressors are rarely required. However, their use during regional anaesthesia for caesarean section is common. Both ephedrine and phenylephrine are equally effective at correcting maternal hypotension following epidural blockade. Phenylephrine is a direct-acting α-adrenoceptor agonist and although it increases maternal blood pressure, vasoconstriction of the uteroplacental blood vessels occurs as part of the generalised vasoconstrictor effect. Ephedrine increases maternal blood pressure more by positive inotropic and chronotropic actions than by peripheral vasoconstriction so uterine blood flow is better maintained when compared with direct α-agonists. At high doses, however, the α-effect of ephedrine is more pronounced and a bolus of ephedrine 10 mg has been associated with an increase in maternal uterine artery resistance.[52] However, other studies, also in humans, reported no significant reduction in placental blood flow when ephedrine 5–15 mg was administered prophylactically by slow intravenous injection.[53] Metaraminol stimulates both α and β receptors but the α-effect is dominant so its main mechanism of action, particularly in large doses, is to increase peripheral vascular resistance.

Thus ephedrine is usually the drug of choice in the treatment or prevention of maternal hypotension following regional blockade although, on balance, evidence suggests that the avoidance of hypotension is more important than the vasoconstrictor used. Most studies using various vasopressors have not demonstrated a negative outcome for the fetus using Apgar scores and umbilical acid-base status.[52] However, a high-risk fetus may be more susceptible to the effects of vasopressors since the uterine arteries in women with pre-eclampsia are more sensitive to adrenaline added to epidural local anaesthetic. In these women ephedrine may be the drug of choice, preferably by infusion, to keep blood concentrations low and to avoid vasoconstriction in uterine blood vessels.

To minimise the incidence of hyotension, a combination of fluid, either colloid or crystalloid, and a vasopressor is often used. Wennberg et al.[54] demonstrated equivalent control of hypotension with either an ephedrine infusion combined with low-volume colloid administration or a more extensive colloid infusion. Whilst many obstetric anaesthetists use volume alone or combined with a vasopressor, others have suggested that the use of a preload is not essential to prevent hypotension following spinal blockade for caesarean section.[55] These authors used a prophylactic infusion of ephedrine titrated against blood pressure but no preload and found no difference in incidence of either hypotension or ephedrine requirements compared with a group receiving a 1000 ml fluid preload. Measures of uteroplacental blood flow were not reported but Apgar scores and cord gas and acid-base data were similar in both groups.

Despite prophylactic measures employed to prevent hypotension and aortocaval compression, epidural analgesia for caesarean section is associated with an incidence of hypotension 14–44%.[56,57] The incidence is greater in mothers undergoing elective caesarean section following 12 hours starvation compared with women receiving epidural analgesia and intravenous fluids in labour.[56] Spinal blockade develops more rapidly than epidural blockade and some authors have suggested that the incidence and severity of maternal hypotension, and therefore of uterine hypoperfusion, is greater.[58] Corke et al.[59] demonstrated an incidence of maternal hypotension of 58% following spinal blockade despite a preload of 5% dextrose in Ringer's lactate of at least 1000–1500 ml. However, others have found no difference and Helbo-Hansen et al.[57] reported a trend towards more frequent hypotension following epidural anaesthesia compared with spinal anaesthesia, 37% versus 31%. Although this did not reach statistical significance it occurred in the presence of a much greater use of prophylactic ephedrine in the spinal group, a 10 mg bolus plus infusion of 50 mg/h compared with a 5 mg bolus in the epidural group.

Hypotension is not uncommon when labour analgesia is managed with intermittent boluses of concentrated local anaesthetic. Although analgesia is achieved rapidly, associated hypotension may lead to fetal acidosis. The use of epidural boluses of less concentrated local anaesthetic has become popular. Fifteen-milligram doses of epidural bupivacaine in volumes of up to 15 ml have been shown to produce little maternal hypotension.[60] The use of epidural infusions results in more consistent analgesia and reduces the need for supplementary top-ups, reducing the cardiovascular instability associated with bolus doses and limiting the fluctuating drug concentrations in the mother and fetus.[40]

Uteroplacental flow is pressure dependent so maternal hypotension may reduce uteroplacental blood flow. This may cause decelerations in fetal heart rate, fetal hypoxia, umbilical arterial acidosis, and neonatal depression on neurobehavioural testing.[56,58,59] The effect of maternal hypotension on the fetus depends predominantly on the absolute systolic pressure and the duration of hypotension. Caritis et al.[58] demonstrated more hypotension with spinal than epidural blockade and this resulted in greater funic acidosis. Following spinal blockade for caesarean section, Corke et al.[59] found that maternal hypotension was associated with greater maternal and fetal acidosis compared with those mothers who did not experience hypotension. However, they used a preload of 5% dextrose in Ringer's lactate. Despite the changes in maternal and neonatal acid-base values, periods of hypotension less than two minutes did not appear to adversely affect neonatal neurobehaviour. Antoine and Young[56] also demonstrated an association between epidural-induced hypotension and fetal lactic acidaemia and funic acidaemia. In a study by Helbo-Hansen et al.,[57] despite the trend towards a higher incidence of hypotension in the epidural group than in the spinal group, the mean umbilical base deficit in the spinal group was greater. This may have been related to the higher doses of prophylactic ephedrine employed in the spinal group despite similar preloads.

Stress response   The pain of labour causes sympathetically mediated vaso-constriction in uterine arteries, reducing intervillous blood flow and so reducing delivery of oxygen to the fetus. Animal studies have shown increased circulating catecholamine levels in response to pain and anxiety, resulting in reduced uterine and placental blood flow and fetal distress. Morishima et al.[61] showed that pain and stress in a pregnant baboon resulted in decreased fetal oxygenation and fetal bradycardia. Effective pain relief led to an improvement in uterine perfusion and in fetal condition. Epidural analgesia reduces plasma catecholamine concentrations by removing pain and blocking sympathetic fibres so uterine blood flow is improved. Shnider et al.[62] demonstrated a reduction in adrenaline concentration by 56% in mothers during labour following the administration of epidural analgesia. Consequently, in the absence of maternal hypotension, epidural analgesia increases intervillous blood flow and exerts a protective effect against progressive metabolic acidosis in both mother and fetus. Furthermore, epidurals are often considered to be positively indicated during labour of a high-risk pregnancy where placental flow is reduced.

Maternal oxygenation and ventilation   The sympathetically mediated vaso-constriction of uteroplacental blood vessels during painful labour may be exacerbated by maternal hyperventilation. Maternal hypocapnia and alkalosis cause uterine vasoconstriction with a reduction in intervillous blood flow and placental gas exchange. This may result in fetal hypoxia and acidosis. Between contractions, the low $PaCO_2$ leads to maternal hypoventilation and the oxygen saturation may fall. Because these changes are mediated by pain, effective epidural analgesia removes the stimulus to hyperventilate, maternal minute ventilation returns to near normal values, $PaCO_2$ tensions rise, and the shifts in acid-base equilibrium are completely abolished. Curtis et al.[63] measured $tcPO_2$ continuously in mothers in labour either with or without epidural analgesia. Those without an epidural showed marked periods of hyperventilation during contractions followed by periods of hypoventilation between contractions, when $tcPO_2$ fell markedly by up to 74 mmHg. In the epidural group there were no such changes in ventilation and $tcPO_2$ was consistently higher. Both Deckardt et al.[12] and Griffin and Reynolds[14] showed a reduction in the incidence of maternal desaturation in women receiving epidural bupivacaine compared with pethidine and nitrous oxide or no analgesia.

It is unclear whether maternal hyperventilation and haemoglobin oxygen desaturation are harmful to the fetus and, if so, whether the improvements that follow epidural analgesia are beneficial to the baby. Deckardt *et al.*[12] demonstrated significantly better neonatal acid-base status following epidural analgesia compared with pethidine and nitrous oxide and suggested this was due to the lower incidence of maternal desaturation in the epidural group. Huch *et al.*[15] demonstrated cardiotocographic changes and fetal hypoxia associated with a reduction in maternal $tcPO_2$. However, most authors have not detected any detrimental effects to the baby.[14,18]

Many obstetric anaesthetists administer supplementary oxygen to the mother before caesarean section under regional anaesthesia. Fox and Houle[64] reported better fetal oxygenation, acid-base status, and time to sustained respiration when mothers breathed 100% oxygen for at least 10 minutes before delivery, compared with mothers who breathed only air. In a later study, Ramanathan *et al.*[65] randomised mothers who had received epidural anaesthesia for caesarean section to breathe air or supplementary oxygen in concentrations of 47%, 74%, and 100%. PaO_2 in maternal blood correlated significantly with PO_2 in umbilical venous and arterial blood. All values increased with increasing inspired oxygen concentration. Mothers who breathed air, and their babies, also demonstrated a metabolic acidosis not seen in the groups receiving supplementary oxygen. However, despite these changes, Apgar scores were similar in all four groups.

Progress of labour Epidural or spinal local anaesthetics have been implicated in the reduction of uterine contractility and loss of the bearing down reflex, thus prolonging the first and second stages of labour and increasing the instrumental and operative delivery rates.[66,67] The reduction in uterine activity demonstrated with local anaesthetics is only transient and may be a result of the supine position or the fluid load rather than the epidural itself. When mothers are correctly positioned with left lateral uterine displacement, epidural analgesia has been shown to have no effect on uterine activity.

Several studies have suggested that the second stage of labour is prolonged by epidural analgesia[66] while others have found no difference.[68] Furthermore, many units employ a policy of waiting for fetal descent before active pushing is commenced in order to minimise the duration of the active phase and in the belief that it increases the chance of a normal delivery. This raises the question of whether a prolonged second stage is harmful to the baby. Pearson and Davies[69] demonstrated a progressive fetal acidosis in the second stage of labour. This was detected even in babies whose mothers received epidural analgesia although prolonged pushing in the group without epidural analgesia was associated with a greater deterioration of fetal acid-base status. In the epidural group, babies born to mothers who pushed during the second stage developed a greater metabolic disturbance than babies whose mothers did not push. Furthermore, delayed pushing in the second stage by women receiving epidural analgesia has been shown not to have any deleterious effect on fetal acid-base balance compared with women allowed to push immediately. It would appear, therefore, that a prolonged second stage of labour is not necessarily harmful to either the mother or fetus in the presence of good epidural analgesia, maternal hydration, and fetal heart rate monitoring to detect fetal hypoxia.[66]

The question remains, however, whether or not epidural analgesia increases the instrumental delivery rate (see Chapter 4). A properly performed low forceps delivery or vacuum extraction has not been associated with adverse neonatal outcome, although mid-pelvis instrumental deliveries have been associated with adverse events. Fortunately, such traumatic deliveries are now rarely performed.

Neuraxial opioids

Epidural opioids have been used in labour since the early 1980s[70] while intrathecal opioids have increased in popularity in the 1990s.[71] Fentanyl and sufentanil are used most commonly during labour. Morphine is rarely used because of its slow onset and high incidence of side-effects. Epidural diamorphine has a longer duration of action than fentanyl but a higher incidence of pruritus. Epidural pethidine has also been used in combination with bupivacaine for pain relief in labour. However, it has a shorter duration epidurally than by intramuscular injection and offers little advantage over the fentanyls.

Pharmacokinetics

The speed and extent to which neuraxial opioids reach the fetal circulation depend on the speed of passage across the dura and/or cerebrospinal fluid and the rate at which they pass into nervous tissue and epidural veins. Any drug absorbed into the systemic circulation is then available for transfer across the placenta. Lipid solubility and molecular weight and shape are the main factors determining passage across the dura. Most opioids are highly lipid soluble (Table 2.2) and pass rapidly into the lipid-rich nerves and spinal cord. Although morphine, diamorphine, and fentanyl have similar molecular weights fentanyl is a thin, elongated molecule rather than the usual globular shape of the other opioids and this ensures more rapid transfer across the dura from the epidural space than either morphine or diamorphine. Highly lipophilic opioids also pass more readily into the bloodstream than hydrophilic drugs. Morphine is more polar than the other opioids and its passage across the dura is relatively slow. This increases the amount available in the epidural space for systemic absorption although its lower lipid solubility means absorption is slower than for other opioids. Once it has crossed the dura and arachnoid, its hydrophilicity favours slow passage from the cerebrospinal fluid into nervous tissue. Rostral spread occurs more readily with morphine compared with the more lipophilic opioids and the incidence of nausea and vomiting and delayed respiratory depression in the mother is greater.

Peak plasma concentrations of fentanyl occur 5–20 minutes after epidural injection. Some investigators have reported blood concentrations after lumbar epidural infusion in the range required for systemic analgesia following continuous intravenous infusion. Others have demonstrated lower peak plasma concentrations of fentanyl after epidural administration compared with the intramuscular route. The differences in these findings are probably dose related. Once in the maternal circulation, passage across the placenta depends on lipid solubility, the proportions to which the drugs bind to plasma proteins, plasma concentrations of these proteins, pH gradient across the placenta, and placental blood flow (see above). F/M ratios reported for fentanyl following epidural analgesia vary. Loftus et al.[72] and Porter et al.[11] reported UV/MV ratios of only 0.37 and 0.34 respectively following epidural fentanyl infusion. Many others have reported values nearer to 1.0 for total drug and slightly higher for free drug[31,32] (Table 2.2).

Sufentanil has been reported as being 5–10 times more potent than fentanyl when used parenterally.[73] When combined with local anaesthetic and used in a dose ratio of 10:1, fentanyl and sufentanil have been shown to provide equally effective analgesia.[74] However, epidural doses much greater than one-fifth to one-tenth of a fentanyl dose are commonly used.[75] Other reports have suggested that the relative potency of sufentanil to fentanyl when given epidurally is more in the order of 3:1.[76,77] Since sufentanil is more lipid soluble than fentanyl, free drug crosses the placenta more readily and some studies have reported greater F/M ratios for sufentanil than for fentanyl. Loftus et al.[72] reported mean UV/MV ratios of 0.37 for fentanyl and 0.81 for sufentanil after epidural administration. This is at odds with the high binding of sufentanil to $(x_1$-acid glycoprotein which suggest that UV/MV ratios should be lower for sufentanil than for fentanyl. Despite this, the low doses of sufentanil required ensure absolute maternal sufentanil concentrations are very low and cord blood concentrations frequently defy measurement. The low fetal plasma concentration is due to a combination of high protein binding in the mother, low maternal dose, and high lipid solubility allowing rapid uptake into fetal tissues, emphasising that blood concentration is not necessarily an accurate guide to fetal load.

Direct effects on the baby

All epidural opioids administered during labour have the potential to produce neonatal depression, since they cross the placenta readily. However, the doses used neuraxially for labour and delivery, particularly via the intrathecal route, are generally small so the effects seen are much less than following systemic administration.

In utero effects   No effects on fetal heart rate variability have been detected following bolus doses of epidural fentanyl.[78] This may be because fetal plasma concentrations are much lower than those achieved after a systemic bolus. However, Cohen et al.[79] demonstrated fetal heart rate changes in 15% of cardiograph tracings after a bolus dose of intrathecal sufentanil 10 µg.

Apgar scores and umbilical acid-base status   The effects of epidural opioids on the neonate are subtle at most. Neither the Apgar score nor umbilical acid-base and gas status is sufficiently sensitive to detect any effects of neuraxial opioids on the neonate.[78] Using a bolus dose of epidural bupivacaine with fentanyl 100 µg followed by an infusion of bupivacaine with fentanyl at 37.5 µg/h, Jones et al.[80] found no difference in the use of naloxone or Apgar scores compared with babies exposed to bupivacaine alone. The mean dose of fentanyl was 357 µg, with one mother receiving 547 µg over a 12-hour period. Carrie et al.[70] reported one baby with a low Apgar score following a bolus of epidural fentanyl but could neither incriminate nor definitely exclude fentanyl as the cause. Using an epidural infusion of either bupivacaine alone or bupivacaine with diamorphine at 0.5 mg/h, Bailey et al.[81] found no difference in Apgar scores or umbilical cord acid-base status.

Neurobehavioural depression   Transient neurobehavioural depression in the newborn has occurred after maternal epidural administration of high-dose alfentanil and sufentanil.[82,83] Heytens et al.[82] gave a bolus of alfentanil 30 µg/kg followed by an infusion at a rate of 30 µg/kg/h and supplementary bolus doses of 30 µg/kg when required. The mean total dose was 199 µg/kg and the authors reported low scores on neurobehavioural testing due to neonatal hypotonia. Capogna et al.[83] used a bolus of sufentanil 80 µg for caesarean delivery and demonstrated low scores for many of the tests of the NACS. Loftus et al.[72] compared placental transfer and neonatal neurobehavioural effects of fentanyl and sufentanil given epidurally for labour analgesia in a dose ratio of 5.7:1. They demonstrated significantly lower NACS 24 hours after delivery in babies whose mothers had received a mean total dose of fentanyl 137 µg compared with bupivacaine alone or with sufentanil 24 µg.

There have been many more reports suggesting no neurobehavioural depression following epidural opioids. Epidural bolus doses of fentanyl 50–100 µg[78] and infusions of up to 400 µg[11] have resulted in similar neurobehavioural scores using the NACS compared with bupivacaine alone. Following epidural fentanyl 50–100 µg for caesarean section, Helbo-Hansen et al.[84] reported some impairment in active tone compared with controls. However, the neurobehavioural scores correlated inversely with dose, suggesting absence of a dose-related effect. Lower doses of alfentanil and sufentanil than those used by Heytens et al.[82] and Capogna et al.[83] are not associated with any adverse neonatal effects. Although Loftus et al.[72] found a higher incidence of low NACS at 24 hours for babies exposed to bupivacaine with fentanyl than those receiving bupivacaine alone, this was not apparent in the sufentanil group. Writer et al.[85] compared continuous epidural analgesia with plain bupivacaine and morphine. Whilst Apgar scores and umbilical cord gas and acid-base status were similar, there were significantly more babies in the morphine group with borderline scores using the ENNS. However, pain relief was also worse in the morphine group and many women required rescue doses of 2-chloroprocaine.

Respiratory depression   There have been many assessments of neonatal respiration following epidural opioids[9,11,75] but few reports of neonatal respiratory depression. Nybell-Lindahl et al.[86] reported neonatal respiratory depression in one baby out of 20 following a bolus of epidural morphine 5 mg in labour. The baby was born one hour and 50 minutes after injection and repeated apnoeic episodes were observed during the first 16 minutes of life. Whether used either during labour or caesarean section, neither fentanyl 100 µg, alfentanil 10 µg/kg + 10 µg/kg/h, nor sufentanil ≤30 µg has resulted in any detectable neonatal effects.[9,78,87] Phillips[75] used bupivacaine combined with sufentanil for pain relief in labour and, despite using a mean dose of sufentanil 78 µg (range 40–151 µg), neonatal Apgar scores and respiratory rate during the first three hours of life were similar to a control group receiving bupivacaine alone. Benlabed et al.[9] examined several indices of respiration in newborns after caesarean delivery. Mothers received epidural anaesthesia using bupivacaine 0.5% with adrenaline 1:200 000, either with or without fentanyl 100 µg. They found no significant differences in neonatal SpO_2, incidence and duration of apnoeic episodes, respiratory rate, minute ventilation or compliance. Porter et al.[11] randomised mothers to receive an epidural infusion in labour of either bupivacaine alone or bupivacaine with fentanyl. Transcutaneous respiratory gas tensions measured continuously in newborns for the first 90 minutes of life demonstrated no differences in either $tcPO_2$ or $tcPCO_2$ between the two groups.

Plasma concentration   Plasma concentrations of fentanyl are low in both mother and baby following epidural fentanyl for labour or caesarean delivery. Whilst large bolus doses of epidural opioids have produced detectable changes in neonatal neurobehaviour,[82,83] neither smaller bolus doses nor epidural infusions achieve sufficiently high concentrations in the fetus to produce clinically detectable changes.[11,78] Fernando et al.[31] studied a combined spinal epidural technique in labour using an initial intrathecal injection of fentanyl and bupivacaine followed by intermittent epidural bolus injections of low-dose bupivacaine with fentanyl 20–30 µg. A mean total dose of fentanyl 105 µg resulted in a mean UV fentanyl concentration of

0.15 ng/ml, the highest value being 0.38 ng/ml. Bader et al.[32] infused bupivacaine 0.125% with fentanyl 2 μg/ml at 10 ml/h up to fentanyl doses of 300 μg for pain relief in labour. The mean UV fentanyl concentration was 0.16 ng/ml and both maternal venous and UV fentanyl concentrations were independent of the duration of infusion. In both studies Apgar scores, umbilical arterial gas and acid-base status, and neurobehavioural scores were within normal limits. Furthermore, no correlation was found between cord fentanyl concentrations and the indices of neonatal welfare.[31] There were, however, no control groups. Porter et al.[11] found no correlation between UV fentanyl concentrations at delivery and indices of either neonatal neurobehaviour or respiration. UV fentanyl concentrations were low, the maximum concentration being 0.24 ng/ml. It would appear that higher concentrations of fentanyl are required to cause neonatal depression. After one or more boluses of fentanyl 150–200 μg, Carrie et al. demonstrated median umbilical arterial concentrations of 0.18 ng/ml (range <0.1–0.25 ng/ml).[70] All except one baby had normal Apgar scores at one minute. This baby had the highest UA fentanyl concentration and an Apgar score of three at one minute and required intubation and treatment with naloxone but the authors could not say definitely that fentanyl was to blame.

The plasma concentration of fentanyl at which respiratory depression may occur in the newborn is also unclear. Fentanyl concentrations of 2–4.6 ng/ml have been associated with respiratory depression in adults as indicated by a 50% depression of the respiratory response to CO_2. However, similar studies have not been performed in the newborn. Studies in the 1960s on the effects of morphine suggested that the fetus may be more susceptible to opioid effects. More recently, some investigators have postulated extreme sensitivity of the newborn to the respiratory effects of fentanyl while others suggest that the susceptibility of infants to postoperative apnoea is similar to that in adults. Following major surgery during which large doses of fentanyl were used, babies have been extubated at plasma fentanyl concentrations of 0.05–0.77 ng/ml. In the study by Porter et al.,[11] the absence of detectable changes in neonatal transcutaneous gas measurements following the use of epidural fentanyl in labour is, perhaps, unsurprising since all UV fentanyl concentrations were ≤0.24 ng/ml, values well below those associated with respiratory depression in adults.

Indirect effects on the baby

Maternal ventilation Maternal respiratory depression may occur following epidural bolus doses of hydrophilic opioids or excessive doses of more lipophilic agents. This may reduce maternal oxygen saturation with potential adverse consequences for the baby. The incidence of respiratory depression, particularly delayed respiratory depression, is greatest for morphine

61

due to its propensity for rostral spread in the cerebrospinal fluid. However, some cephalad spread also occurs with the lipophilic fentanyls. Epidural fentanyl 200 µg has been shown to depress the response of the respiratory centre to CO_2 in healthy adults while sufentanil 50 µg increases end-tidal CO_2. However, most authors, using moderate doses of epidural fentanyl (50–100 µg) and sufentanil (<30 µg), have not demonstrated clinically significant respiratory depression either during or after caesarean section or general surgery. Not surprisingly, several cases of respiratory depression have been reported following the administration of high doses of morphine 1–5 mg directly into the cerebrospinal fluid. Even the lipophilic opioids have caused respiratory depression when used intrathecally. Arkoosh et al.[88] demonstrated depression of the ventilatory response to CO_2 in non labouring parturients following intrathecal sufentanil 10 µg. The incidence of respiratory depression following neuraxial opioids is increased following the use of systemic opioids.

While epidurals using local anaesthetic alone reduce the incidence of maternal oxygen desaturation during labour compared with no analgesia or with nitrous oxide and pethidine (see above), the addition of epidural opioids may reintroduce this problem. Fentanyl combined with bupivacaine increases the incidence of maternal hypoxaemic episodes compared with epidural bupivacaine alone, particularly in the second stage of labour.[14,18] The mechanism for this effect is unclear but, if mothers desaturate during breathholding and pushing, the respiratory depressant effect of epidural fentanyl may reduce their ability to restore oxygen saturation between pushes. Whatever the cause, the incidence of maternal desaturation does not appear to have any detrimental effects on the baby.[18]

Hypotension Mild hypotensive episodes may occur following the use of intrathecal opioids.[79, 89–91] Cohen et al.[79] used sufentanil 10 µg for pain relief in labour and reported an incidence of hypotension of 11–14%. Other investigators have found the incidence of hypotension to be similar following either intrathecal sufentanil 10 µg or epidural bupivacaine 0.25% 12 ml.[89] Vasodilation due to a weak local anaesthetic effect has been excluded as a cause.[90] Other suggested mechanisms include a direct action on spinal opioid receptors, a direct sympatholytic effect at spinal cord level, and a reduction in endogenous catecholamine secretion following the onset of analgesia. The latter suggestion seems unlikely, however, since Ducey et al.[91] reported a significant fall in blood pressure in 21% of mothers receiving intrathecal opioid, using prelabour, third trimester values for comparison. Any episode of maternal hypotension has the potential to reduce intervillous blood flow and adversely affect the baby. However, mild hypotension and/or prompt treatment minimise any effects and no studies have demonstrated adverse neonatal outcome from this effect of intrathecal opioids.

Epidural adrenaline

Epidural adrenaline is sometimes included as part of the test dose to detect intravascular placement of the epidural catheter. Some anaesthetists also combine it with local anaesthetic when establishing and maintaining analgesia for labour or caesarean delivery. Claimed advantages include:

- reduced vascular absorption of some local anaesthetics;
- lower peak plasma levels and reduced risk of local anaesthetic toxicity;
- improved speed of onset of local anaesthetic blockade;
- greater intensity of local anaesthetic blockade;
- improved quality of local anaesthetic blockade;
- prolonged duration of block with lignocaine or mepivacaine.

However, its use in obstetrics is controversial since absorption into the maternal circulation may, potentially, cause:

- reduced uterine activity and force of contraction;
- prolonged duration of labour;
- vasoconstriction of uteroplacental blood vessels;
- adverse effects on maternal and fetal cardiovascular parameters.

These effects are likely to be dose related and occur following systemic absorption from the epidural space. Early studies using high doses of systemic and epidural adrenaline (50–550 µg) have shown a reduction in uterine contractility and a prolonged duration of labour. However, in a number of studies Abboud et al.[92,93] failed to show any reduction in uterine activity or delay in the progress of labour using epidural adrenaline 1:200 000–1:300 000. This supports the view that epidural adrenaline, in doses up to 30 µg and in dilute concentrations of 1:200 000 or less, is unlikely to depress uterine activity.

Results from animal studies investigating the effects of adrenaline on uteroplacental blood flow are similarly conflicting. Intravenous adrenaline 5–100 µg given to pregnant ewes has been demonstrated to decrease uterine blood flow in some studies but to have no such effect in others. Furthermore, in one study epidural adrenaline 55 µg for caesarean section reduced uteroplacental flow, while several others, using less than 100 µg epidural adrenaline with local anaesthetic, failed to demonstrate any significant reduction in uterine and intervillous blood flow in humans.

Any reduction in uteroplacental flow is potentially harmful to the fetus and again, study results are conflicting. Fetal distress has been reported after an intravascular injection of 15 µg in humans. Adrenaline via the epidural route results in lower maternal plasma concentrations than does intravenous injection. Abboud et al.[92,93] reported no adverse effects of small doses (≤40 µg) of epidural adrenaline 1:300 000 or 1:200 000 respectively on fetal heart rate, Apgar scores, neonatal acid-base status, and NACS, when added to either bupivacaine or chloroprocaine for labour and delivery.

The differences in study findings may be due to species and methodological differences, including different routes of administration, doses, and concentrations of adrenaline. On balance, the weight of evidence suggests that epidural adrenaline 5 µg/ml is safe to use via the epidural route for labour and delivery in healthy parturients in that it does not appear to reduce intervillous blood flow provided maternal hypotension is avoided. Women with severe pre-eclampsia, however, are more sensitive to catecholamines, responding with a more marked degree of vasoconstriction. In these women the addition of epidural adrenaline does appear to increase the resistance of uterine blood vessels and in a survey of obstetric anaesthetists' practice, pregnancy-induced hypertension was considered to be the major contraindication to the use of epidural adrenaline.[94]

Clonidine

Clonidine is currently under investigation as an epidural and intrathecal analgesic agent for labour, caesarean section, and postoperative pain relief. It produces analgesia by an α_2-adrenergic action in the dorsal horn of the spinal cord. Most investigations in labour have studied clonidine in combination with bupivacaine since adequate analgesia using epidural clonidine alone occurs only with high doses that are associated with unwanted side-effects. These occur due to α_2-actions throughout the body and include bradycardia, hypotension, respiratory depression, and sedation, the latter being apparent even at very low doses. Whilst epidural bupivacaine combined with clonidine 75–150 µg provides superior analgesia to bupivacaine alone, doses of clonidine equal to or greater than 150 µg intrathecally and 120 µg epidurally are associated with sedation. A dose of clonidine 37.5 µg combined with bupivacaine epidurally avoids unwanted side-effects, but pain scores and duration of analgesia are similar to bupivacaine alone.[95] Consequently it has been suggested that clonidine 75 µg may be an appropriate dose to combine with bupivacaine as a single bolus.[96]

Clonidine crosses the placenta freely and sedation has been observed in the newborn following its use before delivery. However, most studies have shown no effect on either fetal heart rate or Apgar scores when combined with bupivacaine for labour analgesia.

Neostigmine

Neostigmine is another agent currently under investigation for analgesic properties when used intrathecally. Spinal cholinergic and α_2-adrenergic systems are closely linked and analgesia produced by spinal clonidine is enhanced by the cholinergic action of neostigmine and antagonised by the anticholinergic agent atropine. As with clonidine, however, side-effects, particularly nausea, vomiting, and sedation, are marked at analgesic doses.

General anaesthesia for caesarean section

The use of general anaesthesia for caesarean delivery is associated with lower Apgar scores, a greater need for active resuscitation of the neonate, and more admissions to the neonatal unit than following epidural anaesthesia. However, no long-term adverse effects have been reported as long as neonatal resuscitation is provided by trained staff.

Direct drug effects

Thiopentone

Thiopentone is the agent used most commonly for induction of anaesthesia in pregnancy and for caesarean delivery under general anaesthesia. It is a weak acid with a pKa of 7.6 (Table 2.4) and at physiological pH, approximately 60% is unionised. It is 85% bound to albumin (Table 2.4). Thiopentone is also highly lipid soluble and free, unionised drug passes into the brain and placenta within one arm-organ circulation time. Thiopentone has been detected in umbilical venous blood within 30 seconds of maternal intravenous administration.

Following its passage across the placenta, thiopentone has similar effects on the fetus as on the mother, the extent depending on the dose delivered to the fetus and therefore on the induction-to-delivery interval (IDI). If equilibrium was achieved across the placenta the F/M ratio would be around 1.0. However, F/M ratios at the time of delivery vary widely since delivery usually occurs before this point is reached and ratios may be as low as 0.4, thus limiting the neonatal depressant effects. Furthermore, the baby never experiences the profound effects seen in the mother for two reasons. First, on induction rapid redistribution of thiopentone ensures maternal plasma levels fall rapidly and the bolus effects in the mother are short-lived despite a prolonged elimination half-life (Table 2.4). Second, any drug that crosses the placenta passes through the fetal liver and is diluted in the fetal circulation before reaching the brain. It is these factors, and a short IDI that limit the total dose of drug received by the baby.

After intravenous administration of thiopentone maternal arterial and UV blood concentrations equilibrate rapidly across the placenta and the rapid fall in maternal concentration is reflected in a parallel fall in UV

Table 2.4 Pharmacokinetic properties of intravenous induction agents. $T_{1/2\beta}$: elimination half-life

	Protein binding (%)	$T_{1/2\beta}$ (hours)	pka (25°C)
Thiopentone	75–85	4–12	7.6
Propofol	97–98	3–5	11
Ketamine	12	2–4	7.5
Etomidate	76	2–11	4.1

concentration. This led to the belief that there was a "window of opportunity" some time after induction, during which time it was safest to deliver the baby because the drug load to the fetus was least. This is not so because although UV blood concentrations fall soon after induction, the dose received by the baby, and therefore fetal tissue and umbilical arterial concentrations, continue to rise for about 40 minutes after induction. Waiting for the UV concentration to fall would only result in a progressive rise in fetal thiopentone load and tissue concentration.

Propofol

Propofol is not yet licensed for use in obstetric anaesthesia. It is highly lipophilic and protein bound (Table 2.4). It crosses the placenta readily and F/M ratios at delivery have been reported as 0.58–0.76. It is rarely used for caesarean delivery for several reasons. There have been reports of lower Apgar scores following propofol 2.8 mg/kg compared with thiopentone 5 mg/kg, although other reports show no difference. Profound neonatal hypotonia and sedation for more than one hour after delivery have also been reported following induction with propofol for caesarean section. Furthermore, use of propofol 2.5 mg/kg has been associated with an incidence of maternal awareness of up to 40% with the potential for the maternal stress effects described below. Doses greater than this should reduce the incidence but may result in greater neonatal depression.

Ketamine

Although ketamine is much less lipid soluble than thiopentone it crosses the placenta readily. It is a weak base and only 12% is bound to plasma protein (Table 2.4) so F/M ratios tend to be higher than for thiopentone and are often greater than unity. Induction with ketamine 2 mg/kg has been associated with low Apgar scores and inadequate ventilation requiring intubation. Using lower doses, maternal blood pressure, uterine blood flow, and umbilical arterial gas and acid-base status are usually well maintained with cord values similar to those following general anaesthesia with thiopentone. However, low doses may provide inadequate anaesthesia and result in potentially harmful effects to the fetus (see above).

Volatile agents

The effects on the baby of volatile agents used for labour analgesia have been discussed (see pp 38–39). Neither halothane nor the newer agent sevoflurane, however, has been used widely for pain relief but both have been employed for general anaesthesia.

Halothane is now rarely used for maintenance of general anaesthesia in obstetric practice, having been superseded by other inhalational agents, particularly isoflurane. In common with other volatile agents, placental transfer of halothane is rapid, causing a dose-dependent direct neonatal depression. In the mother halothane causes a dose-dependent myocardial depression, reduction in cardiac output, and hypotension. With doses up to 1.5 MAC, uterine vasodilation is sufficient to maintain uteroplacental blood flow and fetal well-being but with higher doses placental blood flow is reduced and fetal hypoxia and metabolic acidosis ensue. The addition of more than 1.5 MAC halothane to nitrous oxide and oxygen improves uterine blood flow and neonatal acid-base status by attenuating the maternal stress response. Similar neonatal outcomes after general anaesthesia for caesarean delivery have been demonstrated using either halothane 0.5%, enflurane 1% or isoflurane 0.75% added to 50% nitrous oxide and oxygen.[97]

There have been a few reports on the use of sevoflurane for general anaesthesia for caesarean delivery. After thiopentone induction, equianaesthetic end-tidal concentrations of isoflurane 0.5% and sevoflurane 1% produced similar changes in maternal heart rate and blood pressure.[98] Indices of neonatal welfare, namely Apgar scores, umbilical gas and acid-base status, and neurobehavioural scores, were also similar in the two groups and in a control group of babies delivered under spinal anaesthesia. Sevoflurane is defluorinated in the liver like the other fluorinated ethers. The extent to which this occurs, around 3%, is much less than methoxyflurane (50–70%) and slightly more than enflurane (2.4%). Since clinical nephrotoxicity in the newborn was never a problem when methoxyflurane was used for pain relief in labour, it is exceedingly unlikely that sevoflurane, used for a short period before caesarean delivery, will prove to have any clinically significant effects on neonatal renal function. Maternal fluoride ion concentrations after the use of sevoflurane for caesarean delivery are well below those associated with polyuric renal dysfunction. The baby receives only a fraction of the sevoflurane to which the mother is exposed and neonatal fluoride ion concentrations at delivery are therefore even lower. Neonatal urinalysis 48 hours after caesarean delivery has been shown to be similar following exposure of the fetus to either isoflurane or sevoflurane.[98]

Opioids

Fentanyl in the doses commonly used for routine caesarean delivery has not been found to adversely affect the fetus although a case of fetal chest wall rigidity has been described following high-dose fentanyl 25 µg/kg intravenously.[99]

Neuromuscular blocking agents

Neuromuscular blocking drugs are fully ionised and cross the placenta very slowly. The small amount of drug that does cross the placenta is usually excreted renally and in the doses used clinically they have no clinical effect on the baby. Only one case of neuromuscular blockade in the newborn has been reported following repeated doses of tubocurare for treatment of status epilepticus in pregnancy.[100]

Indirect drug effects

Maternal stress

During general anaesthesia in the parturient maternal physiology should be kept as near to normal for pregnancy as possible in order to maintain fetal well-being. All induction agents and opioids cross the placenta rapidly and depress the fetus. Whilst a low dose will minimise drug-induced neonatal depression, this advantage is more than outweighed by the detrimental effects associated with light anaesthesia for the mother. Manipulation of the airway and surgical stimulation under inadequate anaesthesia cause increased catecholamine levels in the mother, vasoconstriction of uteroplacental vessels, and a reduction in placental perfusion. Morishima et al.[61] applied a painful stimulus to pregnant baboons and observed a reduction in uterine artery flow, fetal bradycardia, and asphyxia. The fetal condition improved when the stimulus was removed or the mother was anaesthetised with nitrous oxide or a barbiturate. Furthermore, the risk of maternal awareness is not only unpleasant for the mother but may provoke similar distress in the fetus. The effects on the newborn of the anaesthetic agents used for caesarean section under general anaesthesia are reversible and the baby will come to no harm provided adequate resuscitation is provided. It is far more important to ensure correct positioning of the mother and adequate oxygenation and to avoid fluctuations in maternal blood pressure, hyper- or hypoventilation, and maternal stress than to worry excessively over the dose of induction agent received by the baby.

Hypotension

A large fall in maternal blood pressure will reduce placental blood flow profoundly and must be avoided. All induction agents cause maternal vasodilation and myocardial depression and, in so doing, may lower the blood pressure. This is more marked following absolute overdose or following a relative overdose in the presence of hypovolaemia or fixed cardiac output states. Adequate fluid resuscitation is therefore essential before surgery. Aortocaval compression must also be avoided by left uterine displacement, either with a wedge under the right hip or by left tilt of the table. However, provided aortocaval compression is avoided, maternal blood pressure and fetal acid-base status may be better maintained with general anaesthesia compared with regional techniques,[101] and if anaesthesia is required urgently in the presence of severe hypovolaemia, general anaesthesia may provide a more haemodynamic stability.

Maternal oxygenation

It is common practice to administer oxygen at a concentration of 50–100% before delivery of the fetus by caesarean section under general anaesthesia in order to improve fetal oxygenation and acid-base status. Marx and

Mateo[102] administered oxygen during general anaesthesia for caesarean section in concentrations of approximately 30%, 65%, and greater than 90%. Maternal PaO_2 less than 13.3 kPa was associated with a prolonged time to sustained respiration and the lowest fetal oxygen tensions, whilst maternal PaO_2 greater than 40 kPa, achieved by breathing greater than 60% oxygen, produced the shortest times to sustained respiration and the highest neonatal oxygen tensions. In a more recent study oxygen was administered at either 100% with isoflurane or at 50% with nitrous oxide and isoflurane for caesarean section. Babies whose mothers received 100% oxygen not only had higher umbilical venous oxygen tensions but also required less resuscitation and showed a trend towards higher Apgar scores at one minute.[103]

Maternal ventilation

Maternal $PaCO_2$ at term is slightly lower at 4.5 kPa when compared with non-pregnant women, maintaining a gradient for CO_2 excretion across the placenta. Excessive maternal hyperventilation during general anaesthesia reduces $PaCO_2$, causing vasoconstriction of uteroplacental blood vessels and a reduction in placental perfusion. Furthermore, the alkalosis shifts the oxygen dissociation curve to the left, further reducing fetal oxygenation. When maternal $PaCO_2$ falls below 2.9 kPa fetal hypoxaemia occurs and fetal acidosis develops at maternal $PaCO_2$ values of approximately 2 kPa. Normocapnia improves fetal oxygenation, acid-base status, and Apgar scores.

Delivery intervals

Neonatal welfare, as indicated by umbilical gas and acid-base status, is influenced by both the time period from induction of anaesthesia to delivery, the IDI, and the time from incision of the uterus to delivery of the baby, the uterine incision-to-delivery interval (UDI). When regional anaesthesia is used, prolonged IDI does not adversely affect the neonate provided placental perfusion is maintained. Under general anaesthesia however, an IDI of greater than eight minutes has been associated with lower Apgar scores. However, providing hypotension is avoided and uterine displacement is maintained, an IDI of up to 30 minutes is acceptable. The UDI is of greater significance in determining neonatal condition. Under general anaesthesia, a UDI of less than 90 seconds is generally associated with better Apgar scores.

Drugs and breastfeeding

In order for maternal drug administration to affect the baby through breastfeeding, it must be secreted into the breast milk and then absorbed through the infant's gastrointestinal tract. Milk is synthesised in the glandular mammary tissue under the control of prolactin and is secreted by alveolar cells into alveoli. Contractile myoepithelial cells surround the alveoli and contraction of these cells under oxytocin control forces milk from the alveoli into the lactiferous ducts (Fig. 2.5a). Milk is a combination of fat, protein, and carbohydrate, mainly lactose. Colostrum is produced for the first 2–3 days after birth. It has a higher pH and water content than mature milk and is high in protein, low in lactose, and has no fat. Over the next 10 days the proportions change as mature milk is produced, with a lower pH than colostrum. It is high in carbohydrate and fat but has only a little protein.

Drugs that are excreted in breast milk have to pass across the capillary wall, interstitial space, and the secretory mammary cell walls before reaching the duct system (Fig. 2.5b). Only unbound drug is available for transfer from the bloodstream into breast milk. Lipophilic drugs, polar drugs, and ions pass through the endothelial pores by filtration or bulk flow while unbound, lipophilic drugs also diffuse across the endothelial cell wall. Passage of free drug across the mammary cell walls of the alveoli, from interstitium to lactiferous duct, depends on molecular weight, lipid solubility, and pKa and on the pH and concentration gradients between plasma and

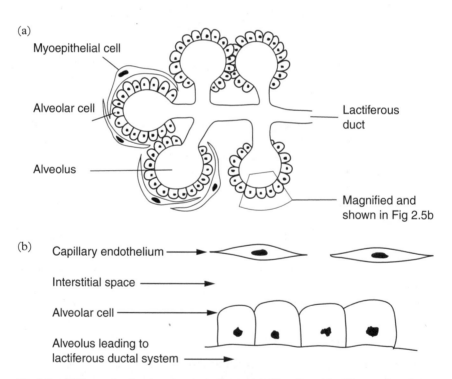

Fig 2.5   Milk production in mammary tissue. (a) Alveoli and lactiferous ductal system. (b) Higher magnification of alveolus wall demonstrating barriers to drug transport

milk. Lipid-soluble, unionised drugs pass freely by diffusion across mammary cell membranes, the main mechanism by which drugs gain access to the milk. Polar drugs bind to proteins in the interstitial fluid and pass via water-filled, protein-lined pores in the mammary cell membrane. Hydrophilic molecules of molecular weight less than 200 Da pass freely via these water-filled channels. A few non-anaesthetic drugs require active transport into milk, for example thiouracil.

Once in the milk, drugs are either free or bound to proteins or fat, depending on their lipid solubility. Because milk contains fat where plasma does not, lipid-soluble drugs may reach a higher concentration in milk than in plasma. In a manner similar to drugs crossing the placenta, the amount of an ionised drug crossing into milk depends on the pKa and the pH gradient. The pH of breast milk is 7.0 so weak bases are more ionised in milk, maintaining a concentration gradient from maternal plasma to milk down which unionised drug may pass. Any alteration in the pH gradient between maternal plasma and breast milk will alter the relative proportions of a drug in each compartment. Because of the high water content of colostrum, hydrophilic drugs are excreted in higher concentration in colostrum than in mature milk.

Even though the maternal milk/plasma ratio (M/P ratio) for drugs may vary from 0.01 to greater than 1.0, the concentration of a drug in breast milk is usually low. The amount of colostrum or milk ingested by the newborn is variable but in the first few weeks is small, further limiting infant exposure to maternal drugs. Furthermore, not all drugs cross the infant gut wall. Clinical drug effects on breastfed infants, therefore, are frequently slight or absent. However, in a breastfeeding mother it is prudent to restrict drug usage to essential drugs only, drugs that are short acting, and those least excreted into milk. Very rarely does a mother need to stop breastfeeding, for example when taking cytotoxic drugs, antithyroid drugs, and radioactive iodine.

There is an abundance of literature on drugs used by or administered to the mother whilst breastfeeding and their effects on the baby. It is beyond the scope of this book to list all the possible effects of all the drugs but Table 2.5 lists some of the drugs used more commonly for anaesthesia and analgesia.

Opioids

The lipophilic and weakly basic nature of opioids permits passage into breast milk. However, although the M/P ratio may reach 2.0, the actual amounts of morphine, diamorphine, and codeine ingested by the baby are small, first-pass metabolism is significant, and these drugs may be used safely in the breastfeeding mother. Pethidine is sometimes avoided because of the prolonged half-life in the newborn (Table 2.2). Fentanyl also passes

71

Table 2.5   Maternally administered drugs and their clinical effects on the baby whilst breastfeeding

	Drug	Potential effects
Opioids	Morphine	None
	Codeine	None
	Diamorphine	None
	Pethidine	Prolonged half-life, may accumulate and cause sedation
	Pentazocine	None
	Fentanyl	None at ≤2 µg/kg
Oral analgesics	Aspirin	Impaired neonatal platelet aggregation, bleeding tendency
		Theoretical risk of Reye's syndrome only
	Paracetamol	None
IV induction agents	Thiopentone	None
	Propofol	None
Volatile agents		No data. Probably none
Benzodiazepines	Temazepam	None
	Nitrazepam	None
	Diazepam	Sedation, lethargy
		Hyperbilirubinaemia
Atropine		Tachycardia, hyperthermia, constipation, urinary retention
H_2-receptor antagonists	Cimetidine	None
	Ranitidine	None
Local anaesthetics	Lignocaine	None
	Bupivacaine	None
Antibiotics	Benzylpenicillin	Small risk of allergic reaction
	Ampicillin	None
	Erythromycin	None
	Gentamicin	None
	Chloramphenicol	Small risk of bone marrow suppression
	Tetracycline	Theoretical risk of tooth discolouration and interference with bone growth
	Sulphonamides	Risk of kernicterus

freely into breast milk and concentrations of 0.4 ng/ml have been reported in colostrum after a maternal dose of 2 µg/kg. However, again, the amount transferred to the baby is minimal and the use of fentanyl should not be a reason to stop breastfeeding. So far, there are no data pertaining to the use of the other fentanyls.

Oral analgesics

Many oral analgesic drugs may be used safely whilst breastfeeding. Since paracetamol is water soluble and weakly acidic, little passes into the baby through the breast milk so, although hepatic metabolism in the newborn is slow, paracetamol is considered safe to use whilst breastfeeding. Aspirin (acetylsalicylate) is a prodrug that is hydrolysed in the maternal gut wall to salicylate. Very little of this active metabolite passes into breast milk (M/P ratio 0.03–0.05) because it is highly charged and protein bound. However, despite this and the lack of evidence to suggest that babies would be at risk from Reye's syndrome, the recommendations are to keep use of this drug to the occasional dose.

No adverse effects have been reported following the use of diclofenac but indomethacin should be avoided since convulsions have been reported in one breastfed infant. It may also be nephrotoxic.

Intravenous induction agents

Both thiopentone and propofol are highly lipophilic and cross into breast milk freely. However, maternal plasma concentrations fall rapidly so the actual dose reaching the milk and being ingested by the baby is negligible and use of these agents in breastfeeding mothers is considered safe.

Volatile anaesthetic agents

It is likely that volatile agents cross into breast milk but no data have been reported following anaesthesia in breastfeeding women. In practice, however, breastfeeding is not a contraindication to their use.

Benzodiazepines

M/P ratios for most benzodiazepines are in the order of 0.1–0.3, although values for diazepam up to 2.7 have been reported. All except diazepam are considered safe for the breastfeeding infant. The half-life of diazepam, however, is more prolonged in the infant than in the adult due to the immature liver and prolonged sedation and lethargy in breastfed newborns have been reported. Furthermore, a single dose to the mother is excreted in milk for up to 10 days. Drug accumulation may occur in the infant and, in the presence of neonatal hyperbilirubinaemia, may cause kernicterus due to precipitation of bilirubin from albumin-binding sites.

Anticholinergic agents

Atropine passes freely into breast milk and may cause tachycardia, hyperthermia, constipation, and urinary retention in the infant. Furthermore, its drying effect may reduce milk production in the mother.

H₂-receptor antagonists

Both cimetidine and ranitidine cross into breast milk and M/P ratios are generally much greater than unity. Although the infant may receive significant doses after repeated use, there are no data to suggest that these may be harmful although, theoretically, ranitidine may be preferable in view of the lower incidence of side-effects and absence of effect on hepatic metabolism.

Local anaesthetics

There are no data suggesting that the use of either lignocaine or bupivacaine is contraindicated whilst breastfeeding. Although both cross the placenta, neither agent has been detected in breast milk following epidural use.

Antibiotics

Antibiotics are frequently administered by the anaesthetist in the perioperative period and mothers may ask us about their safety for the baby whilst breastfeeding. Benzylpenicillin crosses into milk in very small quantities and is not contraindicated whilst breastfeeding. However, it has been known to provoke allergic reactions. Some sulphonamides are highly albumin bound and may displace bilirubin from binding sites, causing kernicterus in neonatal hyperbilirubinaemia. Tetracyclines also cross into milk but are bound to calcium in milk, slowing absorption from the infant gut. No adverse reactions have been reported in the baby although there is the potential for tooth discolouration and interference with bone growth.

Chloramphenicol is usually avoided if possible. Although the M/P ratio is only 0.5 it has the potential to cause bone marrow depression. Aminoglycosides are considered safe since insignificant amounts cross into breast milk and even less is absorbed orally.

References

1 Abboud TK, Khoo SS, Miller F, Doan T, Henriksen EH. Maternal, fetal, and neonatal responses after epidural anesthesia with bupivacaine, 2-chloroprocaine, or lidocaine. *Anesth Analg* 1982;**61**:638–44.

2 Apgar V. A proposal for a new method of evaluation of the newborn infant. *Anesth Analg* 1953;**32**:260–8.

3 Brazelton TB. Effect of prenatal drugs on the behavior of the neonate. *Am J Psychiat* 1970;**126**:1261–6.

4 Rooth G, Lysikiewicz A, Huch R, Huch A. Some effects of maternal pethidine administration on the newborn. *Br J Obstet Gynaecol* 1983;**90**:28–33.

5 Brazelton TB. *Neonatal behavioral assessment scale. Clinics in developmental medicine no. 50.* Spastics International Medical Publications. London: William Heinemann Medical Books, 1973.

6 Scanlon JW, Brown WU, Weiss JB, Alper MH. Neurobehavioral responses of newborn infants after maternal epidural anesthesia. *Anesthesiology* 1974;**40**:121–8.

7 Amiel-Tison C, Barrier G, Shnider SM, Levinson G, Hughes SC, Stefani SJ. A new neurologic and adaptive capacity scoring system for evaluating obstetric medications in full-term newborns. *Anesthesiology* 1982;**56**:340–50.

8 Roberts H, Kane KM, Percival N, Snow P, Please NW. Effects of some analgesic drugs used in childbirth with special reference to variation in respiratory minute volume of the newborn. *Lancet* 1957;**1**:128–32.

9 Benlabed M, Dreizzen E, Ecoffey C, Escourrou P, Migdal M, Gaultier C. Neonatal patterns of breathing after cesarean section with or without epidural fentanyl. *Anesthesiology* 1990;**73**:1110–13.

10 Brice JEH, Moreland TA, Walker CHM. Effects of pethidine and its antagonists on the newborn. *Arch Dis Child* 1979;**54**:356–61.

11 Porter J, Bonello E, Reynolds F. Effect of epidural fentanyl on neonatal respiration. *Anesthesiology* 1998;**89**:79–85.

12 Deckardt R, Fembacher PM, Schneider KTM, Graeff H. Maternal arterial oxygen saturation during labor and delivery: pain-dependent alterations and effects on the newborn. *Obstet Gynecol* 1987;**70**:21–5.

13 Hamza J, Benlabed M, Orhant E, Escourrou P, Curzi-Dascalova L, Gaultier C. Neonatal pattern of breathing during active and quiet sleep after maternal administration of meperidine. *Pediatr Res* 1992;**32**:412–16.

14 Griffin RP, Reynolds F. Maternal hypoxaemia during labour and delivery: the influence of analgesia and effect on neonatal outcome. *Anaesthesia* 1995;**50**:151–6.

15 Huch A, Huch R, Schneider H, Rooth G. Continuous transcutaneous monitoring of fetal oxygen tension during labour. *Br J Obstet Gynaecol* 1977;**84** (suppl 1):1–39.

16 Carstoniu J, Levytam S, Norman P, Daley D, Katz J, Sandler AN. Nitrous oxide in early labor. Safety and analgesic efficacy assessed by a double-blind, placebo-controlled study. *Anesthesiology* 1994;**80**:30–5.

17 Wilkins CJ, Reed PN, Aitkenhead AR. Hypoxaemia after inhalation of 50% nitrous oxide and oxygen. *Br J Anaesth* 1989;**63**:346–7.

18 Porter JS, Bonello E, Reynolds F. The effect of epidural opioids on maternal oxygenation during labour and delivery. *Anaesthesia* 1996;**51**:899–903.

19 Jacobson B, Nyberg K, Grönbladh L, Eklund G, Bygdeman M, Rydberg U. Opiate addiction in adult offspring through possible imprinting after obstetric treatment. *BMJ* 1990;**301**:1067–70.

20 Abboud TK, Swart F, Zhu J, Donovan MM, Peres Da Silva E, Yakal K. Desflurane analgesia for vaginal delivery. *Acta Anaesthesiol Scand* 1995;**39**:259–61.

21 Belfrage P, Boréus LO, Hartvig P, Irestedt L, Raabe N. Neonatal depression after obstetrical analgesia with pethidine. The role of the injection-delivery time interval and of the plasma concentrations of pethidine and norpethidine. *Acta Obstet Gynecol Scand* 1981;**60**:43–9.

22 Rayburn W, Rathke A, Leuschen MP, Chleborad J, Weidner W. Fentanyl citrate analgesia during labor. *Am J Obstet Gynecol* 1989;**161**:202–6.

23 Rayburn WF, Smith CV, Parriott JE, Woods RE. Randomized comparison of meperidine and fentanyl during labor. *Obstet Gynecol* 1989;**74**:604–6.

24 Shnider SM, Moya F. Effects of meperidine on the newborn infant. *Am J Obstet Gynecol* 1964;**89**:1009–15.

25 Kuhnert BR, Linn PL, Kennard MJ, Kuhnert PM. Effects of low doses of meperidine on neonatal behavior. *Anesth Analg* 1985;**64**:335–42.

26 Brackbill Y, Kane J, Manniello RL, Abramson D. Obstetric meperidine usage and assessment of neonatal status. *Anesthesiology* 1974;**40**:116–20.

27 Belsey EM, Rosenblatt DB, Lieberman BA, *et al.* The influence of maternal analgesia on neonatal behaviour: I. Pethidine. *Br J Obstet Gynaecol* 1981;**88**:398–406.

28 Wiener PC, Hogg MIJ, Rosen M. Effects of naloxone on pethidine-induced neonatal depression. *BMJ* 1977;**2**:228–31.

29 Gilbert PE, Martin WR. Antagonism of the convulsant effects of heroin, d-propoxyphene, meperidine, normeperidine and thebaine by naloxone in mice. *J Pharmacol Exp Ther* 1975;**192**:538–41.

30 Chamberlain G, Wraight A, Steer P, eds. *Pain and its relief in childbirth: the results of a national survey conducted by the National Birthday Trust.* Edinburgh: Churchill Livingstone, 1993.

31 Fernando R, Bonello E, Gill P, Urquhart J, Reynolds F, Morgan B. Neonatal welfare and placental transfer of fentanyl and bupivacaine during ambulatory combined spinal epidural analgesia for labour. *Anaesthesia* 1997;**52**:517–24.

32 Bader AM, Fragneto R, Terui K, Arthur R, Loferski B, Datta S. Maternal and neonatal fentanyl and bupivacaine concentrations after epidural infusion during labor. *Anesth Analg* 1995;**81**:829–32.

33 Kleiman SJ, Wiesel S, Tessler MJ. Patient-controlled analgesia (PCA) using fentanyl in a parturient with a platelet function abnormality. *Can J Anaesth* 1991;**38**:489–91.

34 Morley-Forster PK, Weberpals J. Neonatal effects of patient-controlled analgesia using fentanyl in labor. *Int J Obstet Anesth* 1998;**7**:103–7.

35 Hughes SC, Kan RE, Rosen MA, *et al.* Remifentanil: ultra-short acting opioid for obstetric anesthesia. *Anesthesiology* 1996;**85**:A894.

36 de Boer FC, Shortland D, Simpson RL, Clifford WA, Catley DM. A comparison of the effects of maternally administered meptazinol and pethidine on neonatal acid-base status. *Br J Obstet Gynaecol* 1987;**94**:256–61.

37 Morrison CE, Dutton D, Howie H, Gilmour H. Pethidine compared with meptazinol during labour. A prospective randomised double-blind study in 1100 patients. *Anaesthesia* 1987;**42**:7–14.

38 Wilson CM, McClean E, Moore J, Dundee JW. A double-blind comparison of intramuscular pethidine and nalbuphine in labour. *Anaesthesia* 1986;**41**:1207–13.

39 Frank M, McAteer EJ, Cattermole R, Loughnan B, Stafford LB, Hitchcock AM. Nalbuphine for obstetric analgesia. A comparison of nalbuphine with pethidine for pain relief in labour when administered by patient-controlled analgesia (PCA). *Anaesthesia* 1987;**42**:697–703.

40 Abboud TK, Afrasiabi A, Sarkis F, *et al.* Continuous infusion epidural analgesia in parturients receiving bupivacaine, chloroprocaine, or lidocaine–maternal, fetal, and neonatal effects. *Anesth Analg* 1984;**63**:421–8.

41 Scanlon JW, Ostheimer GW, Lurie AO, Brown WU, Weiss JB, Alper MH. Neurobehavioral responses and drug concentrations in newborns after maternal epidural anesthesia with bupivacaine. *Anesthesiology* 1976;**45**:400–5.

42 Covino BG. Comparative clinical pharmacology of local anaesthetic agents. *Anesthesiology* 1971;**35**:158–67.

43 Ala-Kokko TI, Alahuhta S, Jouppila P, Korpi K, Westerling P, Vähäkangas K. Feto-maternal distribution of ropivacaine and bupivacaine after epidural administration for cesarean section. *Int J Obstet Anesth* 1997;**6**:147–52.

44 Rosenblatt DB, Belsey EM, Lieberman BA, *et al.* The influence of maternal analgesia on neonatal behaviour: II. Epidural bupivacaine. *Br J Obstet Gynaecol* 1981;**88**:407–13.

45 Tronick E, Wise S, Als H, Adamson L, Scanlon J, Brazelton TB. Regional obstetric anesthesia and newborn behavior: effect over the first ten days of life. *Pediatrics* 1976;**58**:94–100.

46 Kuhnert BR, Harrison MJ, Linn PL, Kuhnert PM. Effects of maternal epidural anesthesia on neonatal behavior. *Anesth Analg* 1984;**63**:301–8.

47 Kuhnert BR, Kennard MJ, Linn PL. Neonatal neurobehavior after epidural anesthesia for cesarean section: a comparison of bupivacaine and chloroprocaine. *Anesth Analg* 1988;**67**:64–8.

48 Kileff ME, James FM, Dewan DM, Floyd HM. Neonatal neurobehavioral responses after epidural anesthesia for cesarean section using lidocaine and bupivacaine. *Anesth Analg* 1984;**63**:413–17.

49 Corke BC. Neurobehavioural responses of the newborn. The effect of different forms of maternal analgesia. *Anaesthesia* 1977;**32**:539–43.

50 McGuinness GA, Merkow AJ, Kennedy RL, Erenberg A. Epidural anesthesia with bupivacaine for cesarean section: neonatal blood levels and neurobehavioral responses. *Anesthesiology* 1978;**49**:270–3.

51 Writer WDR, Stienstra R, Eddleston JM, *et al.* Neonatal outcome and mode of delivery after epidural analgesia for labour with ropivacaine and bupivacaine: a prospective meta-analysis. *Br J Anaesth* 1998;**81**:713–17.

52 Räsänen J, Alahuhta S, Kangas-Saarela T, Jouppila R, Jouppila P. The effects of ephedrine and etilefrine on uterine and fetal blood flow and on fetal myocardial function during spinal anaesthesia for caesarean section. *Int J Obstet Anesth* 1991;**1**:3–8.

53 Hollmén AI, Jouppila R, Albright GA, Jouppila P, Vierola H, Koivula A. Intervillous blood flow during caesarean section with prophylactic ephedrine and epidural anaesthesia. *Acta Anaesthesiol Scand* 1984;**28**:396–400.

54 Wennberg E, Frid I, Haljamäe H, Norén H. Colloid (3% Dextran 70) with or without ephedrine infusion for cardiovascular stability during extradural caesarean section. *Br J Anaesth* 1992;**69**:13–18.

55 Jackson R, Reid JA, Thorburn J. Volume preloading is not essential to prevent spinal-induced hypotension at Caesarean section. *Br J Anaesth* 1995;**75**:262–5.

56 Antoine C, Young BK. Fetal lactic acidosis with epidural anesthesia. *Am J Obstet Gynecol* 1982;**142**:55–9.

57 Helbo-Hansen HS, Bang U, Garcia RS, Olesen AS, Kjeldsen L. Subarachnoid versus

epidural bupivacaine 0.5% for caesarean section. *Acta Anaesthesiol Scand* 1988;**32**:473–6.

58 Caritis SN, Abouleish E, Edelstone DI, Mueller-Heubach E. Fetal acid-base state following spinal or epidural anesthesia for cesarean section. *Obstet Gynecol* 1980;**56**:610–15.

59 Corke BC, Datta S, Ostheimer GW, Weiss JB, Alper MH. Spinal anaesthesia for caesarean section. The influence of hypotension on neonatal outcome. *Anaesthesia* 1982;**37**:658–62.

60 Shennan A, Cooke V, Lloyd-Jones F, Morgan B, de Swiet M. Blood pressure changes during labour and whilst ambulating with combined spinal epidural analgesia. *Br J Obstet Gynaecol* 1995;**102**:192–7.

61 Morishima HO, Yeh M-N, James LS. Reduced uterine blood flow and fetal hypoxemia with acute maternal stress: experimental observation in the pregnant baboon. *Am J Obstet Gynecol* 1979;**134**:270–5.

62 Shnider SM, Abboud TK, Artal R, Henriksen EH, Stefani SJ, Levinson G. Maternal catecholamines decrease during labor after lumbar epidural anesthesia. *Am J Obstet Gynecol* 1983;**147**:13–15.

63 Curtis J, Shnider SM, Saitto C, *et al.* The effects of painful uterine contractions, position, and epidural anesthesia on maternal transcutaneous oxygen tension (tcPO$_2$). *Anesthesiology* 1980;**53**:S315.

64 Fox GS, Houle GL. Acid-base studies in elective caesarean sections during epidural and general anaesthesia. *Can Anaesth Soc J* 1971;**18**:60–71.

65 Ramanathan S, Gandhi S, Arismendy J, Chalon J, Turndorf H. Oxygen transfer from mother to fetus during cesarean section under epidural anesthesia. *Anesth Analg* 1982;**61**:576–81.

66 Chestnut DH, Vandewalker GE, Owen CL, Bates JN, Choi WW. The influence of continuous epidural bupivacaine analgesia on the second stage of labor and method of delivery in nulliparous women. *Anesthesiology* 1987;**66**:774–80.

67 Thorp JA, Hu DH, Albin RM, *et al.* The effect of intrapartum epidural analgesia on nulliparous labor: A randomized, controlled, prospective trial. *Am J Obstet Gynecol* 1993;**169**:851–8.

68 Phillips KC, Thomas TA. Second stage of labour with or without extradural analgesia. *Anaesthesia* 1983;**38**:972–6.

69 Pearson JF, Davies P. The effect of continuous lumbar epidural analgesia upon fetal acid-base status during the second stage of labour. *J Obstet Gynaecol Br Commonw* 1974;**81**:975–9.

70 Carrie LES, O'Sullivan GM, Seegobin R. Epidural fentanyl in labour. *Anaesthesia* 1981;**36**:965–9.

71 Collis RE, Baxandall ML, Srikantharajah ID, Edge G, Kadim MY, Morgan BM. Combined spinal epidural analgesia with ability to walk throughout labour. *Lancet* 1993;**341**:767–8.

72 Loftus JR, Hill H, Cohen SE. Placental transfer and neonatal effects of epidural sufentanil and fentanyl administered with bupivacaine during labor. *Anesthesiology* 1995;**83**:300–8.

73 Monk JP, Beresford R, Ward A. Sufentanil. A review of its pharmacological properties and therapeutic use. *Drugs* 1988;**36**:286–313.

74 Russell R, Reynolds F. Epidural infusions for nulliparous women in labour. A randomised double-blind comparison of fentanyl/bupivacaine and sufentanil/bupivacaine. *Anaesthesia* 1993;**48**:856–61.

75 Phillips G. Continuous infusion epidural analgesia in labor: the effect of adding sufentanil to 0.125% bupivacaine. *Anesth Analg* 1988;**67**:462–5.

76 Cohen S, Amar D, Pantuck CB, *et al.* Postcesarean delivery epidural patient-controlled analgesia. Fentanyl or sufentanil? *Anesthesiology* 1993;**78**:486–91.

77 Coda BA, Cleveland Brown M, Schaffer R, *et al.* Pharmacology of epidural fentanyl, alfentanil, and sufentanil. *Anesthesiology* 1994;**81**:1149–61.

78 Cohen SE, Tan S, Albright GA, Halpern J. Epidural fentanyl/bupivacaine mixtures for obstetric analgesia. *Anesthesiology* 1987;**67**:403–7.

79 Cohen SE, Cherry CM, Holdbrook RH, El-Sayed YY, Gibson RN, Jaffe RA. Intrathecal sufentanil for labor analgesia – sensory changes, side effects, and fetal heart rate changes. *Anesth Analg* 1993;**77**:1155–60.

80 Jones G, Paul DL, Elton RA, McClure JH. Comparison of bupivacaine and bupivacaine with fentanyl in continuous extradural analgesia during labour. *Br J Anaesth* 1989;**63**:254–9.

81 Bailey CR, Ruggier R, Findley IL. Diamorphine-bupivacaine mixture compared with plain bupivacaine for analgesia. *Br J Anaesth* 1994;**72**:58–61.

82 Heytens L, Cammu H, Camu F. Extradural analgesia during labour using alfentanil. *Br J Anaesth* 1987;**59**:331–7.

83 Capogna G, Celleno D, Tomassetti M. Maternal analgesia and neonatal effects of epidural sufentanil for cesarean section. *Reg Anesth* 1989;**14**:282–7.

84 Helbo-Hansen HS, Bang U, Lindholm P, Klitgaard NA. Neonatal effects of adding epidural fentanyl to 0.5% bupivacaine for caesarean section. *Int J Obstet Anesth* 1993;**2**:27–33.

85 Writer WDR, James FM, Wheeler AS. Double-blind comparison of morphine and bupivacaine for continuous epidural analgesia in labor. *Anesthesiology* 1981;**54**:215–19.

86 Nybell-Lindahl G, Carlsson C, Ingemarsson I, Westgren M, Paalzow L. Maternal and fetal concentrations of morphine after epidural administration during labor. *Am J Obstet Gynecol* 1981;**139**:20–1.

87 Vertommen JD, Vandermeulen E, Van Aken H, *et al*. The effects of the addition of sufentanil to 0.125% bupivacaine on the quality of analgesia during labor and on the incidence of instrumental deliveries. *Anesthesiology* 1991;**74**:809–14.

88 Arkoosh VA, Torjman MC, Montgomery OC, Leighton BL, Norris MC. Does intrathecal sufentanil depress the ventilatory response of CO_2 in the parturient? *Anesthesiology* 1994;**81**:A1147.

89 d'Angelo R, Anderson MT, Philip J, Eisenach JC. Intrathecal sufentanil compared to epidural bupivacaine for labor analgesia. *Anesthesiology* 1994;**80**:1209–15.

90 Mandell GL, Jamnback L, Ramanathan S. Hemodynamic effects of subarachnoid fentanyl in laboring parturients. *Reg Anesth* 1996;**21**:103–11.

91 Ducey JP, Knape KG, Talbot J, Herman NL, Husain FJ. Intrathecal narcotics for labor cause hypotension. *Anesthesiology* 1992;**77**:A997.

92 Abboud TK, Sheik-ol-Eslam A, Yanagi T, *et al*. Safety and efficacy of adrenaline added to bupivacaine for lumbar epidural analgesia in obstetrics. *Anesth Analg* 1985;**64**:585–91.

93 Abboud TK, DerSarkissian L, Terrasi J, Murakawa K, Zhu J, Longhitano M. Comparative maternal, fetal, and neonatal effects of chloroprocaine with and without adrenaline for epidural anesthesia in obstetrics. *Anesth Analg* 1987;**66**:71–5.

94 Holdcroft A. Use of adrenaline in obstetric analgesia. *Anaesthesia* 1992;**47**:987–90.

95 Brichant JF, Bonhomme V, Mikulski M, Lamy M, Hans P. Admixture of clonidine to epidural bupivacaine for analgesia during labor: effect of varying clonidine doses. *Anesthesiology* 1994;**81**:A1136.

96 Eisenach JC, de Kock M, Klimscha W. α_2-adrenergic agonists for regional anesthesia. A clinical review of clonidine (1984–1995). *Anesthesiology* 1996;**85**:655–74.

97 Warren TM, Datta S, Ostheimer GW, Naulty JS, Weiss JB, Morrison JA. Comparison of the maternal and neonatal effects of halothane, enflurane, and isoflurane for cesarean delivery. *Anesth Analg* 1983;**62**:516–20.

98 Gambling DR, Sharma SK, White PF, Beveren TV, Bala AS, Gouldson R. Use of sevoflurane during elective cesarean birth: a comparison with isoflurane and spinal anesthesia. *Anesth Analg* 1995;**81**:90–5.

99 Jarvis AP, Arancibia CU. A case of difficult neonatal ventilation. *Anesth Analg* 1987;**66**:196–9.

100 Older PO, Harris JM. Placental transfer of tubocurarine. *Br J Anaesth* 1968;**40**:459–63.

101 James FM, Crawford JS, Hopkinson R, Davies P, Naiem H. A comparison of general anesthesia and lumbar epidural analgesia for elective cesarean section. *Anesth Analg* 1977;**56**:228–35.

102 Marx GF, Mateo CV. Effects of different oxygen concentrations during general anaesthesia for elective caesarean section. *Can Anaesth Soc J* 1971;**18**:587–93.

103 Piggott SE, Bogod DG, Rosen M, Rees GAD, Harmer M. Isoflurane with either 100% oxygen or 50% nitrous oxide in oxygen for caesarean section. *Br J Anaesth* 1990;**65**:325–9.

3: Pain relief in labour: non-regional

MARK SCRUTTON

The three forms of non-regional analgesia available to women in labour most familiar to anaesthetists are transcutaneous electrical nerve stimulation (TENS), nitrous oxide (Entonox) and systemic opioids, most commonly pethidine in the UK.[1] However, in this era of "Changing Childbirth"[2] it is important that anaesthetists working on the labour ward are familiar with alternative approaches to analgesia that are popular with many mothers and midwives so that they can give informed guidance to women in both the antenatal and labour ward settings.

Psychological methods

Antenatal preparation

Although antenatal preparation in its broadest sense has probably been practised in some form or another for centuries, more recently a number of enthusiasts have emerged claiming spectacular success in reducing pain and improving labour outcomes with specific courses of education and instruction. In *Natural Childbirth*,[3] Grantly Dick Read described a technique for helping women to cope with childbirth using a programme of lectures and physical exercises. He proposed that it was the fear and anxiety born out of ignorance and misinformation in Western society that lead to pain and delayed the progress of labour. He claimed a success rate of over 90% in mothers using his techniques. The Lamaze technique,[4] described by the French obstetrician Dr Ferdinand Lamaze, is another popular method of psychological preparation that many antenatal teachers continue to embrace. Based on breathing exercises requiring such concentration as to distract labouring women from the pain of contractions, Lamaze claimed a success rate of over 90% and commanded considerable media attention. Although there is no doubt that such charismatic individuals can have enormous impact on the women that they look after, their techniques rarely achieve the same success when implemented by others. There are no controlled trials that come close to repeating such results.

Today, most pregnant women have access to some form of antenatal programme designed to prepare them for both childbirth and the immediate postnatal period. Although a number of studies have demonstrated a reduction in analgesic requirements in women attending antenatal classes, this almost certainly reflects an increased ability to cope rather than a reduction in pain itself. In general, there is agreement that antenatal preparation is of overall benefit to pregnant women. However, there may be disadvantages. In the majority of women antenatal preparation alone will not prevent pain and there is evidence that the physiological response to pain may be detrimental to the baby and to the progress of labour. Severe pain and distress cause labouring women to hyperventilate during contractions and this is exacerbated by some of the breathing techniques. As a result, maternal arterial carbon dioxide tension ($PaCO_2$) falls, causing a degree of maternal vasoconstriction and increasing maternal affinity for oxygen.[5] This reduces uterine artery blood flow and delivery of oxygen to the fetus. Between contractions the reduced maternal $PaCO_2$ combined with exhaustion may result in hypoxic episodes due to underventilation or periods of apnoea.[5,6] Some proponents of preparation techniques suggest that pharmacological intervention is never required in childbirth and this can lead to a sense of inadequacy and failure in women who find they can no longer cope once in labour.

Antenatal programmes should include unbiased information on the pros and cons of all forms of analgesia based on scientific research as opposed to anecdotal opinions. Ideally these programmes should include an opportunity to discuss regional techniques with an obstetric anaesthetist. It is much easier to allay fears and anxieties at this stage rather than trying to unpick ill-founded beliefs in the more stressful situation of established labour.

Intrapartum support

Intrapartum support provided by the midwife and, in many cases, a partner may improve labour outcome and reduce analgesic requirements. Once again, the reduction in analgesic requirements may reflect an increased ability to cope rather than an actual reduction in pain. Familiarity with the midwife has been shown to be beneficial and this has led to the development of "team midwifery" in many centres.[7] Unfortunately, financial constraints often limit the ability to provide an effective team midwifery service such that labouring women all too often end up being cared for by an unfamiliar face. Furthermore, increasing workload often limits the amount of psychological support the midwife is able to deliver.

Hypnosis

Hypnosis is an extension of antenatal preparation and has been claimed to reduce pain and improve the outcome of labour. The preparation is extensive, time consuming and can be expensive. Although pain may be reduced in some, efficacy is unpredictable and supplemental analgesia is often required. It is unlikely that hypnosis has any detrimental effect on mother or baby though, once again, techniques relying on breathing exercises may cause hyperventilation, alkalosis, and impairment of placental gas exchange.

Physical methods

Transcutaneous electrical nerve stimulation

Transcutaneous electrical nerve stimulation (TENS) is a popular analgesic technique for the relief of pain in labour despite the fact that studies suggest that its efficacy is limited. TENS is widely available and has the advantage that it can be used not only in labour but also at home during the last few weeks of pregnancy to treat backache and prelabour contractions.

Electrodes are attached with tape or adhesive to the lower back on each side of the spine (Fig 3.1). The electrodes are approximately 10–15 cm², made of conductive rubber and may be reusable or disposable. They are connected to a portable miniaturised current generator that produces electrical pulses. The amplitude of the pulse is variable and can be increased up to 50 mA as required. The preferred pulse duration is 0.05–0.2 ms which can be delivered at a frequency of 1–100 Hz. Two forms of TENS treat-

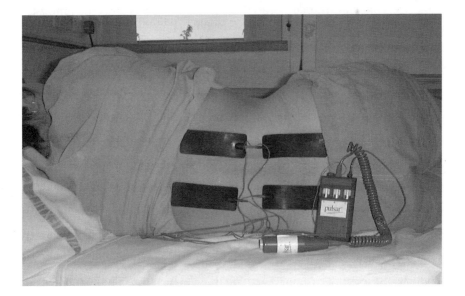

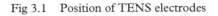

Fig 3.1   Position of TENS electrodes

ment are described. Low-frequency TENS (lo TENS) is delivered at 1–2 Hz and is generally not used in the treatment of labour pain. At this frequency the TENS, often referred to as "acupuncture-like TENS", elicits muscular contractions. With conventional TENS (hi TENS), used most commonly in labour, frequencies of 30–100 Hz cause non-painful electrical paraesthesia over the area of pain.

Once the electrodes are sited, the amplitude is slowly increased until the woman is aware of a strong tingling sensation. This is used as a continuous background stimulus and a separate booster button is pressed to increase the amplitude whenever a contraction occurs. Both background and booster levels are increased as labour becomes more painful and quite powerful stimuli are well tolerated as labour progresses.

Mechanism of action

Ideally TENS electrodes are positioned over the posterior aspect of dermatomes supplied by the posterior primary rami of T10–S4 (Fig 3.1). When electrical stimuli are applied to these mixed nerves, the large myelinated Aβ fibres are stimulated first. This causes activation of collaterals and interneurons in the dorsal horn of the spinal cord that inhibit nociceptive transmission in the smaller Aδ and C fibres at the same level in a mechanism likely to be similar to "closing the gate" as proposed by Melzack and Wall in 1965.[8] TENS may also act by causing descending impulses from cortical centres that inhibit nociceptive afferents. Although there is some evidence from chronic pain states that analgesia persists for some time after cessation of the TENS stimuli, TENS is most effective in labour when used continuously.

There is evidence that lo TENS may act through a secondary endorphinergic mechanism. Studies have demonstrated changes in cerebrospinal endorphin levels in response to lo TENS and that the analgesia produced can be reversed with naloxone. hi TENS is not reversed by naloxone and there is no evidence that it acts through this mechanism.

Efficacy

Enthusiasts report remarkable reduction in labour pain with the use of TENS. Unfortunately this is primarily based on unrandomised trials and anecdotal reports. The majority of randomised controlled trials have produced disappointing results, particularly when comparing TENS to placebo. In placebo-controlled studies, at best only about 10% of women appear to achieve good pain relief requiring no other form of analgesia, although a larger percentage may find it of some help.[9,10] In the 1990 National Birthday Trust survey, 22% of women using TENS found it of some help during labour.[11]

In general, TENS is most effective at reducing the back pain associated with the first stage of labour. Based on this and on experience from the use of TENS in chronic pain, some investigators have suggested that electrodes should be placed over the area of perceived pain rather than the dermatomal levels corresponding to the uterus and perineum. However, although some success has been reported with suprapubic placement of electrodes to treat suprapubic pain, efficacy has not been greatly improved.[12,13]

In a recent systematic review of randomised controlled trials comparing TENS with either sham TENS or no treatment, Carroll *et al.* reported no significant differences in prospective pain outcomes in the 10 studies that were examined.[14] Three studies reported significant differences between active and sham TENS for secondary outcomes. Primary outcomes were defined as any prospective measures of pain made during labour, while secondary outcomes included retrospective assessment of pain and use and timing of any additional pain interventions. The authors concluded that TENS has no significant effect on pain in labour and that alternative interventions should be offered.

Side-effects and complications

TENS appears to be free from significant side-effects and complications for both mother and baby. Some women find the tingling sensation unpleasant or the electrodes irritating. Although TENS has the potential to cause interference on monitors of fetal or maternal heartbeat, modern machines have low current density and filters to prevent this. Despite the fact that retrospective reports have suggested that labour is shortened and neonatal Apgar scores improved with the use of TENS, no such benefits have been reported in prospective clinical trials.

TENS does not restrict mobility but it interferes with some massage techniques and must be removed before epidural siting. Although some maternity units provide TENS free of charge, in the majority of cases mothers must either buy or hire machines themselves, particularly for use outside the delivery unit. This may contribute to the fact that some women who find the technique to be inadequate or ineffective feel cheated by their experience with this mode of analgesia.

In summary, TENS is a safe technique that provides analgesia in no more than 10% of labouring women, may be helpful in 20–30% and can be used at home or on the delivery unit. However, in the majority of women it provides little or no analgesia and is only helpful in early labour, if at all. Nevertheless, it enjoys considerable popularity among many of those who have used it.

Massage

In the 1990 survey by the National Birthday Trust, massage was the most popular form of simple analgesia despite the fact that efficacy was low and supplementary techniques were usually required.[1] Techniques may vary from simple back rubbing to more formal techniques taught in special ante-natal classes or provided by trained masseurs. Lower back massage is often the most effective but techniques involving massage to the abdomen, upper back or indeed any area may provide distraction and relaxation. Although massage has been shown to be efficacious and to reduce further analgesic requirements in a number of trials, the benefit tends to be limited to early labour.

The mode of action of massage is thought to be similar to that of TENS. Cutaneous stimulation of Aβ fibres in the posterior primary rami causes collateral inhibition of nociceptive afferents. Undoubtedly there is also activation of descending cortical inhibitory pathways that supplement this effect.

Massage is safe for mother and baby and although TENS electrodes and epidural catheters may interfere with lower back massage, there are no specific contra-indications. It is a useful simple technique that should be encouraged and involvement of the partner can provide added satisfaction to both parties.

Other Physical Methods

Water baths

Water baths as distinct from water *births* are used as an analgesic and relaxation technique by many women before admission to the delivery unit and during early labour. Often a standard bath will suffice although a larger hot tub or birthing pool allows more mobility and comfort. The mechanism of action is similar to massage with cutaneous stimulation of Aβ fibres inhibiting nociceptive afferents. In a similar manner to increasing the amplitude of TENS, increasing water temperature may improve analgesia as contractions increase in strength. However, there are concerns that increasing maternal temperature may cause fetal tachycardia. This tachycardia may either represent fetal distress or be benign but result in unnecessary obstetric intervention. Both possibilities are best avoided by restricting water temperature to 37°C.

Water baths often restrict mothers to the supine position, which may be detrimental to the progress of labour. Fetal monitoring is restricted and alternative analgesic techniques limited. Both Entonox and pethidine are relatively contraindicated as they may cause dizziness and sedation. Epidural analgesia is contraindicated because of risk of infection and inability to secure the catheter.

Water blocks

The water block technique involves a series of injections of sterile water (0.1–0.5 ml) at 4–6 points over the sacral border in the lower back.[15,16] The injections are usually performed by midwives and have been reported to reduce the back pain associated with labour. The injections are locally irritant and thought to act through the same mechanism as TENS (see above). Although side-effects are minimal, efficacy is limited and the technique is rarely used in this country.[17]

Acupuncture

Acupuncture is offered by a wide variety of practitioners, both medically qualified and lay. Equally varied are the techniques used by individual practitioners. Broadly speaking, these may be divided into "traditional", based on the ancient Chinese teachings and beliefs, and "modern", based on anatomical zones or tender points. Until very recently acupuncture was not used for analgesia in labour by Chinese practitioners because they believed that pain was a natural part of the process, although they did support the use of acupuncture for caesarean section. Despite this, there are a small number of Western enthusiasts who advocate the use of acupuncture in labour both to ameliorate pain and to accelerate the progress of labour. Although these enthusiasts and some of their clients give glowing anecdotal reports, there are no randomised trials to support its efficacy. Apart from the risks associated with infection from needles, reported side-effects are rare.

Although practised by a small number of midwives, acupuncture is not widely available in this country. Private practitioners are expensive and, should the technique fail, mothers may feel cheated.

Abdominal decompression

Abdominal decompression was a technique developed in 1955 by the South African Professor O S Heyns.[18] The technique involved encasing the abdomen in an airtight shell and exposing it to a negative pressure of 20–150 mmHg (Fig 3.2). The negative pressure could be applied intermittently during contractions or continuously throughout labour. Heyns believed that this technique relieved pain, allowed the uterus to contract more efficiently, speeding the process of labour, and improved placental blood flow. He reported success rates of 80–90% although more recent trials fail to show any real benefits. Apart from its lack of efficacy, the equipment was cumbersome and uncomfortable, requiring the mother to remain supine and motionless. The technique has been largely abandoned since the end of the 1960s.

Inhalational agents

Ether and chloroform

When John Snow administered chloroform to Queen Victoria for the birth of Prince Leopold on 7 April 1853, it marked a turning point in the history of obstetric analgesia. Before this time there was widespread belief in professional, religious, and lay circles that pain was both an integral and necessary part of labour. However, ether was in fact the first inhalational

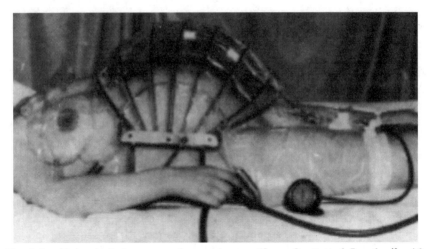

Fig 3.2 Abdominal decompression apparatus (from Scott and Loudon[19] with permission)

agent used for analgesia in labour. In January 1847, six years before the famous royal labour, James Young Simpson, professor of midwifery in Edinburgh, first documented the use of ether in obstetrics when it was given to deliver a dead fetus following an obstructed labour. Although effective, Simpson found ether to have unpleasant side-effects. It had a pungent smell and was irritant to the airways, slow in onset and caused nausea and vomiting.

Chloroform, introduced to obstetric practice at the end of 1847, was more pleasant to breathe, quicker in onset, and rapidly became the agent of choice. Despite the fact that it fell from favour for use in general anaesthesia due to dose-related arrhythmias and hepatotoxicity, it remained popular in obstetric practice where its intermittent administration in low concentrations was felt to balance these side-effects. Nonetheless, the dose administered was hard to control and despite the early recommendation by John Snow to "give the chloroform very gently" such that "complete anaesthesia is never induced in midwifery", loss of consciousness all too often occurred.[20] Furthermore, chloroform reduced uterine contractility and readily crossed the placenta, causing neonatal depression. Despite this, chloroform remained the most commonly used inhalational analgesic in labour until the widespread introduction of nitrous oxide in the 1930s.

Nitrous oxide

History

Nitrous oxide, identified by Joseph Priestly in 1772, was first investigated clinically by Sir Humphrey Davy in 1798. Although Davy noted that breathing nitrous oxide relieved severe toothache, it was not until 1844 that Horace Wells first used it in his dental practice, having been introduced to nitrous oxide at a "laughing gas party". However, following its disastrous therapeutic failure during a demonstration at the Massachusetts General Hospital and the introduction of ether and chloroform, nitrous oxide fell from favour until 1863 when it was reintroduced to dental practice.

Nitrous oxide was first used in obstetric practice in 1880 by Stanislav Klikowitsch, a Polish-Russian physician working in St Petersburg.[21] Klikowitsch noted that nitrous oxide, 80% in 20% oxygen, reduced the crying of labouring women without causing loss of consciousness. He went on to show that, unlike chloroform, it had no depressant effect on uterine activity. However, because of expense in production and difficulty in developing delivery systems, nitrous oxide did not become widely available until the 1930s.

In 1933 Minnitt designed a system for premixing nitrous oxide and air in a 50:50 mixture, simplifying its delivery to the parturient.[22] However, it rapidly became apparent that such mixtures caused hypoxia, delivering as little as 8% oxygen, and were potentially harmful to both mother and fetus. As a result systems were developed to deliver nitrous oxide/oxygen mixtures. Initially delivery systems involved separate sources for oxygen and nitrous oxide because it was believed that nitrous oxide would separate into the liquid phase at high pressures if mixed in a single cylinder with oxygen. However, Tunstall demonstrated in 1963 that, when mixed with 50% oxygen, nitrous oxide did not separate into the liquid phase at a pressure of 2000 lb/in^2 unless the ambient temperature fell to below $-8°C$.[23] In the following decade a number of different concentrations of nitrous oxide in oxygen were assessed resulting in the recommendation by a subcommittee of the Medical Research Council that a 50:50 mixture of nitrous oxide and oxygen provided an adequate degree of analgesia that could be safely administered by unsupervised midwives.[24] Since then this mixture has been marketed as Entonox by the British Oxygen Company and is the most widely used form of nitrous oxide in modern obstetric practice.

Physical properties

Entonox is a mixture of 50% nitrous oxide in 50% oxygen that is supplied in cylinders at a pressure of 137 bar (2000 lb/in^2). At this pressure the two gases "dissolve" into each other, preventing the liquefaction of nitrous oxide. However, the critical temperature for this mixture is $-8°C$. Allowing the Entonox to cool below this temperature will result in separation of the nitrous oxide into liquid form. Such a cylinder will then initially deliver an oxygen-rich mixture until most of the oxygen has been used up whereapon it will deliver a hypoxic concentration of nitrous oxide. More importantly, if stored upright, despite rewarming, the oxygen may remain separated from the nitrous oxide and the same phenomenon may occur. Recommendations have therefore been described to ensure that cylinders that may have been cooled inappropriately are first stored for at least 24 hours in the horizontal position at a temperature of greater than 10°C and then inverted several times before use.[24] Similarly, precautions must be taken to prevent cooling of pipeline supplies.

As an inhalational anaesthetic agent nitrous oxide has low potency but it provides analgesia in subanaesthetic doses (Table 3.1). Analgesia is rapid in onset due to the low blood gas solubility coefficient (Table 3.1). It is rapidly eliminated from the lungs between contractions such that there is minimal accumulation in mother or fetus even during prolonged use in labour. Entonox is delivered from a cylinder via a pressure-reducing valve and then self-administered through a demand valve using either a face mask or mouthpiece (Fig 3.3).

Table 3.1 Characteristics of inhalational agents used in labour

	MAC %	Blood/gas sol. Coeff at 37°C	Inspired % for analgesia in labour
Ether	1.9	12	Unmeasured
Chloroform	0.5	10	(0.2–0.9)*
Nitrous oxide	105	0.47	50
Trichloroethylene	0.17	9	0.35–0.5
Methoxyflurane	0.2	13	0.35
Enflurane	1.68	1.9	0.25–1.25
Isoflurane	1.15	1.4	0.2–0.75
Desflurane	6.0	0.42	1–4.5
Sevoflurane	2.0	0.6	Not reported

*Historically often delivered in unmeasured concentrations

Efficacy

Before the recommendations made by the Medical Research Council in 1970, nitrous oxide was available in concentrations of up to 80% in oxygen. Trials at and before this time had suggested that analgesic efficacy was greater in the more concentrated mixtures – particularly 70% or more. However, at these higher concentrations the incidence of loss of consciousness became unacceptably high. As a result, only the 50% mixture (Entonox) is now available for general use in labour. Studies examining the efficacy of Entonox have produced mixed results and although some of the earlier studies reported effective analgesia in over 60% of users, more recent placebo-controlled trials are disappointing. Even in early labour, when enthusiasts claim it to be most effective, a recent double-blind placebo study has shown it to be ineffective.[26]

Although overall analgesic efficacy is clearly limited, Entonox has compared favourably with other forms of non-regional analgesia such as TENS. Comparisons with methoxyflurane and trichloroethylene have shown little

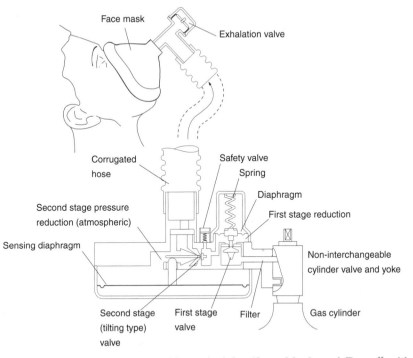

Fig 3.3   The Entonox valve: working principles (from Moyle and Davey[25] with permission)

difference in efficacy. More importantly, it is now well documented that Entonox is more effective than pethidine in doses of up to 150 mg.[27] Despite this evidence and the well-recognised detrimental side-effects to mother and baby (see below), pethidine is all too frequently offered to women who find Entonox inadequate. This should be discouraged and women who require further analgesia should be offered epidural or spinal analgesia which has been consistently demonstrated to be more effective.

A number of strategies have been used in attempts to improve the efficacy of Entonox. The simplest yet most important way to optimise the analgesia provided by Entonox is careful instruction of the parturient. Inhalation must begin at the start of the contraction in order to try to attain analgesic levels as the contraction peaks. As soon as the contraction starts to wane, inhalation should stop. Nitrous oxide is then eliminated as the contraction fades and the mother has minimal hangover between contractions. The distraction provided by the technique itself and the need to concentrate on taking regular deep breaths of Entonox during the contraction almost certainly contribute to the success of this technique.

The time from starting to inhale Entonox to peak analgesic efficacy is about 45–60 seconds. If the parturient begins to inhale at the start of her contraction, the peak of the contraction often occurs before maximal analgesic effect has been achieved. In order to reduce the time to peak analgesic efficacy, a number of groups have given supplementary continuous low-flow Entonox via nasal prongs.[28,29] This background administration of Entonox allows analgesic levels to be attained more quickly. The nasal prongs are well tolerated and studies suggest that analgesia is improved and is preferred by the parturient. Other strategies to improve analgesia include supplementation with low doses of volatile anaesthetics such as enflurane or isoflurane (see below).

Side-effects

A proportion of mothers report feeling dizzy, unpleasantly light-headed or out of control when using Entonox and nausea and vomiting are common. A small percentage may even lose consciousness although this is unusual with Entonox alone. Reassurance and the appropriate timing of inhalation with contractions can often overcome some of these side-effects. However, if unrelieved, the side-effects will resolve rapidly once Entonox is withdrawn.

Of greater concern has been the effect of Entonox on maternal ventilation. During contractions mothers tend to hyperventilate while breathing Entonox. The high inspired concentration of oxygen that results maintains good arterial oxygen levels that are potentially beneficial to the baby, particularly if there is fetal distress. However, hypocapnia often occurs and may decrease oxygen transfer across the placenta by causing vasoconstriction and increasing the affinity of maternal haemoglobin for oxygen. Between contractions, hypocapnia combined with any residual sedative effects of Entonox may increase the incidence of maternal hypoventilation and arterial oxygen desaturation. The evidence for this latter complication is equivocal. In women receiving no analgesia, hyperventilation and hypocapnia caused by the pain of contractions may precipitate similar periods of hypoventilation and desaturation between contractions.[6] Studies comparing Entonox with placebo show no difference in the incidence of desaturation in those using Entonox.[26] Conversely, in studies comparing Entonox with epidural analgesia, desaturation appears more common in those using Entonox. Epidural analgesia alleviates the pain of contractions, preventing hyperventilation and subsequent hypoventilation.[30] Hence, although desaturations may be more common in those using Entonox than in those with epidurals, there is no good evidence to suggest that the use Entonox causes more desaturations than normal labour without analgesia.

Entonox has no documented effect on the progress or outcome of labour. Comparison of Apgar scores and more complex neonatal outcome measures show no detrimental effects on the baby. Two studies have suggested that children born to mothers using Entonox are 2–4 times more likely to develop amphetamine or opioid dependency later in life.[31,32] However, these studies have been heavily criticised and further research is required to address this disturbing suggestion.

Prolonged use of nitrous oxide interferes with methionine synthetase activity which may lead to the development of megaloblastic anaemia and subacute combined degeneration of the spinal cord. Neither complication has been recorded in obstetric use. These side-effects have, however, been described in those using Entonox as a drug of abuse. Although Entonox abuse is unlikely to occur in mothers using it appropriately in labour, unsupervised access allows potential for this to occur among care providers.

In the 1980s much attention was focused on the pollution caused by the use of volatile anaesthetic agents and nitrous oxide. There was concern that chronic exposure to low background levels of these agents might cause health problems among medical staff. Despite the fact that prospective studies have failed to support these suggestions, much time and money have been spent developing complex scavenging systems to reduce pollution. Nitrous oxide is difficult to scavenge from the apparatus used by labouring mothers and maintaining minimal ambient levels depends on efficient labour ward ventilation systems. Current standards in the UK require ambient nitrous oxide levels to be below 100 ppm although it has been shown that midwives and other obstetric care providers are frequently exposed to higher levels.[33]

Other agents

Trichloroethylene (Trilene) was introduced into obstetrics in the 1940s, replacing the more toxic chloroform. As with nitrous oxide, it provides analgesia at subanaesthetic concentrations. Although a potent anaesthetic agent, it has a relatively high blood gas solubility resulting in slow onset of analgesia but gradual accumulation and hence improved analgesia as labour progresses (Table 3.1). Inspired concentrations of 0.35–0.5% provided similar analgesic effects to Entonox and were delivered using portable vaporisers. Although popular with midwives in the UK, the Central Midwives Board withdrew approval for its use in labour in 1993 and it is no longer available.

Methoxyflurane, another potent volatile anaesthetic agent with low blood gas solubility, was introduced in 1960 (Table 3.1). Administered in a concentration of 0.35% in air, analgesia was of slower onset than Entonox but improved as methoxyflurane accumulated during the course of labour. Analgesia is similar to Entonox but nausea and vomiting may be less common in mothers using methoxyflurane. Although popular in the United States, it failed to displace trichloroethylene in the UK. Methoxyflurane is partially metabolised in the liver, producing elevation of serum inorganic fluoride ions. Though not reported in obstetric use, renal failure related to high fluoride levels has been documented following

91

prolonged methoxyflurane use in general anaesthesia. This concern, combined with the lack of any demonstrable advantage over Entonox has led to its withdrawal from obstetric use.

Isoflurane and enflurane have both been investigated in obstetric practice. At subanaesthetic concentrations, 0.75% and 1% respectively, studies suggest that analgesia is superior to Entonox but at the expense of increased maternal sedation.[34,35] At lower concentrations sedation is reduced but analgesia is no longer better than Entonox. In general, the additional apparatus required for delivering these combinations is cumbersome, expensive and therefore not generally available to labouring women. However, one group has demonstrated that isoflurane will form a stable gas mixture with Entonox at pressures of 137 bar and can therefore be delivered from the same cylinder or gas supply.[36]

The newer volatile agents desflurane and sevoflurane both have low blood gas solubilities and offer the theoretical advantage that speed of onset and elimination should be rapid. The use of desflurane has been investigated and shown to provide similar analgesia to Entonox but with an increased incidence of amnesia.[37] However, the cost of desflurane, the complex vaporiser required for its delivery, and its lack of significant therapeutic advantage make widespread use unlikely. Sevoflurane has not been investigated in obstetric practice but may become a potential therapeutic alternative or adjunct to Entonox if its cost is reduced.

Despite being in obstetric use for over a century and the introduction of many alternative inhalational agents, nitrous oxide in the form of Entonox remains the most popular inhalational analgesic agent used in labour. Though placebo-controlled trials suggest analgesic efficacy is limited, Entonox undoubtedly helps many mothers to cope with labour and has minimal detrimental side-effects.

Systemic opioids

History

Opioids have been used for analgesia in labour for hundreds of years often as an incidental component of a complex potion. The Greeks and Romans used opium which in some cases was mixed with mandragora, a plant extract containing hyoscine. Historical texts from the 16th and 17th centuries report the use of many elaborate herbal concoctions, used topically or taken orally, some of which contained opioids. However, it was not until the early 20th century that techniques deliberately employing the analgesic effects of the opioids gained major attention.

"Twilight sleep" was an analgesic technique developed in Germany first described in 1902. A single dose of morphine was followed by intermittent doses of hyoscine titrated until the labouring woman became subdued. Its main effect was to cause profound sedation and in about 95% of cases mothers had no recollection of the experience of labour or childbirth. Side-effects were severe and as with most systemic opioids, the quality of analgesia was poor. Hyoscine caused hallucinations and delirium often necessitating physical restraint. These complications were minimised by nursing the woman in a quiet, darkened room, making monitoring difficult. Neonatal depression was frequent. A physician was required to administer the drugs, making hospital admission mandatory and leading to a campaign for more hospital admissions among its enthusiasts.[38] Although attempts were made to standardise the technique and broaden its application, the severe side-effects led to its growing unpopularity within the medical profession. Some attempts were made to improve the cocktail by adding barbiturates but generally such changes only increased the dangers and since the end of the 1930s the technique has been largely abandoned.

Pharmacology

An *opiate* is defined as a drug that is derived from opium which itself is an extract of the poppy, *Papaver somniferum*. Such drugs include morphine, codeine, and thebaine. An *opioid* is defined as any drug that has agonist and/or antagonist activity at an opioid receptor and embraces the naturally occurring opioid peptides and synthetic opioid bases.

Opioid Receptors

Evidence that several different subtypes of opioid receptor existed came from studies demonstrating "cross-tolerance" among opioids in animal experiments. Martin *et al.* demonstrated the existence of three receptor subtypes, μ, κ, and σ, named after the drugs that bound to them, morphine, ketocyclazocine, and SKF 10,047 (N-allylnormetazocine).[39] The σ-receptor is no longer considered a true opioid receptor as it has no affinity for the opioid antagonist naloxone. However, in 1977 Lord *et al.* proposed the existence of a fourth receptor, δ.[40] Opioid receptors are coupled to guanine nucleotide G proteins and cause inhibition of neural transmission either by potassium channel activation (μ and δ) or by inhibition of voltage-dependent calcium channels (κ and δ).

The three accepted opioid receptor subtypes have been further divided and it is likely that more will be identified in future (Table 3.2). μ-receptors have been subdivided into three groups. μ_1-receptors are present predominantly in the brain and mediate analgesia and sedation centrally. μ_2-receptors mediate analgesia in the dorsal column of the spinal cord. Other μ_2-receptors are thought to be responsible for respiratory depression and for decreasing motility in the gastrointestinal tract. Most recently, a third μ-receptor has been described that selectively binds both

Table 3.2   Opioid receptor classification and localisation of analgesic action (adapted from Pasternak [41] with permission)

Receptor	Receptor subtype	Analgesia	Other
μ	μ$_1$	Supraspinal	Euphoria
			Dependence
	μ$_2$	Spinal	Respiratory depression
			Gastrointestinal effects
	M6G	Spinal/supraspinal	
κ	κ$_1$	Spinal	Psychotomimesis
			Sedation
	κ$_3$	Supraspinal	
δ	δ$_1$	Supraspinal	
	δ$_2$	Spinal/supraspinal	
σ*		Supraspinal	Dysphoria

*No longer classified as a true opioid receptor

diamorphine and morphine-6-glucuronide, a potent metabolite of morphine.[42] Two κ-receptors have been identified, κ$_1$ and κ$_3$, both mediating analgesia primarily at the spinal level. However, dysphoria is a common side-effect of κ-agonists, limiting their clinical application. Two δ-receptors have been described mediating analgesia, particularly effective at the spinal level. A growing numbers of new receptor subtypes are likely to be identified and debate continues concerning their physiological roles.

Drugs that bind to opioid receptors are grouped into three categories: agonists, partial agonists, and antagonists (Table 3.3). Agonists such as morphine and fentanyl bind to opioid receptors and, in large doses, cause profound analgesia. Partial agonists such as buprenorphine and pentazocine are incapable of producing profound analgesia at high doses, having a low maximum effect. Some partial agonists such as buprenorphine have a very high affinity for opioid receptors despite low efficacy and may therefore act as antagonists by displacing molecules of higher efficacy but lower affinity from receptors. κ-receptors are unable to mediate as profound analgesia as μ-receptors. Hence opioids that bind principally to κ-receptors may

Table 3.3   Actions of opioid drugs at different receptors

	μ-receptors	κ-receptors
Pethidine	++	+
Morphine	+++	+
Meptazinol	+/-	+
Pentazocine	+/-	+
Nalbuphine	-	+
Fentanyl	+++	??
Buprenorphine	+/-	-
Naloxone	- -	-

Key: + agonist, +/- partial agonist, - antagonist

94

appear to be partial agonists because they have low maximum effects. Pure antagonists such as naloxone bind with high affinity to opioid receptors but have no efficacy.

Pharmacokinetics

The opioids in common use have molecular weights between 200 and 500. They all contain a basic nitrogen atom that can accept a proton in acid solution, becoming ionised and hydrophilic. However, the non-ionised moiety is able to cross lipid membranes most rapidly. Hence high lipid solubility enhances speed of onset and increases the volume of distribution. Morphine possesses two hydroxyl groups that reduce the lipophilicity of the molecule and slow the rate at which it crosses lipid membranes. In the related molecule, diacetyl morphine (diamorphine/heroin), these groups are substituted with more lipophilic acetyl groups allowing rapid passage of the molecule across the blood–brain barrier and faster onset of action. Pethidine and other phenylpiperidine derivatives such as fentanyl and sufentanil are also more lipid soluble than morphine and have a more rapid onset of action.

Hydrophobic drugs are highly protein bound in the plasma. Basic drugs such as the opioids are principally bound to the acute-phase protein α_1-acid glycoprotein. Maternal levels of α_1-acid glycoprotein are higher than fetal and this to some degree reduces placental transfer of the drug to the fetus, though not enough to prevent the neonatal side-effects (see below). One important exception is fentanyl which is bound to several protein fractions including albumin. Albumin concentrations are higher in fetus than mother and may result in a greater burden of fentanyl in the newborn.

Morphine is conjugated in the liver to produce morphine-3-glucuronide and, to a lesser extent, morphine-6-glucuronide, both of which are excreted in the urine. Morphine-6-glucuronide has profound analgesic activity mediated through its own μ-receptor subtype (Table 3.2) and may accumulate in renal failure. Pethidine is dealkylated in the liver to produce its principal metabolite, norpethidine. Both molecules are then hydrolysed, conjugated, and eliminated in the urine. Norpethidine produces analgesia and sedation, is proconvulsant and has a prolonged half-life in both mother (17–25 h) and the newborn (62 h).

Pharmacodynamics

Opioids produce analgesia by actions in at least three primary sites: the periaqueductal grey matter, the nucleus raphe magnus, and the dorsal horn of the spinal cord, principally in the superficial layers of the spinal grey matter, laminae I, II, and III (Fig 3.4).

Stimulation of opioid receptors in the periaqueductal grey matter activates descending inhibitory pathways passing via the nucleus raphe magnus and relayed down to the dorsal horn cells of the spinal cord. Analgesia

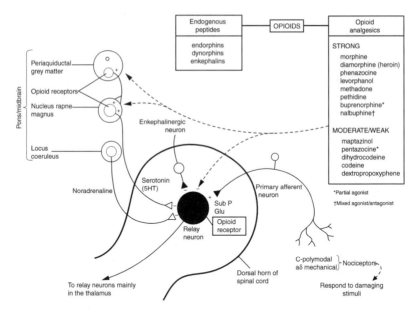

Fig 3.4 Simplified scheme of pain pathways and sites of opioid modulation (from Neal[43] with permission)

results from serotoninergic and noradrenergic inhibition of the dorsal horn relay neurons. Interruption of the descending pathways has been shown to attenuate the analgesic response to systemic opioids. In the dorsal horn itself there are opioid receptors on the relay neurons that inhibit the transmission of nociceptive stimuli. Systemic (intramuscular or intravenous) opioids act primarily within the central nervous system at a supraspinal level. As a result, the dose of drug required to produce *effective* analgesia by this route would cause unacceptable sedation and respiratory depression in both mother and neonate. Administration of opioids by the spinal or epidural route greatly enhances their analgesic efficacy and allows administration of much smaller doses, minimising undesirable side-effects.[44]

Pethidine (Meperidine)

Pethidine was introduced in the 1930s and has since become the most commonly used and widely investigated systemic opioid in labour. Developed in Germany during the First World War as a substitute for morphine which was unavailable in Germany due to an Allied embargo, pethidine was promoted for its analgesic and spasmolytic properties. It became very popular among midwives and labouring women many of whom, unaware of its addictive properties, became dependent on the drug. It was not until the Dangerous Drugs Act of 1949 that its use became restricted.

Possession and administration of pethidine by midwives is now regulated under the Medicines Act 1968 and the Misuse of Drugs Regulations 1983, although it was made legally available to midwives in 1950. Widespread availability and ease of administration has resulted in the continued use of systemic pethidine in labour despite overwhelming evidence of its lack of efficacy and detrimental effects on both mother and baby.

Pethidine is commonly administered by the intramuscular route in doses of 50–100 mg, 3–4 hourly. There is some evidence that superior analgesia is achieved by deltoid injection as absorption from the gluteus muscle may be reduced in labour. Intravenous administration in boluses of 25–50 mg, 1–2 hourly, or as continuous infusion have been investigated in an attempt to improve quality of analgesia.[45] Better analgesia has been reported using these techniques but the side-effect profile appears unchanged. Improved efficacy has also been reported with patient-controlled analgesia (PCA) in doses of up to 0.25 mg/kg and lockout times of 10 minutes.[46] However, other evidence suggests that pethidine consumption may be increased and neonatal depression more common.[47]

Efficacy

Despite many anecdotal reports and a number of retrospective trials suggesting that pethidine provides satisfactory analgesia, the overwhelming majority of prospective trials continue to report that pethidine is, at best, a poor analgesic in labour.[48] Studies that describe good analgesic results from the use of pethidine invariably base their clinical assessment on the reports of independent observers or retrospective questioning of mothers after delivery. Independent observers base their judgement on the fact that the parturient appears quieter and thus sedation, which is potentially harmful for the mother and may detract from her experience of birth, has become confused with analgesia. Mothers asked to score their pain retrospectively 24 hours after delivery report significantly less pain than when interviewed during labour. Direct questioning during labour reveals that though they may feel more sleepy, there has been little or no improvement in pain. Accurate assessment of pain in labour and the effect of analgesic intervention can only be made by the parturient herself at the time of labour.

On the stepladder of obstetric analgesia there is a general belief among childbirth educators and mothers that harmless, non-invasive techniques come first (psychological preparation and support, massage, warm baths, TENS, etc.), followed by nitrous oxide and then finally, if stronger analgesia is required, pethidine or epidural. However, evidence suggests that pethidine is no more effective than the non-invasive techniques and nitrous oxide. Indeed, in a number of studies both TENS and nitrous oxide have been shown to produce superior analgesia to pethidine.[27,49] Pain scores have even been shown to increase after administration of pethidine although this may be put down to ineffective analgesia in the face of progressing labour.

Pethidine has been compared with several other systemic opioids. On each occasion it was hoped that the alternatives would supply superior analgesia with improved side-effect profiles. However, in the vast majority of cases, analgesia was similar and side-effects little altered. These comparisons will be discussed under the individual drugs (see below). No randomised trials have compared pethidine with placebo. Though in the past such trials have been considered unethical, the evidence now suggests that the analgesic efficacy of pethidine is little better than that of a placebo while the side-effects are considerably more serious.

There have been a number of attempts to improve the efficacy of pethidine by administering it in combination with other drugs. In general, such combinations have only increased sedation, amnesia, and dysphoria while having little impact on analgesia.

When compared with epidural analgesia in randomised trials, pethidine invariably produces clinically inferior analgesia.[50,51,52]

Effects on the mother

The central side-effects of pethidine are sedation and dysphoria. In a national survey of pain relief in childbirth, the principal criticisms of mothers given pethidine were that it made them feel confused, out of control, and sleepy while failing to relieve their pain.[1] However, some women reported that although their pain remained unaffected, pethidine made them less concerned about it.

As described above, alkalosis caused by hyperventilation associated with pain causes a reduction in uterine blood flow and impairs placental gas exchange. The administration of pethidine exacerbates this problem as it provides minimal reduction of the pain, so failing to prevent hyperventilation during contraction, and yet causes a degree of sedation between contractions that exacerbates the periods of hypoventilation.[30]

Pethidine increases the incidence of nausea and vomiting and delays gastric emptying. Residual gastric volumes of over 700 ml have been recorded in women who have received pethidine in labour despite being kept nil by mouth.[53] In the event of unplanned general anaesthesia, such women are undoubtedly at increased risk of pulmonary aspiration. An antiemetic such as metoclopramide, which promotes gastric emptying, will reduce these side-effects but is unlikely to prevent them altogether. As a result, all parturients using or planning to use pethidine should be kept strictly nil by mouth throughout labour.

Effect on the progress of labour

There are no randomised controlled trials to suggest that opioids in general or pethidine in particular have any effect on the progress of labour. However, a number of groups have suggested that pethidine slows the progress of labour. In the first half of the 20th century many believed that pain was an essential component of labour and that all forms of pain relief, including the opioids, prolonged it. A mechanism for this effect was never clarified although intravenous morphine has been shown to reduce maternal oxytocin levels in early labour and a number of animal studies have demonstrated that opioid administration delays parturition.[54] Despite this, it is unlikely that the doses of morphine or pethidine used in humans would be sufficient to affect the progress of labour. Thornton et al. showed that the administration of pethidine caused no change in fetal oxytocin production whereas epidural analgesia appeared to increase it.[55] Though it had been suggested that fetal oxytocin may influence the onset and duration of labour, high levels of cystine aminopeptidase, an enzyme that rapidly degrades oxytocin in the placenta, work against significant feto-maternal transfer.[56]

Other groups have suggested that rather than slowing labour, pethidine may actually accelerate it. Many midwives believe that pethidine is the analgesic of choice in early labour for this very reason. Though never proven, a number of rather tenuous explanations have been proposed. Pajntar et al. demonstrated that pethidine given in the active phase of labour was associated with an increase in contractility of the body of the uterus but a concomitant decrease in the contractility of the cervix.[57] They suggested that this explained how pethidine might accelerate the progress of labour by facilitating cervical dilation. A second suggestion was put forward by Milwidsky et al. who demonstrated that pethidine in therapeutic concentration stimulates urokinase, plasmin, and collagenase activity in vitro.[58] They proposed that these enzymes were responsible for degrading cervical collagen and elastin leading to accelerated cervical effacement and dilation during labour. However, none of these changes has ever been shown to correlate with the duration of the active phase of labour.

In summary, there is no good evidence that pethidine, or indeed any parenteral opioid, has any effect on the progress or duration of labour.

Effects on the baby

Pethidine is a weakly basic piperidine derivative which is 20–30 times more lipophilic than morphine although it has only about one-third the lipophilicity of methadone and one-thirtieth that of fentanyl. This degree of lipophilicity allows pethidine to diffuse rapidly across the placenta such that it can theoretically approach transplacental equilibrium in a single circuit, although equilibrium deeper into the fetal compartment may take considerably longer. Rate of diffusion is not limited by permeability but is dependent on the rate at which it is delivered to the placenta and removed into the fetus: flow-dependent transfer. Morphine, which is less lipophilic, diffuses more slowly across the placental membrane and its transfer is therefore partially limited by permeability.

Pethidine is principally bound to α_1-acid glycoprotein (30–60%). At term, levels of this protein tend to be higher in the maternal than the fetal circulation and, in theory, favour distribution of pethidine into the maternal compartment. However, this relatively weak binding appears to have little effect in practice. pH gradients across the placenta may be of greater importance. As a weak base, pethidine is ionised to a greater extent in the more acidic milieu of the fetal circulation. Thus, a certain degree of ion trapping may occur on the fetal side of the placenta, increasing fetal uptake of the drug. In the normal situation, the pH of the fetal circulation is only slightly more acidic than that of the mother and therefore the disparity in concentration of free drug is not great. However, in the compromised fetus, acidosis may increase and ion trapping become more significant, resulting in increased fetal pethidine levels and concomitant side-effects (see below).

The neonatal side-effects of pethidine, respiratory depression in particular, are most severe if the dose delivery interval is 2–3 hours.[59,60] This is due to gradual distribution of pethidine and norpethidine into the fetal compartment that leads to persistent transplacental passage of pethidine into the fetus for some time after maternal plasma concentrations have started to fall. This continuous increase of total fetal dose of pethidine, together with a progressive rise in fetal norpethidine levels, can result in long-lasting neonatal depression and is of course augmented by repeated maternal dosing traditionally occurring 3–4 hourly.

The neonatal side-effects of pethidine are compounded by the production of its active metabolite norpethidine. Both mother and fetus are able to metabolise pethidine to norpethidine and, in the baby, most of the norpethidine probably results from its own N-dealkylation. Norpethidine has analgesic activity but is considerably less potent than pethidine. However, it causes more repiratory depression and has proconvulsant properties. The half-lives of pethidine and norpethidine in the mother are approximately four and 20 hours respectively but in the neonate are 13 and 62 hours.[61,62] These prolonged half-lives probably explain why some of the behavioural changes observed in exposed neonates persist for several days after delivery.

Intrauterine effects of pethidine on the fetus

Changes have been observed in fetal heart rate pattern (reduced variability), fetal breathing movements and muscular activity, fetal EEG activity, and fetal scalp oxygen tension following parenteral administration of pethidine. The bearing that these changes may have on fetal well-being is unclear but it is likely that changes in fetal heart rate may result in unnecessary intervention. Impaired fetal acid-base balance may also occur following maternal administration of small doses of pethidine and persist after delivery.

Early neonatal effects

Maternal administration of pethidine causes neonatal respiratory depression which is worst after a dose delivery interval of about three hours and particularly after repeated maternal doses.[59-61] This respiratory depression results in decreased Apgar scores, depressed oxygen saturations, and increased arterial carbon dioxide tensions.[59,63,64] Even in the absence of clinically obvious respiratory depression at the time of birth, more subtle changes in respiratory patterns may occur in the first few days of life. Hamza *et al.* studied a group of babies whose mothers had received infusions of pethidine in labour. When compared with a control opioid-free group, Apgar scores were not depressed and in quiet sleep the groups were indistinguishable. However, in active sleep SaO_2 levels <90% and apnoeic episodes were more common in the pethidine group.[65]

Neurobehavioural studies of babies exposed to pethidine *in utero* are difficult to design and interpret due to the multitude of factors that affect early neonatal behaviour. However, babies exposed to pethidine *in utero* are sleepy, less able to develop suckling skills, and take longer to establish breastfeeding. Large doses of pethidine given to mothers result in impaired thermoregulation in the newborn and may increase the need for medical intervention in the early hours of life.

The effects of pethidine on the baby can be rapidly reversed immediately after delivery with 60–100 µg/kg of intramuscular naloxone, an opioid antagonist. This dose of naloxone in the newborn appears to have a clinical effect for up to 48 hours and reverses the neurobehavioural effects of pethidine without any apparent harm.[66] Although naloxone has a slightly prolonged half-life in the newborn, it is shorter than that of pethidine (three hours compared with 20 hours approximately) and therefore needs to be given intramuscularly in a large dose to have a significantly prolonged effect. Naloxone is less able to antagonise the effects of the longer acting norpethidine than those of pethidine. Respiratory support with bag and face mask or even intubation and ventilation may be required in addition to naloxone, particularly when the narcotic effect of pethidine is superimposed on any other cause of fetal compromise. However, in babies of sickle cell patients or chronic drug abusers who have been exposed *in utero* for a prolonged period to excessive doses of pethidine or other opioids, naloxone may cause severe withdrawal reactions, including convulsions and coma, and should therefore be avoided.

Late effects

As with nitrous oxide (see above), some evidence has emerged that babies of mothers who received pethidine during labour might be more liable to develop drug addiction problems later in life. In a comparison of the intrapartum care of mothers of 200 opioid addicts with that of unaffected siblings, Jacobson *et al.* showed that the mother was more likely to have had

101

pethidine during labour in the addict group.[32] Although the control group was poorly matched and the study was retrospective, it does raise the possibility of a particularly disturbing long-term side-effect of an ineffective drug that remains in such widespread use.

Contraindications and drug interactions

All systemic opioid drugs licensed for use in labour have some degree of sedative action and may potentiate sedation caused by other drugs that may have been given (e.g. benzodiazepines, anti-epileptic drugs, magnesium sulphate, and some antidepressants). Furthermore, if large doses of parenteral opioids have been given in labour, subsequent institution of effective epidural analgesia may result in heavy maternal sedation. As a result, prior administration of systemic opioid agonists is considered by some to be a relative contraindication to the use of epidural opioids.

In parturients considered to be at increased risk of requiring caesarean section, epidural analgesia should be preferred to pethidine, in part because of the gastrointestinal changes mentioned above but also because of the rapidity with which an effective epidural block can be extended in the event of an emergency caesarean section. In pregnancy-induced hypertension, pethidine is ineffective in preventing surges in blood pressure caused by the pain of uterine contraction. Its use may also worsen acid-base balance in an already compromised fetus. Pethidine is unsuitable for use in severe pregnancy-induced hypertension because its active metabolite, norpethidine, has proconvulsant properties. Renal impairment, which is often associated with pregnancy-induced hypertension, reduces the clearance of norpethidine, increasing the likelihood of this complication.

The use of pethidine is absolutely contraindicated in parturients taking monoamine oxidase inhibitors (MAOIs).

Other agents

Although pethidine remains the most widely used systemic opioid in obstetric analgesia, many alternatives have been investigated over the years. The aim has been to try to reduce the side-effects and to improve the analgesia. Although several alternatives have drawn a small number of enthusiastic supporters, this enthusiasm has been largely based on anecdotal reports.

Morphine and diamorphine

Although probably the first opioid to be used as an analgesic in labouring women, recent evidence of the lack of efficacy of pethidine has led to the re-examination of the role of morphine. Incremental intravenous doses provide an insignificant reduction in overall pain score measured during labour.[67] Neonatal side-effects are similar to pethidine and sedation in the mothers may be profound. The use of morphine via any route confers no advantage and causes similar side-effects to pethidine.

Though systemic diamorphine is used enthusiastically in a small number of units, there is little information comparing it with other opioids. Its increased lipid solubility suggests that it might reach the sites of action more quickly than morphine. However, there is no information about its efficacy or side-effect profile compared with pethidine or morphine but it is unlikely to offer any great improvement.

Meptazinol

Meptazinol is a mixed opioid agonist/antagonist which produces analgesia at the κ-receptor and has some cholinergic side-effects. It enjoys popularity in a small number of units where it is believed to be superior to pethidine. It is given in doses of 100–150 mg IM every 2–4 hours and has approximately one-tenth the potency of morphine and a slightly shorter duration of action. In high doses it can cause dysphoria, which reduces its potential for abuse, and its antagonist properties may cause withdrawal in parturients dependent on μ-agonists. It rarely causes respiratory depression although there is some theoretical concern that should respiratory depression occur, this may be only partially reversed by naloxone. This complication has never been reported in obstetric use. When compared with pethidine, some studies have demonstrated slightly better pain relief with meptazinol. Side-effect profiles are similar although vomiting is more common with meptazinol.

Pentazocine

Pentazocine is a mixed μ-agonist/antagonist and a κ and σ-agonist of about one-third the potency of morphine that enjoyed popularity in the early 1970s. As with many such alternative opioids, it was deliberately synthesised to minimise its potential for abuse – large doses causing dysphoric side-effects. It is presented as a racemic mixture of which the l-isomer alone has analgesic activity mediated through the κ₁-receptor. Although it does cause some sedation, there is a ceiling to this effect at larger doses. It is irritant on intramuscular or subcutaneous administration. For analgesia in labour it has been given in a dose of 40 mg IM every 2–4 hours. However, there is no evidence that it provides superior analgesia to pethidine and it has fallen from favour because of its relatively short action and the need for repeated doses which provide diminishing analgesia and occasional dysphoria.

Nalbuphine

Nalbuphine is a mixed μ-agonist/antagonist and a κ-agonist with clinical effects similar to pentazocine. It is a more potent μ-antagonist than pentazocine but causes analgesia mediated primarily by the κ-receptor. It is approximately equipotent to morphine and is given in doses of 10–20 mg IM in labour. Once again, its perceived advantage is that as a competitive antagonist it has a ceiling effect and might therefore be less likely to cause excessive maternal or fetal respiratory depression. However, κ-mediated sedation is a common side-effect and it can cause dysphoria, though less so than pentazocine. Once again, there is little evidence that nalbuphine is more efficacious than pethidine and it has never gained popularity in the UK.

Fentanyl

Fentanyl is a highly lipid-soluble phenylpiperidine derivative acting primarily on μ-receptors that is approximately 80–100 times as potent as morphine. Its lipid solubility results in a rapid onset of action but although its duration of action is shorter due to rapid redistribution, its terminal half-life – approximately eight hours – is longer than that of morphine or pethidine. Fentanyl is principally bound to albumin, favouring transplacental transfer, and when used repeatedly during labour, fetal/maternal ratios have been shown to rise to about 0.7 or more.

Although more commonly used and thoroughly investigated when given by the epidural or spinal routes, fentanyl has been used systemically in labour. In an unblinded study of 105 women, Rayburn et al. showed that fentanyl given intravenously (50–100 µg/h) produced similar analgesia to intravenous pethidine (25–50 mg/h).[68] Maternal nausea, vomiting, and sedation were worse in the pethidine group and although neonatal side-effects were reported as similar, naloxone was given more frequently in the pethidine group. In a previous study, the same group had reported that intravenous fentanyl given in a cumulative dose of 50–600 µg titrated according to maternal needs to 137 women caused no hazards to mother or baby.[69] However, they did observe a transient decrease in fetal heart rate variability in the 30 minutes immediately following fentanyl administration.

Unfortunately, most other information about systemic fentanyl in labour consists of case reports of its use in women in whom, for various reasons, epidural analgesia was contraindicated. Although there are no prospective double-blind trials comparing intravenous fentanyl with pethidine, it is unlikely that the former will provide significantly better analgesia by this route.

Remifentanil

Remifentanil is an ultrashort-acting opioid analgesic agent recently introduced into anaesthetic practice that is still in the process of establishing a suitable clinical niche. Remifentanil produces rapid onset and offset of profound analgesia but equally profound sedation and muscle rigidity. It has been hoped that remifentanil may be a suitable drug for intravenous PCA in labour. Unfortunately, although fast in onset, its peak effect is not seen until about 80 seconds after injection, when the intensity of contraction pain is declining. Therefore respiratory depression is a significant possibility limiting its use for labour analgesia. It has, however, been used to facilitate the siting of an epidural in a distressed parturient.[70]

Tramadol

Tramadol is a weak μ-agonist that has been prescribed in labour in doses of 50–100 mg, four hourly. Once again, its proposed advantage was that it had been reported to have few of the detrimental side-effects associated with other opioids. Evidence concerning maternal and fetal side-effects is conflicting and tramadol has no clear advantages over pethidine.

Non-steroidal anti-inflammatory drugs

Pethidine has been compared with intramuscular injections of ketorolac. Although ketorolac produced fewer maternal and neonatal side-effects, analgesia was inferior. It is unlikely that non-steroidal anti-inflammatory drugs will gain popularity for analgesia in labour because of the perceived risk of adverse effects on the fetal circulation, in particular vasoconstriction and premature closure of the ductus arteriosus.

Summary

Systemic opioids in general and pethidine in particular have been widely investigated and in randomised controlled trials shown to be consistently ineffective. Although Entonox, TENS, and the other non-invasive techniques may only provide a minimal degree of analgesia, they are generally safe and help many women to cope with their experience of childbirth. Should such techniques prove inadequate, regional analgesia remains the only effective alternative. While debate may remain in other areas, many senior midwives, obstetricians, and anaesthetists now agree that systemic pethidine has no place in modern obstetric analgesia.

References

1 Steer P. The methods of pain relief used. In: Chamberlain G, Wraight A, Steer P, eds. *Pain and its relief in childbirth: the results of a national survey conducted by the National Birthday Trust*. London: Churchill Livingstone, 1993:49–67.

2 Department of Health. *Changing childbirth*. London: HMSO, 1993.

3 Read GD. *Natural childbirth*. London: Heinemann, 1933.

4 Lamaze F. *Painless childbirth: psychoprophylactic method* (trans. Celestin CB). London: Burke Publishing Company, 1958.

5 Huch R. Maternal hyperventilation and the fetus. *J Perin Med* 1986;14:3–17.

6 Reed PN, Colquhoun AD, Hanning CD. Maternal oxygenation during normal labour. *Br J Anaesth* 1989;62:316–18.

7 Keirse MJNC, Enkin M, Lumley J. Support from caregivers during childbirth. In: *The Cochrane pregnancy and childbirth database. The Cochrane collaboration and update software*, 1995, Issue 1.

8 Melzack R, Wall PD. Pain mechanisms: a new theory. *Science* 1965;150:971–8.

9 Harrison RF, Woods T, Shore M, Mathews G, Unwin A. Pain relief in labour using transcutaneous electrical nerve stimulation (TENS). A TENS/TENS placebo controlled study in two parity groups. *Br J Obstet Gynaecol* 1986;93:739–46.

10 Thomas IL, Tyle V, Webster J, Neilson A. An evaluation of transcutaneous electrical nerve stimulation for pain relief in labour. *Aust NZ J Obstet Gynaecol* 1988;**28**:182–9.

11 Wraight A. Coping with pain. In: Chamberlain G, Wraight A, Steer P, eds. *Pain and its relief in childbirth: the results of a survey conducted by the National Birthday Trust.* Edinburgh: Churchill Livingstone, 1993;79–92.

12 Robson JE. Transcutaneous nerve stimulation for pain relief in labour. *Anaesthesia* 1979;**34**:357–60.

13 Bundsen P, Ericson K, Peterson L-E, Thiringer K. Pain relief in labor by transcutaneous electrical nerve stimulation. Testing of a modified stimulation technique and evaluation of the neurological and biochemical condition of the newborn infant. *Acta Obstet Gynecol Scand* 1982;**61**:129–36.

14 Carroll D, Tramer M, McQuay H, Nye B, Moore A. Transcutaneous electrical nerve stimulation in labour pain: a systematic review. *Br J Obstet Gynaecol* 1997;**104**:169–75.

15 Ader L, Hansson B, Wallin G. Parturition pain treated by intracutaneous injections of sterile water. *Pain* 1990;**41**:133–8.

16 Trolle B, Moller M, Kronborg H, Thomsen S. The effect of sterile water blocks on low back labor pain. *Am J Obstet Gynecol* 1991;**164**:1277–81.

17 Ranta P, Joupilla P, Spalding M, Kangas-Saarela T, Hollmen A, Joupilla R. Parturients' assessment of water blocks, pethidine, nitrous oxide, paracervical and epidural blocks in labour. *Int J Obstet Anesth* 1994;**3**:193–8.

18 Heyns OS. Abdominal decompression in the first stage of labour. *J Obstet Gynaecol Br Emp* 1959;**66**:220–8.

19 Scott DB, Loudon JDO. A method of abdominal decompression in labour. *Lancet* 1960;**i**:1181–3.

20 Snow J. In: Richardson BW, ed. *On chloroform and other anaesthetics: their actions and administration.* London: John Churchill, 1858:250.

21 Klikowitsch S. Ueber die therapeutische Wirkung des Stickoxyduls bei einigen Krankheiten. *St Petersburger Medicin Wochenschr* 1880;**15**:117–18.

22 Minnitt RJ. Self-administered analgesia for the midwifery of general practice. *Br J Anaesth* 1934;**11**:148–52.

23 Tunstall ME. Effect of cooling on pre-mixed gas mixtures for obstetric analgesia. *BMJ* 1963;**ii**:915–17.

24 Cole PV, Crawford JS, Doughty AG, *et al.* Specifications and recommendations for nitrous oxide/oxygen apparatus to be used in obstetric analgesia. *Anaesthesia* 1970;**25**:317–27.

25 Moyle JTB, Davey A. Equipment for the inhalation of oxygen and Entonox. In: Ward C, ed. *Ward's anaesthetic equipment.* London: WB Saunders, 1998:86.

26 Carstoniu J, Levytam S, Norman P, Daley D, Katz J, Sandler AN. Nitrous oxide in early labor. Safety and analgesic efficacy assessed by a double-blind, placebo-controlled study. *Anesthesiology* 1994;**80**:30–5.

27 Holdcroft A, Morgan M. An assessment of the analgesic effect in labour of pethidine and 50 per cent nitrous oxide in oxygen (Entonox). *J Obstet Gynaecol Br Commonw* 1974;**81**:603–7.

28 Arthurs GJ, Rosen M. Self-administered intermittent nitrous oxide analgesia for labour. Enhancement of effect with continuous nasal inhalation of 50 per cent nitrous oxide (Entonox). *Anaesthesia* 1979;**34**:301–9.

29 Davies JM, Willis BA, Rosen M. Entonox analgesia in labour. A pilot study to reduce the delay between demand and supply. *Anaesthesia* 1978;**33**:545–7.

30 Griffin RP, Reynolds F. Maternal hypoxaemia during labour and delivery: the influence of analgesia and the effect on neonatal outcome. *Anaesthesia* 1995;**50**:151–6.

31 Jacobsen B, Nyberg K, Eklund G, Bygdeman M, Rydberg U. Obstetric pain medication and eventual adult amphetamine addiction in offspring. *Acta Obstet Gynaecol Scand* 1988;**67**:677–82.

32 Jacobsen B, Nyberg K, Gronbladh L, Eklund G, Bygdeman M, Rydberg U . Opiate addiction in adult offspring through possible imprinting after obstetric treatment. *BMJ* 1990;**301**:1067–70.

33 Mills GH, Singh D, Longan M, O'Sullivan J, Caunt JA. Nitrous oxide exposure on the labour ward. *Int J Obstet Anesth* 1996;**5**:160–4.

34 McGuinness C, Rosen M. Enflurane as an analgesic in labour. *Anaesthesia* 1984: **39**:24–6.

35 McLeod DD, Ramayya GP, Tunstall ME. Self-administered isoflurane in labour. A comparative study with Entonox. *Anaesthesia* 1985;**40**:424–6.
36 Tunstall ME, Ross JAS. Isoflurane, nitrous oxide and oxygen analgesic mixtures [letter]. *Anaesthesia* 1993;**48**:919.
37 Abboud TK, Swart F, Zhu J, Donovan MM, Peres da Silva E, Yakal K. Desflurane analgesia for vaginal delivery. *Acta Anaesth Scand* 1995;**39**:259–61.
38 Pitcock CD, Clark RB. From Fanny to Ferdinand: the development of consumerism in pain control during the birth process. *Am J Obstet Gynecol* 1992;**3**:1–8.
39 Martin WR, Eades CG, Thompson JA, Huppler RE, Gilbert PE. The effects of morphine- and nalorphine-like drugs in the nondependent and morphine dependent chronic spinal dog. *J Pharmacol Exp Ther* 1976;**197**:517–32.
40 Lord JAH, Waterfield AA, Hughes J, Kosterlitz HW. Endogenous opioid peptides: multiple agonists and receptors. *Nature* 1977;**267**:495–9.
41 Pasternak GW. Correlating the molecular biology and pharmacology of opioid receptors. Proceedings of the 2nd Annual Therapeutic Developments in Chronic Pain. Annapolis MD, 1998.
42 Brown GP, Yang K, King MA, *et al.* 3-Methoxynaltrexone, a selective heroin/morphine–6beta-glucuronide antagonist. *FEBS Lett* 1997;**412**:35–8.
43 Neal MJ. Opioid analgesics. In: Neal MJ (ed) *Medical pharmacology at a glance.* Oxford: Blackwell Science, 1997.
44 Justins DM, Knott C, Luthman J, Reynolds F. Epidural versus intramuscular fentanyl. Analgesia and pharmacokinetics in labour. *Anaesthesia* 1983;**38**:937–42.
45 Isenor L, Penny-MacGillivray T. Intravenous meperidine infusion for obstetric analgesia. *J Obstet Gynecol Neonatal Nurs* 1993;**22**:349–56.
46 Robinson JO, Rosen M, Evans JM, Revill SI, David H, Rees G. Self-administered intravenous and intramuscular pethidine. A controlled trial in labour. *Anaesthesia* 1980;**35**:763–70.
47 Rayburn W, Leuschen MP, Earl R, Woods M, Lokovic M, Gaston-Johansson F. Intravenous meperidine during labor: a randomised conparison between nurse and patient controlled administration. *Obstet Gynecol* 1989;**74**:702–6.
48 Olofsson C, Ekblom A, Ekman-Ordeberg G, Hjelm A, Irestedt L. Lack of analgesic effect of systemically administered morphine or pethidine on labour pain. *Br J Obstet Gynaecol* 1996;**103**:968–72.
49 Harrison RF, Shore M, Woods T, Mathews G, Gardiner J, Unwin A. A comparative study of transcutaneous electrical nerve stimulation (TENS), entonox, pethidine + promazine and lumbar epidural for pain relief in labor. *Acta Obstet Gynecol Scand* 1987;**66**:9–14.
50 Thorp JA, Hu DH, Albin RM, *et al.* The effect of intrapartum epidural analgesia on nulliparous labour: a randomised controlled, prospective trial. *Am J Obstet Gynecol* 1993;**169**:851–8.
51 Ramin SM, Gambling DR, Lucas MJ, Sharma SK, Sidawi JE, Leveno KJ. Randomized trial of epidural versus intravenous analgesia during labor. *Obstet Gynecol* 1995;**86**:783–9.
52 Robinson JO, Rosen M, Evans JM, Revill SI, David H, Rees GAD. Maternal opinion about analgesia for labour. A controlled trial between epidural block and intramuscular pethidine combined with inhalation. *Anaesthesia* 1980;**35**:1173–81.
53 Holdsworth JD. Relationship between stomach contents and analgesia in labour. *Br J Anaesth* 1978;**50**:1145–8.
54 Russell JA, Gosden RG, Humphreys EM, *et al.* Interruption of parturition in rats by morphine: a result of inhibition of oxytocin secretion. *J Endocrinol* 1989;**121**:521–36.
55 Thornton S, Charlton L, Murray BJ, Davison JM, Bayliss PH. The effect of early labour, maternal analgesia and fetal acidosis on fetal plasma oxytocin levels. *Br J Obstet Gynaecol* 1993;**100**:425–9.
56 Landon MJ, Copes DR, Shiells EA, Davison GM. Degradation of radiolabelled vasopressin (125I-AVP) by the human placenta perfused in vitro. *Br J Obstet Gynaecol* 1988;**95**:488–92.
57 Pajntar M, Vlentincic B, Verdenik I. The effect of pethidine hydrochloride on the cervical muscles in the active phase of labour. *Clin Exp Obstet Gynecol* 1993;**X**:145–50.
58 Milwidsky A, Finci-Yeheskel Z, Mayer M. Direct stimulation of urokinase, plasmin and collagenase by meperidine: a possible mechanism for the ability of meperidine to enhance cervical effacement and dilation. *Am J Perinatol* 1993;**10**:130–4.

59 Shnider S, Moya F. Effects of meperidine on the newborn infant. *Am J Obstet Gynecol* 1964;**89**:1009–15.

60 Belfrage P, Boreus LO, Hartvig P, *et al.* Neonatal depression after obstetrical analgesia with pethidine: the role of the injection-delivery time interval and of the plasma concentrations of pethidine and norpethidine. *Acta Obstet Gynecol Scand* 1981;**60**:43–9.

61 Kuhnert BR, Kuhnert PM, Philipson EH, *et al.* Disposition of meperidine and normeperidine following multiple doses during labor. II. Fetus and neonate. *Am J Obstet Gynecol* 1985;**151**:410–15.

62 Kuhnert BR, Kuhnert PM, Tu ASL, *et al.* Meperidine and normeperidine levels following meperidine administration in labour. I. Mother. *Am J Obstet Gynecol* 1979;**133**:904–8.

63 Taylor ES, von Fumetti HH, Essig EL, Goodman SN, Walker LC. The effects of demerol and trichloroethylene on arterial oxygen saturation in the newborn. *Am J Obstet Gynecol* 1955;**69**:348–51.

64 Koch G, Wendel H. Effect of pethidine on the post natal adjustment of respiration and acid-base balance. *Acta Obstet Gynecol Scand* 1968;**47**:27–37.

65 Hamza J, Benlabed M, Orhant E, Escourrou P, Curzi-Dascalova L, Gaultier C. Neonatal pattern of breathing during active and quiet sleep after maternal administration of meperidine. *Pediatr Res* 1992;**32**:412–16.

66 Weiner PC, Hogg MJ, Rosen M. Effects of naloxone on pethidine induced neonatal depression. *BMJ* 1977;**2**:228–31.

67 Olofsson C, Ekblom A, Ekman-Ordeberg G, Granstrom L, Irestedt L. Analgesic efficacy of intravenous morphine in labour pain: a reappraisal. *Int J Obstet Anesth* 1996;**5**:176–80.

68 Rayburn WF, Smith CV, Parriot JE, Woods RE. Randomised comparison of meperidine and fentanyl during labour. *Obstet Gynecol* 1989;**74**:604–6.

69 Rayburn WF, Rathke A, Leuschen MP, Chleborad J, Weidner W. Fentanyl citrate analgesia during labour. *Am J Obstet Gynecol* 1989;**161**:202–6.

70 Brada SA, Egan TD, Viscomi CM. The use of remifentanil infusion to facilitate epidural catheter placement in a parturient: a case report with pharmacokinetic simulations. *Int J Obstet Anesth* 1998;**7**:124–7.

4: Regional analgesia and anaesthesia

MICHAEL PAECH

Regional analgesia and anaesthesia are cornerstones of obstetric anaesthetic practice and they are being used increasingly in many countries. Not only is there accumulating evidence of greater efficacy and safety compared to alternatives but the role and acceptance of regional blocks has expanded with continuing developments and improvements in the pharmacological armamentarium, equipment, monitoring, and clinical management.

Caesarean section (CS) is the most common surgical procedure performed in established pregnancy and in most developed countries is used for 10–25% of deliveries. Central neuraxis block provides effective anaesthesia with significant maternal and fetal advantages over general anaesthesia and enables parents to experience the joy of childbirth and immediate interaction with their infant. Similarly, regional anaesthesia confers advantages for most surgical procedures throughout pregnancy, especially postpartum.

Regional analgesia provides the best pain relief in labour, is widely used, and is readily converted to anaesthesia if required. In addition to effectively and safely alleviating suffering, it may reduce maternal and perinatal morbidity in a variety of obstetric or medical situations.

Indications for regional anaesthesia and analgesia (Box 4.1)

Surgery during pregnancy

Epidural or spinal anaesthesia are usually the preferred options for surgery during pregnancy, including CS (see later under "Practical procedures"). Although regional block has no advantage over general anaesthesia with respect to fetal development or avoidance of postoperative abortion in early pregnancy, it is recommended because serious maternal risks (such as gastric aspiration or hypoxia) can be minimised. Also, the potential for drug-induced teratogenetic or developmental fetal effects is less and better early postoperative recovery and analgesia result.

Box 4.1   Indications and contraindications to Regional Analgesia and Anaesthesia

Indications
Surgery during pregnancy
Labour analgesia
Anticipated difficult or operative delivery (e.g. multiple pregnancy, breech presentation, premature fetus)
Obstetric disease (e.g. severe pre-eclampsia)
Maternal disease (e.g. specific cardiac, respiratory, muscular, neurological and metabolic disorders; morbid obesity)

Contraindications
Refusal to consent
Clinical bleeding (e.g. coagulopathy, severe thrombocytopenia or other haematological disorder)
Uncorrected hypovolaemia

Relative contraindications
LA allergy
Local or systemic infection
Major haemorrhage
Anticoagulation and severe pre-eclampsia-induced thrombocytopenia
Maternal disease (e.g. specific cardiac and neurological disorders)

Labour analgesia

Ideally, regional analgesia in labour should be available on demand but provision of an efficient 24-hour service is strongly determined by socioeconomic and medicopolitical factors, especially the availability of medical expertise, cost, and community demand. Epidural and combined spinal-epidural analgesia provide the most effective labour analgesia and few would disagree with the 1992 statement of the American Society of Anesthesiologists and College of Obstetricians and Gynecologists that "Labor results in severe pain for most women. There is no other circumstance where it is considered acceptable for a person to experience severe pain amenable to safe intervention, while under a physician's care".

Complicated obstetrics

Regional analgesia produces excellent delivery conditions and can be advocated for complicated obstetric cases, especially where difficult or operative delivery is anticipated.[1,2] Interference with spontaneous internal rotation of the presenting part and with maternal expulsive power is best avoided, so techniques which minimise motor block are recommended, followed by augmentation of neural block if instrumental or operative delivery is required.

Pre-eclampsia, fetal growth restriction, prematurity, and breech delivery complicate multiple pregnancy. Malposition and poorer outcome for the second twin are common and anaesthesia may be required for version, fetal extraction, and breech or operative delivery.

Regional analgesia avoids the effects of systemic opioids on the premature fetus, obtunds premature bearing-down reflexes, prevents delivery through an undilated cervix, and creates good conditions for intrauterine manipulation and controlled delivery. The time between deliveries is reduced and the condition of the second twin likely to improve.[3] Regional anaesthesia is also preferable for CS, because although aortocaval compression may be difficult to manage and the mean cephalad spread of subarachnoid local anaesthetic (LA) is greater than in singleton pregnancy, deterioration of neonatal condition secondary to longer uterine incision-to-delivery interval is less likely.

Breech presentation accounts for 3.5% of term fetuses and many are delivered by CS, because perinatal mortality corrected for prematurity and abnormalities is four times higher with vaginal delivery. Vaginal breech delivery would not be considered in many units unless conducted under regional analgesia, which provides the benefits of an alert, comfortable, and cooperative parturient.[4] A controlled delivery can improve neonatal outcome and epidural or spinal anaesthesia is indicated for CS to minimise the neonatal impact of more difficult and prolonged delivery, especially now that potent tocolytics such as glyceryl trinitrate are available as an alternative to volatile anaesthetic agents.

Despite the difficulty of obtaining prospective data, similar considerations apply in the preterm fetus. Epidural analgesia with high doses of LA may arguably increase the risk of assisted delivery, but does not increase neonatal retinal haemorrhage and epidemiologically has been associated with a significant reduction in neonatal death in low birthweight infants. A combined spinal-epidural technique has been recommended for operative delivery of the preterm infant, because the cephalad extension of spinal anaesthesia tends to be less than with an equivalent dose in a term pregnancy.

Maternal disease (see Chapter 6)

Pre-eclampsia complicates about 3% of pregnancies and provided appropriate contraindications are observed, regional analgesia in labour is advantageous to both mother and baby.[5] Reduction in plasma catecholamine levels and fall in peripheral vascular resistance reduces blood pressure (BP) fluctuations associated with pain and contractions and improves intervillous blood flow. Circulatory responses to epidural analgesia are similar to those of normal parturients. For CS, slowly established epidural anaesthesia gives better maternal haemodynamic stability than general anaesthesia and avoids potential airway problems. Vasodilator or magnesium sulphate therapy may intensify falls in BP; however, response to vasopressor drugs is normal. Spinal block has traditionally been avoided in pre-eclampsia, but recent studies suggest that haemodynamic responses are usually similar to epidural anaesthesia and that spinal anaesthesia remains a valuable option.[6]

Regional analgesia is indicated on the basis of reduced maternal morbidity in a variety of medical conditions, especially certain cardiac, respiratory, muscle, and metabolic disorders. Pain relief leads to less sympathetic activity and lower circulating catecholamine levels, resulting in circulatory stability and less cardiac work. Gradual, modest reduction in peripheral resistance (using techniques which avoid administration of large LA boluses and sudden significant changes in afterload) improves cardiac output in regurgitant valvular conditions and favours the balance of myocardial oxygen supply to demand in myocardial ischaemia. Elective assisted delivery, avoiding the Valsalva manouevre (and elevated intrathoracic pressure), is beneficial. Although regional blocks must be used with caution for CS in parturients with stenotic valvular lesions, cardiomyopathy, severe myocardial ischaemia and pulmonary hypertension, for labour regional analgesia (using opioids, low-dose LA, and preferably drug delivery by infusion) is usually the method of choice.

Regional analgesia benefits parturients with conditions such as severe asthma, cystic fibrosis, myasthenia gravis, and myotonic dystrophy. Respiratory work from pain-induced hyperventilation is less, the depressant effects of systemic opioids avoided, and ability to clear secretions enhanced. In diabetics, epidurals reduce catecholamine and 11-hydroxycorticosteroid levels, resulting in better maternal glucose control and placental perfusion. At CS, hypotension may worsen fetal acidosis but neonatal outcome is comparable to that of non-diabetic parturients if hypotension is aggressively treated.

Advantages for obese parturients include reduction of cardiopulmonary stress and better oxygenation in labour. For CS, the considerable hazards of general anaesthesia in this group are avoided and excellent postoperative analgesia in surgically difficult patients who are at increased risk of respiratory, infective, and thromboembolic complications can be provided. Although careful consideration is required, epidural analgesia may control surges of intracranial pressure and benefit parturients with some neurological disorders (for example, cerebral arteriovenous malformations and aneurysms or space-occupying lesions). In those with high spinal cord injuries, regional block is important in blocking autonomic hyperreflexia in response to labour pain.

Contraindications to regional anaesthesia and analgesia

The role of regional analgesia and anaesthesia in obstetrics is under constant re-evaluation. In certain parturients and situations where epidural or spinal techniques were once considered absolutely contraindicated, blocks are now used with caution or even recommended. In each individual case, however, the obstetric anaesthetist must consider the underlying pathophysiology, current medical condition, obstetric needs, and other relevant factors before discussing with the patient the advantages, disadvantages, and risks. Consultation with medical colleagues is often appropriate.

There are now few absolute contraindications to a regional block apart from patient refusal. Only in exceptional circumstances, however, would an epidural or spinal be considered in the face of severe uncorrected hypovolaemia or evidence of clinical bleeding from thrombocytopenia or coagulopathy.

Local anaesthetic allergy

LA allergy is almost always a misdiagnosis and true allergy is very rare.[7] Even if the situation cannot be clarified, regional block may be feasible with alternative drugs. Despite drawbacks such as nausea and a brief duration of action, subarachnoid pethidine produces spinal block for CS and compares favourably with hyperbaric lignocaine for postpartum sterilisation. Intraspinal clonidine and opioid provide excellent analgesia in early labour, although are less reliable when labour is more advanced. Intrathecal neostigmine is being evaluated.

Local or systemic infection

Although uncommon, both localised and systemic infection create concern about the risk of superficial epidural site infection and, more seriously, epidural abscess or meningitis secondary to microbial inoculation or direct or haematogenous spread. An area of infected skin should not be traversed but in the presence of minor folliculitis or acne, preparatory and subsequent cleansing with potent antiseptics can dramatically reduce skin flora. Regional blocks in a clinically septic patient may worsen haemodynamic instability and considerable caution should be exercised. Prospective data from surgical patients with remote infected sites suggest epidural catheterisation does not confer a high risk. This is supported by an apparent absence of serious complications when it is employed in parturients with low-grade fever or chorioamnionitis, especially if they are systemically well and receiving antibiotics.[8]

Epidural blood patching after dural puncture is not associated with changes in immunological status, infection or neurological function in

113

human immunodeficiency virus (HIV) positive women. Retrospective studies in parturients with recurrent herpes simplex virus (HSV) infection suggest that blocks are safe provided the skin site is lesion free, although caution with intraspinal morphine is required (see "Herpes simplex virus reactivation" below). In the rare situation of active viral infection such as varicella pneumonia or primary HSV, careful consideration is necessary.

Obstetric haemorrhage and hypovolaemia

If regional analgesia and anaesthesia are not avoided in the presence of haemorrhage and significant uncorrected hypovolaemia, cardiac output may deteriorate because of sympathectomy-induced peripheral venous pooling and impairment of physiological compensatory mechanisms. In addition, with abruptio placenta, impaired coagulation (and the risk of intraspinal haematoma) must be considered. However, regional blocks remain a safe option if adequate resuscitation has occurred, blood and rapid infusion systems are readily available, and the patient's condition is stable. In elective cases where hypovolaemia is an anticipated risk (for example, CS for anterior placenta praevia), regional anaesthesia appears safe provided patient selection is sensible.[9] Potential advantages are reduced blood loss and thromboembolic complications, although consent should be obtained for both blood transfusion and general anaesthesia if required.

Risk of intraspinal haematoma

Fear of epidural, subdural or subarachnoid haematoma is a major deterrent to regional blockade and the exceptionally low incidence of this complication in obstetrics (two cases in over 900 000 blocks in two combined series)[10,11] attests to the clinical value of heeding traditional contraindications such as full anticoagulation, severe thrombocytopenia, and coagulopathy. Nevertheless, laboratory and clinical research and prospective audit now support the safety of regional analgesia and anaesthesia in many pregnant women who might previously have been denied its benefits.[12,13] With adequate assessment, preparation, treatment and planning, parturients on drugs with anticoagulant activity (aspirin, subcutaneous heparin) and some with minor bleeding disorders or thrombocytopenia are candidates. Most tertiary units do not preclude regional blocks in parturients who have been on aspirin therapy or prophylactic low-dose heparin provided other risk factors (for example, severe pre-eclampsia-induced thrombocytopenia or liver disease) are excluded. In some countries even subcutaneous heparin prophylaxis is not discontinued, although in light of a 1998 US Federal Drug Administration bulletin reporting haematoma in patients receiving low molecular weight heparin, caution seems justified.

The decision to use epidural or spinal block in those with pre-eclampsia-induced or immune thrombocytopenia and specific haemotological conditions must be based on individual assessment, using consultation and informed consent[14]. In the most common familial bleeding disorder encountered, type 1 von Willebrand's disease, the safety margin is increased by a rise of factor VIII complex levels of over 200% during pregnancy. Many units allow pre-eclamptic parturients with platelet counts of about 75 000 × 10⁹ /dl or more to receive regional block, based on evidence from thromboelastography that overall clotting function is likely to be undisturbed[14] and provided coagulation abnormalities and clinical bleeding are absent. Despite many thrombocytopenic parturients having unknowingly received central neuraxis blocks without adverse consequences, there appears to be only one report of a haematoma in this subgroup. An argument can be made for small-gauge spinal needle techniques, based on the 1–15% incidence of venous trauma with epidural insertion.

Medical disorders

Insufficient data are available for most medical conditions to allow comparison of maternal and fetal morbidity and mortality with regional analgesia or anaesthesia versus alternatives. Multidisciplinary evaluation and individual risk-benefit assessment are essential to optimal management. In general, however, the benefits of regional analgesia in labour are considered to outweigh the problems associated with labour-induced haemodynamic and respiratory changes, provided LA doses are titrated slowly and haemodynamic disturbance minimised with opioid and infusion techniques. At CS, block-induced sympathectomy and concurrent direct drug effects alter heart rate, preload, and afterload and circulatory instability or myocardial ischaemia are justifiably major concerns in some cardiac or cardiorespiratory conditions.[15] These include primary and secondary pulmonary hypertension, fixed or limited cardiac output states[16,17] (severe valvular stenosis, hypertrophic obstructive and peripartum cardiomyopathy), and bidirectional shunts[18] (Eisenmenger's syndrome). Although spinal anaesthesia is best avoided in severe disease (New York Heart Association class III or IV), slowly titrated epidural block has been used successfully. In severe respiratory and muscular disease, the effects of high sensory block and some intercostal muscle impairment on respiration and the ability to cough must be considered. Traditionally, spinal anaesthesia has been avoided in pre-eclampsia on the basis of increased vasomotor reactivity and rapid haemodynamic changes but this attitude is overly restrictive. The response of mild or moderate pre-eclamptic parturients to regional anaesthesia is similar to, and may be less marked than, normal women, while vasopressor responses are not significantly exaggerated. Spinal anaesthesia for CS is not contraindicated, especially if resuscitation and stabilisation have been achieved.

Central nervous system pathology may increase some risks associated with regional, so block delivery should occur in specialist centres. Needle insertion into an area of spinal pathology (arteriovenous malformation, spinal cord tumour, neurofibromatosis) is clearly inadvisable, as is breach of the dura in those with raised intracranial pressure. However, although transient increases in intracranial pressure occur during injection, epidural analgesia established by an experienced anaesthetist assists control of pain-induced pressure elevations. In parturients with intercurrent neurological disease such as multiple sclerosis, where postpartum deterioration is common, regional block does not appear to exacerbate disease but informed consent is clearly essential.

Effects of regional analgesia and anaesthesia on the baby

Regional analgesia and anaesthesia have a variety of potential effects on the fetus and neonate (see Chapter 2).[19,20] These include foetotoxic drug effects and the implications of drug administration and physiological changes associated with the block in early pregnancy, effects on uteroplacental blood flow, fetal acid-base status, and respiratory gas exchange. Alteration of neonatal stress responses, direct and indirect effects of analgesic or anaesthetic drugs and physiological changes, and drug effects on the breastfed infant must also be considered. Assessments of well-being include interpretation of fetal heart rate patterns, Apgar scores, fetal and neonatal acid-base status, neurobehavioural scoring, and perinatal morbidity and mortality. Fetal effects can be viewed as direct (for example, placental drug transfer) or indirect (for example, the consequences of alterations to maternal physiology and placental exchange functions or maternal biochemistry and psychology). During labour, uterine contractions intermittently reduce uteroplacental blood flow and oxygen content of the intervillous space or cause umbilical cord compression. Fetal reserve is good. The well term and premature fetus tolerate such changes and transplacental drug effects, although acidaemia develops and an acute fall in fetal heart rate is likely to indicate fetal hypoxia.

The effect of epidural analgesia is complex but has potential impact on uteroplacental and fetal blood flow, uterine tone and activity, maternal physiology and hormone responses, as well as direct fetal drug effects.[19,20] Avoiding aortocaval compression is critical and supine positioning must be avoided at all times, including during vaginal examination, fetal blood sampling, instrumental delivery, and transfer to the operating room. Aortic compression may go undetected and because uterine blood flow is not autoregulated, even mild falls in maternal blood pressure may reduce placental perfusion. When parturients turn from left lateral to a supine position, only some fetal heart rate patterns deteriorate but in almost all cases fetal scalp capillary pH, transcutaneous oxygen tension, and cerebral oxygenation fall.

Opioid effects

Opioids are safe to use in early pregnancy. Morphine has both basic and weakly acidic groups, low lipophilicity and weak α_1-acid glycoprotein binding. Pethidine is a weakly basic, α_1-acid glycoprotein-bound piperidine derivative, which is almost 40 times more lipophilic than morphine but 20 times less so than fentanyl. Transplacental transfer of pethidine is rapid and increased in the presence of acidosis by ion trapping. Both pethidine and its metabolite norpethidine have markedly prolonged half-lives in the neonate, accumulating for many hours. Repeated doses of systemic pethidine produce significant neonatal depression but limited evaluation of restricted doses of epidural pethidine in labour has not identified adverse effects. Fentanyl is mainly albumin bound and, like the even more lipophilic sufentanil, has rapid placental transfer. Despite early equilibration, neither accumulate significantly in the fetus or alter neonatal neurobehavioural scores.

The placenta probably acts as a depot for lipophilic opioids and in conjunction with rapid maternal drug redistribution, this leads to very low or undetectable umbilical venous and arterial levels which show no correlation with fetal outcome. In labour, subarachnoid fentanyl and prolonged epidural fentanyl infusion have no effect on fetal heart rate variability, Apgar scores,or umbilical blood gas values. Cumulative fentanyl doses up to 400 µg do not depress neonatal respiration, although may be associated with transient effects on tone. Before CS, 50–100 µg of epidural fentanyl with LA does not depress the term neonate, alter respiratory parameters or patterns of breathing or affect neurobehaviour.

Local anaesthetic effects

LAs, which are weak bases of intermediate to high lipophilicity and variable α_1-acid glycoprotein binding, are safe to use in early pregnancy. Maternal or fetal pharmacological effects are only likely in the presence of toxic levels. The foetomaternal drug ratio is mainly determined by transplacental binding, with highly bound LAs having the lowest ratios (for example, ropivacaine 0.2 versus lignocaine 0.5–0.6). Chloroprocaine, which is very rapidly metabolised by plasma esterase, is barely detectable in cord blood. All LAs undergo flow-dependent transfer according to the transplacental concentration gradient of the freely diffusable unionised component. Equilibration of free bupivacaine between maternal and fetal compartments occurs in about 40–60 minutes and fetal levels rise with increasing duration of maternal administration. Systemic accumulation of lignocaine exceeds that of bupivacaine, increasing the risk of maternal toxicity and fetal effects with repeated or continuous epidural lignocaine administration during labour.

Fetal myocardial uptake of bupivacaine does not account for reduction in fetal heart rate variability or the transient deceleratory changes seen within

20 minutes, suggesting indirect mechanisms. Fetal electrocardiogram waveform analysis indicates that bupivacaine tends to increase rate (probably indirectly), without altering myocardial conduction. Double-blind studies indicate no important changes in fetal heart rate or neurobehavioural scores from LA anaesthesia, bolus versus infusion administration during labour, nor any difference between bupivacaine and lignocaine.

Other drug effects

Clonidine produces fetal abnormalities in some animal species but is considered safe in pregnancy based on limited clinical data. Its role in obstetrics remains unclear. Epidural clonidine in doses of less than 100 μg may reduce the fetal heart rate without influencing outcome. Sufentanil 10 μg or clonidine 75 μg added to epidural LA for CS results in similar neonatal neurobehavioural effects.

Epidural adrenaline increases the fetal equilibration rate of bupivacaine without reducing fetal exposure and its clinical effects are unimportant in healthy parturients.

Indirect effects on placental blood flow and uterine tone

LAs potentially alter uteroplacental flow by influencing arterial tone or extrinsic myometrial compression. The effect of LA on myometrial activity is considered later. During labour, plasma catecholamine levels rise with pain and anxiety and in animal models this may cause fetal asphyxia secondary to uterine artery vasoconstriction. Catecholamine levels fall after epidural analgesia and radioisotope studies suggest that intervillous blood flow improves. Doppler flow velocimetry both in labour and in association with regional anaesthesia for CS shows little change, providing maternal cardiac output is maintained. In pre-eclamptic parturients, however, where intervillous blood flow may be reduced by as much as 50%, epidural analgesia may dramatically improve flow.[21] In the presence of high plasma levels of LA following paracervical block or accidental intravenous injection, vasoconstriction may occur. The opioids and clonidine have no significant effect on uterine flow or myometrial tone.

Under normal conditions, neither epidural adrenaline (25–100 μg), which has mainly maternal β-sympathomimetic action, nor unintentional intravenous injection of 15 μg in a test dose, significantly alters intervillous blood flow. However, if resistance within the maternal placental circulation is high, as little as 40 μg of epidural adrenaline may transiently increase uterine resistance, sometimes resulting in deceleratory fetal heart rate changes.[22] Thus, plain LA is preferably for all epidural blocks associated with severe pre-eclampsia or fetal growth retardation secondary to abnormalities of uteroplacental flow.

Fetal heart rate abnormalities are common following subarachnoid opioids for labour analgesia, but are usually transient and infrequently require intervention. They are thought to result from increases in uterine tone as pain relief leads to a large fall in circulating adrenaline levels, with loss of its tocolytic effect.

The fetal implications of changes in maternal temperature are considered under "Shivering and temperature regulation" on p 164. Normal labour has a mild but potentially detrimental effect on fetal biochemistry, with a cumulative fetal acidaemia dependent on the duration of labour and, in particular, maternal pushing. This acidaemia is abolished by epidural analgesia in the first stage of labour and diminished during the expulsion phase. Epidural analgesia also protects against maternal hyperventilation, serving to maintain fetal haemoglobin saturation by preventing reduction in maternal oxygen tension associated with between-contraction hypoventilation.

Regional anaesthesia for caesarean section: fetal outcome

Regional anaesthesia for CS avoids general anaesthesia-related drug depression and a significant fall in intervillous blood flow, while optimising maternal oxygenation. A variety of neonatal benefits ensue. These include higher Apgar scores, earlier establishment of sustained respiration, less neonatal resuscitation in both full-term and premature infants, higher early neurobehavioural scores (especially for alertness, tone, sucking, and overall responsiveness), better preservation of the neonatal stress response to extrauterine life, and improved outcome in the breech baby.

Nevertheless, maternal hypotension from regional anaesthesia may exacerbate fetal acidaemia, and in a large epidemiological study the frequency of neonates with a pH <7.10 (biochemical evidence of significant asphyxia) was significantly higher with regional anaesthesia.[23] Greater acidaemia associated with spinal anaesthesia may reflect either more severe hypotension or increased vasopressor drug requirement. Transient hypotension (<2 minutes) does not harm the healthy fetus, whereas prolonged hypotension of five minutes or more or profound falls of systolic BP (70 mmHg or less) may lead to fetal heart rate changes, acidaemia, and lower Apgar scores or neurobehavioural impairment. With good cardiovacsular management, neonatal acid-base status is similar after epidural and spinal anaesthesia. When CS is performed for fetal distress, either a spinal block or extension of an epidural block produces greater improvement in biochemical parameters (from those at the time of decision), and higher Apgar scores, than general anaesthesia.[24]

Fetal oxygenation and biochemical health are optimised by maternal oxygen administration and a short uterine incision-to-delivery interval, because delays of greater than three minutes under spinal anaesthesia are associated with increased fetal acidosis and lower Apgar scores. Administration of 5%

119

dextrose is of no benefit and, when excessive, causes acidaemia, reduced fetal oxygenation, and neonatal hypoglycaemia.

Regional analgesia and anaesthesia: breastfeeding

Preliminary series have found that epidural analgesia does not influence the percentage of women reporting difficulty with breastfeeding. Infant sucking behaviour is similar to controls having no labour analgesia and better than that of parturients who receive intravenous fentanyl, even if the epidural solution contained fentanyl.

No adverse effects on lactation or feeding have been associated with regional anaesthesia for CS and some data suggest breastfeeding is more readily established than after general anaesthesia. After spinal anaesthesia, three days of epidural bupivacaine analgesia results in a greater volume of breast milk and gain in infant weight than non-steroidal anti-inflammatory (NSAID) analgesia.[25] Breastfed infants of mothers receiving intravenous pethidine (and its metabolite norpethidine), in contrast to those exposed to morphine, may develop subtle neurobehavioural changes on the third and fourth days after CS. Little information is available on either the pharmacokinetics of breast milk drug transfer or the clinical impact of the smaller doses of opioid required for intrathecal and epidural analgesia in this setting.

Effects of regional analgesia and anaesthesia on labour and delivery

Regional analgesia and duration of labour

A number of physiological and pharmacological factors related to labour pain and epidural analgesia can influence uterine contractility and the progress of labour. *In vitro* and *in vivo* studies show that pain relief (with reduction of the tocolytic effect of circulating catecholamines) has a variable and relatively unimportant effect on uterine activity. Epidural analgesia is usually associated with no change in the number of uterine contractions and increased fundal dominance (increased intrauterine pressure in the upper segment) during contractions. Occasionally transient increases in tone are reported and uterine hyperactivity is a postulated explanation for unexpected fetal heart rate decelerations in the presence of unaltered maternal haemodynamics. The effect of individual LAs varies, although only plasma LA levels well above the normal clinical range (for example, following accidental intravenous injection or paracervical block) increase uterine tone. Epidural adrenaline 15 µg or more may transiently reduce activity due to its β-sympathomimetic action, but has no significant effect on the progress of labour.[26] Untreated hypotension or aortocaval compression also reduce activity, as does intravenous preloading with crystalloid 500–1000 ml. This causes a transient but significant reduction in uterine tone for about 20 minutes, possibly due to release of atrial natriuretic hormone or a fall in oxytocin levels.[27]

How these factors interact and impact clinically varies.[28] There does not appear to be any effect from epidural analgesia on the rate of cervical dilation or on standard labour curves during established labour. Preliminary investigation of combined spinal-epidural analgesia suggests no significant effect on labour progress. Epidurals have been associated with an increased duration of the first stage of labour in retrospective or non-randomised studies, which are confounded by selection bias. Although randomised controlled trials have the greatest potential to identify an effect from epidural analgesia, few have been attempted. The two main hallmarks of good clinical research, randomisation and blinding, are difficult to apply. Blinding of analgesic technique is impossible (which predisposes to bias and tends to overestimate treatment effect) and it is unethical to compel parturients to maintain their allocated treatment (epidural versus non-epidural analgesia) throughout labour. Analysis of compliant participants is confounded by postrandomisation selection bias and intention-to-treat analysis (of all in the allocated group irrespective of the type of analgesia ultimately received) is preferable but often flawed by high dropout or crossover rates. Prospective, randomised trials have produced inconsistent results, although meta-analysis found epidural analgesia resulted in a clinically modest increase in labour duration, of the order of 45 minutes in the first stage and 15 in the second.[29] The results of two even more recent and well-conducted randomised trials are consistent with this.[30,31]

Several mechanisms have been proposed by which epidurals might increase the duration of the second stage of labour (and also instrumental delivery).[28] In animals, oxytocin is released in response to distention of the pelvic floor (Ferguson's reflex) but in humans neither the relevance nor magnitude of this response is clear, nor is it known if regional analgesia blocks the response. However, oxytocin infusion during the second stage in nulliparous parturients receiving epidural analgesia reduces the duration of the expulsive phase and non-rotational instrumental deliveries.[32] The maternal urge to bear down is reduced in 50% of women receiving 0.25% bupivacaine, although this is less likely when low-dose LA-opioid solutions are used. While it has been postulated that dense neural block prevents effective maternal expulsive efforts and delays rotation of the presenting part on the pelvic floor, a large prospective study found that small pelvic outlet capacity was associated with both use of epidurals and persistent posterior position, but that epidural analgesia itself was not independently associated with malposition.[33]

It is argued that, compared with assessment of fetal descent, the only importance of length of second stage is as a marker for other obstetric problems. Only the time spent actively pushing influences progressive fetal acidaemia and some studies suggest that delaying maternal expulsive efforts until the fetal head has descended to at least below the ischial spines will reduce the incidence of forceps delivery. The American College of Obstetricians and Gynecologists now recommends that, providing monitoring indicates fetal well-being, prolongation of the second stage under epidural analgesia be defined as three hours for nulliparous women and two hours for parous women.

In summary, the evidence for an effect on the duration of first-stage labour is unclear and although it may be slightly increased, this probably varies with individual circumstances. Similarly, any increase in the duration of the second stage is small and probably of little significance to fetal outcome.[28,29]

Effect of regional analgesia on instrumental delivery and caesarean section rates

During the 1970s and 1980s the incidence of CS in many countries rose dramatically (for example, in the USA from 5% to 24%). This attracted much attention in the health care industry and community and although the increase is partly attributable to factors such as increases in primiparity, maternal age, multiple delivery, and birth weight, 75% has been ascribed to changes in medical practice. The use of regional analgesia in labour has also increased and retrospective studies have identified a strong association with assisted delivery or CS (based on dystocia or failure to progress but not fetal indications). A causal relationship is difficult to establish, however, because almost all available data are confounded by selection bias. Women who receive an epidural are, for a variety of reasons, a subpopulation at greater risk of complicated labour and delivery. Even allowing for independent obstetric risk factors which increase the likelihood of epidural analgesia (nulliparity, premature rupture of the membranes, induction of labour, malposition, multiple pregnancy, and medical factors such as pre-eclampsia), patient factors such as increased maternal age, a prolonged latent phase of labour or more severe early pain are also associated with both request for regional block and assisted delivery. Furthermore, labour management and outcome (diagnosis of dystocia, active management of labour policy, and threshold for intervention) vary with public versus private obstetric care, unit policy, and indeed dramatically between individual obstetricians. In addition, regional analgesic techniques are not generic, with a range of delivery methods, drugs, doses, and management strategies used.[34]

When high concentrations of LA are used, epidural analgesia is associated with high rates of instrumental delivery in nulliparous women and the relationship persists for outlet forceps and vacuum delivery, but not rotational forceps, with current techniques.[29] Infusion or patient-controlled epidural analgesic delivery systems minimise LA administration and motor block, as does combination of opioid and LA. Some studies suggest this leads to more vaginal deliveries but problems such as failure to adequately standardise obstetric management mean caution should be exercised before ascribing outcome differences to epidural technique.

Many obstetricians and midwives continue to advocate discontinuation of epidural analgesia in the second stage of labour. Withholding top-ups in the second stage does not make spontaneous delivery more likely and only increases the severity of maternal pain.[35] However, well-conducted randomised trials demonstrate that late discontinuation of a 0.125% bupivacaine epidural infusion, which frequently produces dense motor block, decreases the incidence of instrumental delivery compared to continuation. In contrast, a 0.0625% bupivacaine-fentanyl infusion is equally effective and can be continued without an impact, although good analgesia is difficult to obtain.[36] Further data supporting the opinion that regional blocks in labour have little effect on instrumental delivery come from observational studies of delivery outcome in maternity units during time periods when epidural drug doses were reduced.

Midcavity forceps are used infrequently these days and a meta-analysis of epidural versus non-epidural analgesia found no increase in instrumental delivery for dystocia.[29] Following a study by Thorp et al., published in 1993,[37] which reported no difference in forceps delivery but a highly significant increase in CS for dystocia in nulliparous women receiving epidural analgesia, the focus of debate has shifted to the impact on delivery by CS. Thorp's study has attracted much debate and criticism, especially on the grounds of investigator bias and inadequate labour management guidelines. These authors attributed the remarkable impact of epidural analgesia to its commencement in early labour, but subsequent studies demonstrate that the timing of epidural placement is not important and that withholding regional analgesia until beyond 5 cm cervical dilation is unjustified.[34]

Despite the difficulties faced in conducting randomised trials discussed previously, several recent studies have attempted to address this issue. One of the first involved 1330 women of mixed parity and reported more instrumental and CS deliveries with epidural analgesia compared with systemic opioid analgesia but failed to detail the specific delivery method and, because of high crossover rates, could not exclude selection bias and the likelihood of distortion of the results.[38] Several further studies from the same unit had improved methodology or reduced crossover rates between groups but compliance with group allocation continued to pose problems.[39] On intention-to-treat analysis, these latest trials indicate that neither epidural nor CSE analgesia has any significant effect on the incidence of forceps delivery or CS.[30,31] Further prospective randomised studies are in progress.

A less rigorous method of assessing the impact of epidural analgesia on labour outcome is analysis of impact data. Under steady-state conditions, the effect of removing or introducing an epidural service, or greatly increasing epidural utilisation, is audited.[40] These studies show no significant change in the rate of operative delivery and statistical modelling of large patient populations has not identified epidural analgesia as an independent risk factor. Obstetric labour management, operative delivery criteria, and the obstetrician's practice patterns have been identified as the most important determinants of labour progress and outcome. Obstetricians' individual CS rates vary in homogeneous populations from 6.5% to 41% and show no relationship with rate of use of epidural analgesia in labour. In a unit where 42% of both public and privately insured parturients received an identical method of epidural analgesia, CS rate for dystocia was found to be 0.5% versus 14% respectively.[41] In a study of low-risk parturients delivered by 11 obstetricians, the only factor accounting for a variation in CS rate between 10% and 32% was the obstetrician.[42] Several interventions, including active management of labour, protocols for the diagnosis of dystocia and strict criteria for intervention, and staff education, may significantly reduce CS rates, even as epidural service utilisation increases.

Whether epidural or CSE analgesia alters delivery mode remains debatable. The strongest evidence to date suggests no significant effect compared with parenteral opioid. Indeed, if any effect occurs, it is minimal compared to that of materno-fetal and obstetric factors and currently there is no justification for withholding regional analgesia at any time.[34]

Consent

While the moral and legal arguments for gaining consent before treatment are not generally disputed, there are many practical issues which create confusion and provoke disagreement between clinicians. Litigation for "minor" complaints (postdural puncture headache, pain during surgery under regional block) is more common in obstetric anaesthesia. The obstetric anaesthetist must be prepared to disclose and discuss such problems, with a view to obtaining informed consent from both an ethical and a legal perspective.[43-45]

The philosophical principles on which consent is based are those of autonomy (the right of informed patients to follow a self-chosen plan voluntarily) and beneficence (the physician's primary duty is to help or at least do no harm). Valid ethical consent requires that the patient has sufficient relevant information on which to base a decision, the opportunity to express their opinion, and an assurance that their wishes will be respected. Informed consent is a process of good communication between patient and doctor, poor patient rapport creating an atmosphere of high medicolegal risk. Women who initially refuse to have a CS performed under regional anaesthesia, for example, will usually comply if the advantages are explained and their apprehensions (for example, fear of painful insertion and backache) allayed. A dilemma may arise, however, when the patient's decision conflicts with the anaesthetist's perception of their duty of benefi-cence. An example is the woman who is assessed as having a difficult airway but who adamantly refuses regional anaesthesia for surgery, despite a strong recommendation. The risks and benefits of each anaesthetic option should be presented openly, although at times specific or numeric data supporting the recommendation may be lacking or difficult to provide. In any setting, if safe and reasonable alternatives exist (in the above case, awake intuba-tion), these must be discussed and the patient's final decision respected. Although the anaesthetist has the right to refuse care in an elective situa-tion, their ethical obligation is to at least make alternative arrangements and ethical opinion leans towards requiring a reluctant physician to provide care if the situation is an emergency.

"Therapeutic privilege" describes the practice of withholding certain information in order to benefit the patient. This is very unlikely to be justi-fiable in the obstetric population, where surveys suggest most parturients desire detailed information. Expressed consent is more appropriate than implied and although oral consent is valid, it may be difficult to prove in the absence of written documentation. It can be argued that a written consent form is largely irrelevant to the process of informed consent and surveys suggest most anaesthetists do not obtain written consent for regional anal-gesia in the presence of labour pain or medications. A preprinted written consent form becomes very complicated in attempting to cover both elec-tive and emergency situations but a limited checklist may act as a prompt and alternative to individualised notation regarding the topics discussed. The notation approach provides more convincing evidence that discussion occurred, although the depth of discussion, and what is disclosed, may vary according to the level of risk, the circumstances, and local expectations.

Community expectations about disclosure are changing, with a move away from medical paternalism (the doctor discloses and does what they think is best). In 1991, English surgical patients appeared most interested in routine aspects of their perioperative care.[46] In 1993, Australian patients had higher expectations of detailed information[47] and in 1996 the majority of surgical patients in a New Zealand survey considered a "minimal" infor-mation leaflet withheld too much information compared with more detailed versions.[48] A recent survey of Canadian parturients noted a desire to discuss all epidural complications, especially serious events such as convulsions, paralysis, and effects on the baby.[49]

Legal requirements with respect to informed consent vary from country to country but are based on either the "professional standard" (the standard of care consistent with responsible contemporary practice), the "reasonable person standard" (which requires disclosure of all information to the extent that it would satisfy the hypothetical reasonable person) or the "patient need" or "subjective person" standard, which emphasises the autonomy of the patient and the requirement to tailor disclosure to the individual's particular wants and needs of relevance to their decision making. Unfortunately, the anaesthetist must decide if a risk is material to a particular patient, being guided especially by patient preferences and questions and by their clinical experience. Essential elements include explanation of the procedure, its risks and benefits; the opportunity for inquiries to be answered, and patient cooperation during the procedure.

Obtaining consent for epidural analgesia in labour in distressed parturients who may be affected by drugs is difficult and may not be legally valid.[45] Recall is affected by the timing of discussion. Parturients in active labour have poor recall, one-third not even remembering that risk explanation occurred. Previous antenatal education and written information or verbal discussion improve recall of intrapartum discussion about epidurals during labour, with risks such as headache, pruritus, and nerve damage frequently remembered.[50] Other factors such as formal education, prior experience, communication skills, and current pain levels may also influence recall. During labour, the anaesthetist is unlikely to face problems in most legal systems provided discussion occurred and the parturient was cooperative. Assessing competence to consent for research is also fraught with difficulty in this setting but informed consent should be easy to understand, presented in a relaxed, non-coercive manner and must address common concerns such as increased risk and fear for the baby's safety. It is preferably obtained antenatally and reconfirmed during labour.

The patient who has made a directive in advance poses special problems. An example is the parturient with a birth plan stating that she does not want an epidural "under any circumstances, even if I ask for it", but then, distressed with pain, requests it. It can be argued that the new request is temporary and that she should be encouraged to manage without. On the other hand, she has every right to change her mind and her decision made when not in pain is unlikely to be legally binding. It has been argued that an informed decision can only be made when the parturient knows the nature and degree of pain.[45] A judgement must be made as to her competency, the opinion of her partner and support persons canvassed, and ultimately the anesthetist should act in what he or she perceives to be the patient's best interest. Although the right of choice in the obstetric setting deserves promotion and implementation, the individual should also take responsibility for the consequences of their decision.

Regional analgesia for pain relief during labour and delivery

Overview

Subarachnoid cocaine was used for pain relief in parturients in Switzerland before 1900, caudal anaesthesia introduced in Germany in 1909 and paracervical block in 1926. In 1927 in Italy, injection of the sympathetic chain at the third lumbar level was noted to relieve labour pain and the Italian surgeon Dogliotti published his experience with lumbar and thoracic epidural anaesthesia for surgery in 1931. Continuous techniques were subsequently introduced, starting with spinal in 1940, caudal in 1942 and then lumbar epidural analgesia in 1949. Continuous caudal block through malleable needles and rubber catheters was popular until supplanted by the lumbar approach after about 1960. With advances in the quality and safety of regional techniques, they have become increasingly popular, because pain relief is superior to all alternatives. The ability to cope, feeling relaxed and aware are often cited as benefits, so if a service is readily available, 30–90% of parturients will opt for regional blocks.

An understanding of obstetric pain mechanisms and pathways is essential (Fig 4.1), as are appropriate standards of equipment, assistance, and

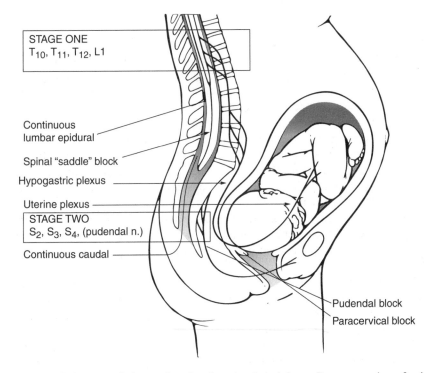

Fig 4.1   Pain transmission and regional analgesia in labour. Representation of pain fibres responsible for transmission of pain in the first stage of labour (T10, T11, T12, L1) as opposed to the second stage (S2, S3, S4). Location for various regional techniques for pain relief (from McDonald JS. Associated pain management problems of parturition. In: Bonica JJ, McDonald JS, eds. *Principles and practice of obstetric analgesia and anesthesia*, 2nd edn. Malvern, USA: Williams and Wilkins, 1995, with permission)

127

monitoring. Prospective audit suggests that with sound education, technique, drug selection, and attention to prevention and management of serious complications, the safety of obstetric regional analgesia continues to improve.[51] Outmoded techniques (for example, caudal analgesia with large doses of LA for contraction pain) or failure to place an intravenous cannula (which contributed to a death reported in the 1991–93 Report on Confidential Enquiries into Maternal Deaths in the United Kingdom) cannot be condoned. Further information is becoming available about the association between regional analgesia and various postpartum sequelae. The question as to whether epidurals in labour increase postpartum backache has been resolved by several recent prospective studies, which indicate no significant association (see Chapter 8). Furthermore, epidurals do not appear to be associated with a higher incidence of difficulty with breastfeeding.

Lumbar epidural analgesia

Technique

Epidural analgesia is popular,[52] although provision of an epidural service is not always feasible, so there is considerable international, national, and regional variability in availability and utilisation. A European survey found about 15% of parturients received an epidural in labour, whereas 27% did so in the United Kingdom. In a large UK survey, failure to provide an epidural was identified as the most frequent cause of anxiety and disappointment during labour.[53] A mean reduction in contraction pain score of at least 80–90% can be expected and 80–90% of parturients report effective analgesia, albeit "excellent" or "good" in three-quarters during the first stage and two-thirds during the second stage of labour. In experienced hands (with adjustment of epidural solutions and parturient position and catheter manipulation or resiting as required), only 5% experience inadequate analgesia. Approaches such as the double-catheter technique (insertion of lumbar and caudal catheters) or supplementary single-shot caudal analgesia are now rarely used.

Epidural and combined spinal-epidural analgesia necessitate interventions such as intravenous access and regular maternal haemodynamic monitoring, although routine continuous fetal heart rate monitoring is controversial,[54] and many units use criteria based on obstetric and medical indications alone. Midwifery or anaesthetic monitoring of dermatomal spread can be useful, especially in assessing inadequate blocks, but as yet is not routine.

For labour analgesia, epidural catheters are usually inserted between the second and fourth lumbar vertebrae. Although two of three studies suggest that aortocaval compression is more likely in the flexed left lateral decubitus position, the parturient's position during insertion (sitting versus lateral) is usually determined by her or the anaesthetist's preference. Skin preparation with chlorhexidine is preferred as it is a more effective antiseptic than iodine. Accumulating evidence supports the superiority of a loss of resistance to saline (versus air) technique in reducing accidental dural punctures and avoiding air-induced complications.[55] Ease of use, complication rates, and patient comfort are similar for 16 and 18 gauge epidural needles.[56] Multiholed catheters inserted 3–5 cm are preferable to terminal eye catheters because unsatisfactory blocks (unilateral block and clot obstruction) are fewer and replacement less often required. Blood is more easily aspirated through a multiholed catheter, so that in the event of accidental intravascular catheter placement, the risk of intravenous injection is reduced. A disadvantage is the potential for multicompartment (epidural, subdural, subarachnoid) block, although this is very uncommon. Catheter movement (out more frequently than in) can be reduced by changing the parturient's position before securing the catheter to the skin or by tunnelling or suturing the catheter when prolonged catheterisation is anticipated.

Epidural solutions and intermittent bolus epidural analgesia

The choice of epidural solutions should be tailored to the epidural delivery technique, obstetric and medical considerations, and the parturient's desires.[57] The majority of women in our unit request that their pain be made tolerable, with 30% seeking pain-free labour and 10% only a minor reduction in intensity. The use of minimum effective doses of LA should optimise safety (reduced risk of accumulative or acute LA toxicity; slower onset and restricted spread of spinal block after inadvertent subarachnoid injection). Excellent epidural analgesia can be obtained with bupivacaine at dose rates of 5–15 mg/h and accidental intravenous boluses of 25 mg or less are unlikely to cause serious toxicity.

Bupivacaine, which has a long duration of action and minimal plasma accumulation or tachyphylaxis with repeat dosing, has been the LA of choice. The addition of adrenaline increases the duration of boluses and improves infusion analgesia, at the expense of intensifying motor block. It is best avoided where placental function is compromised and in maternal cardiac disease. Lignocaine 1–2% (the latter with adrenaline to reduce systemic absorption) is suitable for instrumental delivery. Recently, chiral LAs have been developed as pure enantiomers, rather than as racemic mixtures. The new long-acting amide LA, ropivacaine, is an S-enantiomer and levo- or S-bupivacaine appears promising, although the first obstetric studies are only recently reported. Their pharmacological properties are similar to bupivacaine, although toxicity potential is less.[58] Ropivacaine, which has been commercially available in many countries since 1996, results in less motor block than bupivacaine at equivalent concentration, with meta-analysis of initial comparative trials suggesting less motor block at a 2.5 mg/ml (0.25%) concentration and better neonatal neurobehavioural scores.[59] Determination of minimum (median effective) local anaesthetic analgesic concentration in labour suggests ropivacaine is less potent than bupivacaine,[60,61] and thus it has yet to be confirmed that ropivacaine offers any clinical advantage with respect to motor block at commonly used epidural concentrations (of 0.125% or less).

Although 0.25% bupivacaine alone is effective for intermittent bolus administration, the high incidence of profound lower limb weakness is not ideal and, with the exception of some European trials, lower concentrations have poor reliability unless delivered by infusion or patient-controlled techniques. Continuous infusion of 0.08–0.125% bupivacaine at 12.5–20 mg/h is effective but dense motor block is common. When used alone, epidural opioids (for example, pethidine 50 mg, fentanyl 200 µg or sufentanil 30 µg) are effective in early labour, but unsatisfactory later and repeat doses may affect the fetus.

Addition of opioids to epidural solutions allows a reduction in local anaesthetic dose, without compromising analgesia. Several studies using up-down sequential allocation have now identified minimum local anaesthetic concentrations for local anaesthetics alone or in combination with opioid. Lengthy clinical experience with the addition of opioid to LA shows it to be safe and beneficial.[52,57,62] Mild opioid-induced pruritus (incidence about 25% with sufentanil and fentanyl, 3% with pethidine) is a disadvantage, but unpleasant sensory and motor numbness, shivering, and possibly urinary catheterisation and hypotension are reduced. Most parturients retain good mobility (with 80% capable of walking), are more satisfied, and impact on labour is minimal. Moreover, analgesia is improved in those experiencing an early desire to push, perineal pain or backache.

Bupivacaine 10–15 mg, combined with opioid, gives 80% of parturients good pain relief in early labour within 20 minutes. For anaesthetist or midwife-administered intermittent bolus epidural analgesia, 0.1–0.125% bupivacaine plus either fentanyl 2–5 µg/ml, pethidine 2.5 mg/ml, diamorphine 0.25 mg/ml or sufentanil 1 µg/ml is more effective than each individual drug alone. Analgesia is similar in quality and duration to larger doses of 0.25% bupivacaine (60–90 minutes), with less muscle weakness and numbness, greater maternal satisfaction and, in some studies, more spontaneous deliveries when compared to plain bupivacaine boluses.[63] No benefit is conferred by routinely adding opioid to bupivacaine concentrations of 0.25% or more but the additional fentanyl produces dose-dependent LA dose sparing, which in early labour is best achieved using 3 µg/ml.[64]

Clonidine is an α_2-adrenergic agonist with potent intraspinal analgesic properties, a history of safe obstetric use as an antihypertensive, and no effect on uteroplacental blood flow. Although a reduction in fetal heart rate is seen with doses above 100 µg, fetal outcome is unchanged and maternal motor block and respiratory depression absent. Epidural clonidine and opioid results in effective analgesia in early labour, similar to that of LA and opioid, although onset is slower and quality lower in late labour. When clonidine is combined with LA and opioid, there is a modest improvement in analgesia, LA dose sparing and longer subarachnoid analgesia, although dose-finding studies are in progress to determine if side-effects such as maternal sedation and hypotension can be avoided. The latter are minimised if epidural bolus doses are limited to 75 μg, or infusion to 25 μg/h. Whether clonidine will establish a role in epidural analgesia in the future remains uncertain, pending further investigation.[65]

Continuous infusion and patient-controlled epidural analgesia

Two alternative methods of maintaining pain relief are continuous infusion epidural analgesia and patient-controlled epidural analgesia (PCEA). Infusions provide more uniform pain relief and better haemodynamic stability than intermittent top-ups, while potentially reducing staff workload and lowering drug utilisation.[62] Dedicated syringe or infusion pumps are programmed at rates of 6–15 ml/h (depending on the epidural solution) to maintain sensory block to at least the umbilicus (T10 dermatome). Initial infusion rates can be based on the extent of initial bolus spread and the desired dose rate, but often require adjustment or supplementation with boluses of similar or more concentrated solution to meet individual variability in response and treat inadequate analgesia. Although plain bupivacaine 0.08–0.125% at dose rates of 12.5–20 mg/h is effective, mobility is significantly improved after LA dose reduction achieved by adding opioids such as fentanyl 1–3 μg/ml, sufentanil 0.5 μg/ml or diamorphine 25–50 μg/ml. At a sufentanil:fentanyl ratio of 1:2, sufentanil produces better analgesia and greater bupivacaine sparing with similar side-effects, although this is probably because the potency ratio of these drugs is 1:4.5. At a ratio of 25:2, diamorphine results in lower pain scores compared with fentanyl when infused with bupivacaine 0.125% at 7.5 ml/h.

Although popular, infusion of 0.125% bupivacaine and opioid is inappropriate. Indeed, most parturients achieve good analgesia in early labour with infusions of much lower concentration (0.015–0.04% bupivacaine plus opioid, with or without adrenaline, at 10–15 ml/h). This is consistent with the 95% confidence limit for the minimum effective analgesic concentration for bupivacaine combined with fentanyl 3 μg/ml in early labour of 0.045%. This figure increases as labour progresses but analgesia equivalent to 0.125% bupivacaine is consistently obtained with 0.0625% bupivacaine (with opioid), while delivering less drug and significantly reducing motor block. Unfortunately, even low concentration of LA given by infusion leads to inability to stand or walk in at least a fifth of parturients after two or three hours and prolonged periods lying in one lateral position should be avoided to minimise unilateral block.

Obstetric patient-controlled epidural analgesia has been reviewed recently.[66] Solutions similar to those chosen for infusions are suitable (for example, 0.0625% bupivacaine with 2 µg/ml fentanyl). Although a concurrent background infusion may reduce supplementation rates, a demand-bolus only method (for example, 4–5 ml at a 10–15-minute lockout; total bupivacaine delivery 4–8 mg/h) gives excellent pain relief with minimal motor block and potential for ambulation. Compared with infusions, PCEA either further reduces staff intervention or supplementation or reduces total bupivacaine administration by 25–50%. The safety of PCEA is well established, with over 2750 parturients enrolled in clinical trials without mishap. Haemodynamic stability is similar to that with infusions and the absence of postural hypotensive effects in parturients who self-administer while walking has been demonstrated. The mean cephalad level of sensory block is similar to alternative approaches and the very low rates of LA use and small bolus doses required make toxicity or high spinal block after inadvertent subarachnoid injection highly unlikely. Parturients who benefit particularly are those requesting regional analgesia in early labour, those wishing to maximise feelings of control during childbirth, those who want the flexibility of titrating solution to meet their individual needs at different times during labour, and those keen to retain good mobility and to ambulate. The technique is less suitable when epidural analgesia is established near the end of labour and in parturients who are exhausted or uninterested in assuming responsibility for drug administration. A limitation to the introduction of PCEA services during labour has been the expense, bulkiness, and unsuitability of many sophisticated electronic pumps. The development and availability of purpose-designed devices, including inexpensive disposable and user-friendly ambulatory pumps, has the potential to greatly broaden the availability of PCEA.

Combined spinal-epidural analgesia

Combined spinal-epidural analgesia (CSE) in labour is now widely used, continues to increase in popularity and, in some units, has superseded epidurals as the routine approach to regional analgesia during labour. It combines the advantages of initial subarachnoid (spinal) analgesia with the flexibility of an epidural.[67,68] Compared with epidural analgesia, CSE has a more rapid onset (good analgesia in 90% within five minutes)[69] and produces at least comparable, and, arguably in late labour, better analgesia. Additional advantages are minimal motor weakness and reduced maternal and fetal drug exposure. Disadvantages include more frequent and intense pruritus (up to 60% with sufentanil and 30% with fentanyl) and the inevitable risk of postdural puncture headache (PDPH).

Fine pencil-point spinal needles (for example, the 27 gauge modified Whitacre) are recommended, usually in a needle-through-epidural-needle approach in the sitting position, which allows rapid identification of subarachnoid placement and reduces failure to identify cerebrospinal fluid to about 5%. Spinal analgesia is achieved with subarachnoid opioid, with or without bupivacaine. After the spinal needle is withdrawn, an epidural catheter is inserted. Catheter position should be tested before subarachnoid analgesia begins to wane (usually 90–180 minutes later, depending on the stage of labour and drug combination).

Fentanyl and sufentanil are popular opioids, with dose-response studies suggesting an effective dose in 95% (ED_{95}) of about 20–25 µg for fentanyl and 6–8 µg for sufentanil. Bupivacaine 5 mg alone produces excessive motor block, but 2.5 mg added to opioid allows over 90% of parturients to remain weight bearing and significantly increases the duration of effective analgesia. Preliminary dose-response data suggest 1–1.5 mg of spinal bupivacaine or 2 mg of ropivacaine may be optimal and current research is designed to investigate drug combinations that maximise the duration of initial spinal analgesia. In nulliparous parturients in early labour a combination of bupivacaine 2.5 mg, sufentanil 10 µg and adrenaline 200 µg produces analgesia for a mean of three hours (Fig 4.2),[70] and 30 µg of clonidine with sufentanil 2.5 mg produces longer analgesia than sufentanil 5 µg alone.[71] Evidence that clonidine potentiates subarachnoid bupivacaine, but not ropivacaine requires confirmation.

Experience in one hospital, involving several thousand parturients, suggests serious complications are uncommon, although meningitis has been

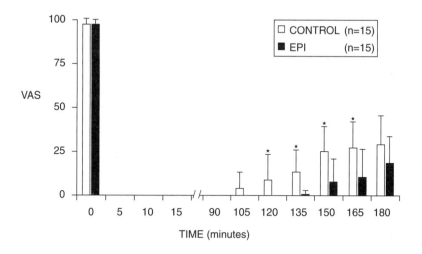

Fig 4.2 The addition of epinephrine to intrathecal bupivacaine and sufentanil for ambulatory labour analgesia. Visual analogue scores (VAS) over time (in minutes) after the intrathecal administration of the study solution (open columns represent 2.5 mg bupivacaine plus sufentanil 10 µg and closed columns the same combination with the addition of adrenaline 200 µg). Data represent mean ±SD. * $P < 0.05$ (from Campbell DC et al.[70] with permission)

Table 4.1   Regimens for regional analgesia for labour and delivery

Drug	Dose	Comment
Epidural analgesia: intermittent bolus		
Bupivacaine	0.25% 6–10 ml	More motor block
	0.125% 10–15 ml	Effective for < 50%
	0.1-0.125% + opioid 10–15 ml	Effective for 80–90%
Ropivacaine	2 mg/ml 8–12 ml	Similar to 0.25% bupivacaine 6–10 ml
	1 mg/ml + opioid 10–15 ml	
Fentanyl	2–5 µg/ml	
Sufentanil	0.5–1 µg/ml	
Diamorphine	0.25–0.5 mg/ml	
Pethidine	2.5 mg/ml	
Adrenaline	1: 400–800 000	Increases duration/motor block
Clonidine	75–100 µg + opioid (or +LA)	Effective adjunct. Role unclear
Epidural analgesia: continuous infusion at 10–15 ml/h		
Bupivacaine	0.02–0.04% + opioid + adrenaline	
	0.06–0.08% + opioid	More reliable
	0.125%	Increased motor block
Ropivacaine	0.08–1 mg/ml + opioid	Potency ratio to bupivacaine 0.6
	2 mg/ml at 6–8 ml/h	
Fentanyl	1–2 µg/ml;	
Sufentanil	0.5 µg/ml	
Diamorphine	25 µg/ml	
Adrenaline	1: 800,000	May improve efficacy
Clonidine	25 µg/h	May improve efficacy. Role unclear
Epidural analgesia: patient-controlled 4–6 ml bolus; 10–15 minute lockout		
Bupivacaine	0.0625% + opioid	Infusion unnecessary
Ropivacaine	1 mg/ml + opioid	Limited investigation
Adrenaline	1:400–800 000	Increases motor block
Clonidine	4.5 µg/ml	May improve efficacy. Role unclear
Spinal analgesia (including combined spinal-epidural analgesia)		
Bupivacaine	1–2.5 mg	
Ropivacaine	1–2 mg	
Fentanyl	20–25 µg	
Sufentanil	5–7.5 µg	

reported and further large series are required to document complication rates.[67] Severe respiratory depression may also occur after subarachnoid opioids, with an estimated frequency of one in 5000 for spinal sufentanil. Currently, most reviewers support the selected, rather than routine, use of CSE analgesia, on the grounds that it has more side-effects, higher cost and lacks prospective safety data compared with an epidural.[66-68]

Continuous spinal analgesia

Continuous spinal analgesia is infrequently used in obstetrics, because of concern about complication rates and the substantial risk of PDPH associated with catheter placement.[72,73] Claims that PDPH rate is lower following intrathecal catheterisation and with subarachnoid opioid analgesia have not been satisfactorily substantiated. Some countries have commercial spinal microcatheters available and after accidental puncture with an epidural needle, the option of inserting the epidural catheter into the subarachnoid space for labour analgesia appears to be increasingly popular. The benefits of a spinal catheter, namely continuous but accurate and titratable drug placement (usually solutions as for spinal analgesia with CSE analgesia), are attractive. Low doses of LA, opioid, and possibly adrenaline or cloni- dine can be administered intermittently, by infusion or even by patient- controlled technique. Continuous spinal analgesia is particularly valuable in cases where location of the epidural space is likely to be very difficult or hazardous. Examples include patients with musculoskeletal deformities involving the lumbar spine, vertebral canal deformities, severe idiopathic scoliosis, previous spinal surgery and in whom haemodynamic changes associated with epidural analgesia are poorly tolerated, such as those with severe pulmonary hypertension and certain congenital cardiac anomalies or conduction disorders.

Lumbar sympathetic and paracervical block

Bilateral paravertebral lumbar sympathetic block and paracervical block[74] are infrequently used in most countries (although in some European coun- tries 10–12% of deliveries are managed with paracervical and pudendal blocks). Lumbar sympathetic and paracervical blocks effectively relieve contraction pain, which is mediated via sympathetic afferents passing through the paracervical plexus to the 10–12th thoracic and first lumbar nerve roots. Lumbar sympathetic block, usually at the L2 level, may be technically difficult and has a limited duration. Paracervical block is more straightforward and performed by injecting submucosal LA into the vaginal fornices lateral to the cervix. Subsequent analgesia is superior to that from intramuscular pethidine, with 40–80% of parturients experiencing good relief for 60–90 minutes.

The proximity of the uterine vessels to the uterine sympathetic plexus results in a high risk of inadvertent intravascular injection or rapid systemic absorption of LA and other complications which include laceration, haematoma, abscess, and sacral neuropathy. The major disadvantage of paracervical block is a 10–70% incidence of fetal bradycardia (onset 2–20 minutes and duration 4–12 minutes) and intrauterine death. Brady- cardia reflects fetal hypoxaemia and acidosis and is thought to follow umbilical artery vasoconstriction and high fetal blood levels of LA. Recent trials in selected women have been able to reduce, but not eliminate, this event (incidence 2–4%). Paracervical block should not be used in the com- promised or premature fetus and meticulous technique using lignocaine or chloroprocaine, with a guarded needle, avoidance of aortocaval compres- sion and continuous fetal heart rate monitoring are recommended.

135

Regional anaesthesia for instrumental delivery

Regional techniques suitable for instrumental delivery include epidural, spinal and combined spinal-epidural anaesthesia, pudendal nerve block, and local perineal infiltration. The latter may be adequate for episiotomy and low outlet forceps or vacuum delivery. The condition of the parturient and fetus, the likelihood of successful vaginal delivery, and whether an epidural catheter is providing effective pain relief influence the technique selected. In all cases except minor infiltration, resuscitation facilities must be readily available, an intravenous cannula in place, and fluids, oxygen, vasopressors, and a means to displace the gravid uterus available.

Pudendal nerve block

Pudendal nerve block for low instrumental delivery is now almost exclusively performed by obstetricians and has been largely superseded by neuraxial regional block where epidural services are available. The pudendal nerve (anterior roots of sacral nerves S2, 3, and 4) is somatic and supplies the lower vagina and perineum, although these areas also receive innervation from ilioinguinal, genitofemoral, and posterior femoral cutaneous nerves. A bilateral transvaginal pudendal block is safer, less painful, and more successful than the transperineal approach. The nerve is blocked as it passes behind the ischial spines adjacent to the lateral vaginal wall before it divides and additional perineal infiltration is advisable. The recommended approach is to use a guarded needle and 1% lignocaine with adrenaline (or 3% 2-chloroprocaine) 10–15 ml each side, as close proximity of the pudendal vessels makes intravascular injection a hazard. Failure of the block is common and complete analgesia is achieved in only 40–50% of parturients.[74]

Epidural, spinal, and combined spinal-epidural anaesthesia

Effective epidural analgesia in labour can be readily converted to epidural anaesthesia for instrumental delivery by administration of an appropriate dose of more concentrated LA. In the absence of a contraindication to adrenaline, 2% lignocaine with adrenaline 1:200 000 8–10 ml (preferably alkalinised with 8.4% sodium bicarbonate 1 ml to increase efficacy and speed of onset) through a mid or low lumbar catheter is a suitable combination which rapidly provides good sacral anaesthesia. In North America 3% 2-chloroprocaine is popular. Other alternatives are 0.5% bupivacaine and 7.5 mg/ml ropivacaine. Spinal analgesia from a combined spinal-epidural is usually adequate for a simple lift-out delivery.

If an epidural catheter is not in place or adequate sacral anaesthesia cannot be established, subarachnoid or caudal epidural block are alternative approaches. The latter is now rarely used because of a 5–10% failure rate, a high risk of serious maternal local anaesthetic toxicity (approximately one in 100 in a recent non-obstetric series), and several well-publicised cases of accidental injection into the fetal head. Low spinal anaesthesia ("saddle block" from 1 ml hyperbaric 0.5% bupivacaine in the sitting position) is suitable for urgent instrumental delivery. If rotational or midcavity forceps delivery is anticipated, it is prudent to use the lateral position or a larger dose, aiming for sensory anaesthesia to the umbilicus (T10).

Unless instrumental delivery appears straightforward, current obstetric practice is to either proceed immediately to CS or to conduct a trial of instrumental delivery in an operating area with full facilities. Here a combined technique provides greater flexibility. A low spinal block (T10–S5) with, for example, 1–1.5 ml hyperbaric 0.5% bupivacaine sitting provides good haemodynamic stability and excellent conditions for assisted vaginal delivery, while surgical anaesthesia to T4 may be obtained rapidly by administration of epidural LA if instrumental delivery is deemed too hazardous or fails. Both 1.5–2% lignocaine with adrenaline and 3% 2-chloroprocaine (with or without alkalinisation) usually extend the block within five minutes.

Regional anaesthesia for elective caesarean section

Advantages and principles of regional anaesthesia for caesarean section

Between 1970 and 1996, the Confidential Enquiries into Maternal Deaths in England and Wales (more recently, the UK), the most comprehensive national audit of anaesthetic-related mortality, described 214 maternal deaths directly related to anaesthesia, of which only 14 were associated with regional blocks. In the 1982–84 report the comment was made that, where possible, epidural anaesthesia should be preferred to general anaesthesia for CS. Between 1991 and 1993, seven of eight maternal deaths directly attributed to anaesthesia and all deaths associated with CS followed complications of general anaesthesia. A review of anaesthesia-related maternal deaths in the USA from 1979 to 1990 noted that, although anaesthetic-related mortality declined in the latter section of that time, the estimated risk of death associated with general anaesthesia between 1985 and 1990 was over 16 times that of regional anaesthesia.[75] Analysis of US obstetric malpractice claims shows general anaesthesia is more frequently associated with severe injuries and results in higher payments.

Maternal and fetal considerations and ultimately patient preference will determine the type of anaesthetic used for elective CS and indications and contraindications to regional anaesthesia have been considered. Nevertheless, epidural and spinal anaesthesia are the foundation of modern obstetric anaesthesia for CS and in many major centres up to 95% of all CS are conducted under regional block. In the UK in the early 1990s, only 50% were so conducted, emphasising the importance of continuing to document and promote this approach.[76] The maternal and fetal benefits of regional anaesthesia for CS extend beyond safety. In conjunction with documentation of these advantages and improvements in the quality of intraoperative conditions, both anaesthetic and community attitudes and expectations are changing and refusal of awake CS is uncommon. Common patient fears include pain during surgery and subsequent back pain, fear of needle placement and of seeing or hearing during surgery. Discussion and education can allay anxiety and psychological preparation for this unique experience is critical. Regional anaesthesia permits active participation in childbirth and early infant bonding, while accompanied by a partner or a support person, with most parturients finding the experience more satisfying than delivery under general anaesthesia. Average blood loss during surgery is less, neonatal resuscitation less likely to be required, high-quality postoperative pain relief available, and maternal postoperative morbidity reduced (Box 4.2).[76]

Patient preparation includes a fasting period for solids of at least six hours and prophylaxis against acid aspiration. Regimens vary, the pharmacological armamentarium including histamine$_2$-receptor antagonists (for example, ranitidine 150 mg orally in two doses six hours apart and at least one hour before surgery), non-particulate antacid (for example, 0.3 molar sodium citrate 30 ml) given no more than 30 minutes before surgery; and prokinetic drugs such as metoclopramide 10 mg intravenously (although mainly for its antiemetic effect and increase in lower oesophageal sphincter tone). The respiratory effects of regional anaesthesia are consistent with a restrictive ventilatory defect, including reduction in peak expiratory flow, forced vital capacity and forced expiratory volume in one second. These changes are of insufficient magnitude to lower maternal arterial oxygen ten-

---

Box 4.2   Benefits of regional anaesthesia for the parturient

Safety
- Lower maternal mortality
- Reduced postoperative morbidity
- Less neonatal resuscitation

Maternal satisfaction
- Awake, alert mother accompanied by a support person
- Immediate maternal bonding with infant
- Earlier establishment of breastfeeding
- High-quality postoperative intraspinal opioid analgesia
- Better early postoperative recovery

---

sion. Oxygen via a face mask (8 l/min) or nasal prongs (4 l/min) is routinely given, despite it being difficult to document any clinical improvement in outcome for the healthy, term fetus. Profound bilateral surgical anaesthesia and prevention of hypotension (discussed in the section on hypotension on p 160) are the keys to a satisfactory outcome for both mother and baby.

Local anaesthesia and nerve block

Local infiltration, with or without abdominal nerve block, is a technique reserved for exceptionally rare situations in developed countries. Few data are available.[77] Indications might include failed intubation where regional block is also impossible or contraindicated (severe juvenile rheumatoid arthritis, severe uncorrected kyphoscoliosis, spinal muscular atrophy). The skin, subcutaneous tissue, muscle, and posterior rectus sheath are infiltrated in turn as the abdomen is opened, the line of the uterine incision infiltrated, and solution injected intraperitoneally. Large volumes of LA are necessary (60–100 ml), mandating the use of dilute solutions such as 0.5% prilocaine or lignocaine with adrenaline. Bilateral block of the ilioinguinal nerves using 5–10 ml of 0.25–0.5% bupivacaine is an additional strategy that reduces postoperative analgesic requirement. Nevertheless, even with planning and gentle handling of tissues, intraoperative pain remains likely and when available, alternative techniques are preferred.

Epidural anaesthesia

Technique

In the UK and Australasia and to a lesser extent in North America and Europe, epidural anaesthesia has been the favoured method for elective CS. Although the epidural may be placed with the patient in either the lateral or sitting position, most prefer the latter in the obese parturient when bony landmarks cannot be palpated. Potential benefits of injecting LA through the epidural needle (minor complications appear similar with 16 and 18 gauge needles) before threading a catheter include better spread of solution and block reliability (although study results are inconsistent) and fewer venous cannulations and paraesthesiae. Bolus injection through the needle does not produce surgical anaesthesia more rapidly than an incremental approach, however, and is arguably less safe with respect to serious LA toxicity or total spinal block and results in more frequent haemodynamic events requiring intervention. In many countries there is no suitable test dose to detect both subarachnoid and intravenous placement and many drugs and techniques (for example, air with Doppler monitoring) have been evaluated. The routine use of test doses remains controversial and the concept of "every dose is a test dose" with selective use of specific drugs, having a thorough understanding of their limitations and risks, is commended.

Test dosing is only one of several useful measures for preventing or detecting aberrant catheter placement;[78] 15–25 ml of LA administered slowly, in divided doses, through a lumbar epidural catheter with the patient in the left lateral position results in bilateral spread and minimises the risk of aortocaval compression.

Epidural solutions

Several LA solutions are appropriate. Plain lignocaine should be avoided because of unsatisfactory block and greater risk of accumulative LA toxicity. Lignocaine 1.5–2% with adrenaline 1:200 000 is a good choice, conferring a moderately rapid onset (sensory block to T4 in 10–20 minutes). Both onset and quality are improved by alkalinisation or warming of LA to 38°C and by administration in the lateral position; 3% 2-chloroprocaine works more rapidly but has disadvantages such as postoperative back pain and antagonism of epidural opioid analgesia. Bupivacaine 0.5% has a slow onset of about 30 minutes. Ropivacaine 7.5 mg/ml may prove a safer alternative to bupivacaine in situations where avoidance of adrenaline is advisable (for example, severe pre-eclampsia or maternal cardiac disease). The addition of an epidural opioid such as fentanyl 50 μg is highly recommended. This significantly reduces the risk of intraoperative pain and nausea, without significant maternal or fetal effects.[79,80]

Management

Fewer than one in 200 elective epidural blocks prove inadequate after surgery is commenced and maternal pain during surgery occurs in less than 10%.[51] Nevertheless, all patients should be forewarned of this possibility and complaints of intraoperative pain heeded and managed. The upper and lower levels of the block must be tested and documented before the start of surgery. If loss of light touch extends above T5, intraoperative pain is very unlikely, even if intraspinal opioid is omitted;[81] motor block of the abdominal muscles and lower limbs and vasodilated, warm, dry feet should also be indicative. Initial evaluation of intraoperative pain during awake CS requires checking of the pain intensity and the level of anaesthesia, exclusion of surgical or epidural complications and, when possible, determination of aetiology.[79,80] Pain may result from inadequate anaesthesia (upper or lower sensory level inadequate or block asymmetric or patchy), visceral input (peritoneal pain mediated by the greater splanchnic nerve may occasionally require T1 block and large nerve roots such as L5 and S1 may remain incompletely blocked), subcostal or referred shoulder tip pain (from subdiaphragmatic fluid, mediated by the phrenic nerve C3–5), or precordial pain (often of uncertain origin but rarely associated with venous air emboli, gastric reflux or myocardial ischaemia). Visceral pain is reduced by preoperative epidural opioid and lignocaine alkalinisation and is less likely if the uterus is not exteriorised by the obstetrician. It may be amenable to supplemental analgesia with intravenous opioid, inhaled nitrous oxide, local wound ufiltration or intravenous ketamine (5 mg boluses to a maximum of 20 mg), although maternal sedation, respiratory depression, and amnesia are potential consequences. If these measures do not adequately control pain, conversion to general anaesthesia should be considered.

The most common maternal side-effects during regional anaesthesia for CS are nausea and shivering, discussed later under "Immediate complications". Maternal blood pressure must be checked immediately, as nausea (with or without sweating, pallor, vomiting, and signs of cerebral hypoperfusion) is often the first indication of hypotension and responds rapidly to vasopressor therapy.

Spinal anaesthesia

Advantages and disadvantages

During pregnancy, drug requirements for spinal anaesthesia are reduced by about 30% from early in the first trimester, probably because of hormonal effects on neuronal sensitivity. Spinal anaesthesia or a combined approach (CSE) performed in a low lumbar interspace below the termination of the spinal cord (usually L2) has increased in popularity compared with epidural

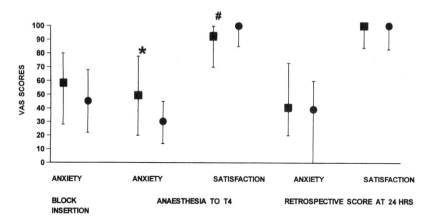

Fig 4.3   Maternal anxiety and satisfaction with epidural or spinal (combined spinal-epidural) anaesthesia for caesarean section. Visual analogue scores (VAS): 0 = not anxious or completely dissatisfied and 100 = as anxious as imaginable or completely satisfied. Values represent median and interquartile range for anxiety or satisfaction at the time of commencing anaesthesia, on establishment of anaesthesia, and for an overall intraoperative rating performed 24 h postpartum. Squares represent epidural anaesthesia and circles represent combined spinal-epidural anaesthesia. * P = 0.01, # P = 0.04, both epidural anaesthesia versus combined spinal-epidural anaesthesia, Wilcoxon ranked sum test (from Davies SJ et al.[82] with permission)

techniques. Advantages of spinal anaesthesia include a faster onset (except compared with epidural chloroprocaine), reliability, improved intraoperative conditions, reduced postoperative sequelae, and some minor maternal advantages for elective CS.[82-85] Indirect costs are reduced due to a shorter stay in the operating unit. Shivering is less common and severe and maternal presurgical anxiety reduced (possibly because of the rapid onset of dense block). Furthermore, the risk of LA toxicity is almost eliminated.

Potential disadvantages include an increased likelihood of fall in cardiac output after preloading alone, and thus higher ephedrine requirements to maintain circulatory stability, and PDPH. PDPH has been dramatically reduced by the introduction of small-gauge non-cutting spinal needles. Pencil-point needles of 24 gauge or less are associated with an incidence of severe headache of less than 1%, a rate comparable with that following epidural accidental dural puncture.

Technique and solutions

Patient variables such as height and weight have little influence on the spread of solution and although there is some correlation with body mass index, interindividual variability is too great to allow clinical dose adjustment. Techniques involving patient positioning in both the lateral and sitting positions should be mastered, because the latter may be useful in obesity or scoliosis and the former in parturients needing urgent delivery for footling breech or cord prolapse where upright positioning is inadvisable.

Surgical anaesthesia to T5 is obtained within 5–15 minutes with bupivacaine 10–15 mg (using hyperbaric 0.5% or 0.75% bupivacaine in 8.25% dextrose). Hyperbaric lignocaine 5% (60–80 mg) is disadvantaged by short duration (45–60 minutes), less predictable distribution and concerns over transient radicular irritation (see below "Regional anaesthesia for retained placenta"). Hyperbaric bupivacaine is recommended because of its reliable spread to the midthoracic level and appropriate duration of action. Isobaric plain 0.5% bupivacaine compares favourably with hyperbaric bupivacaine, although may occasionally produce unexpectedly high block, especially when injected in the sitting position, due to slight hypobaricity in cerebrospinal fluid at body temperature. Injection of hyperbaric solutions in the right (versus left) lateral position produces a more uniform block, after repositioning to left pelvic tilt. The incidence of intraoperative visceral pain is dose related and lower (at similar sensory block level) when larger LA doses have been administered. When injected while sitting, 10 mg of hyperbaric bupivacaine produces less satisfactory results than 12.5 mg, while 12 mg in the lateral position (followed by turning to supine with left uterine displacement) is reliable in achieving bilateral spread and results in fewer cervical blocks than 15 mg. Satisfactory anaesthesia is also obtained with high volume 0.125% and 0.25% plain bupivacaine in appropriate dose.

To reduce the incidence of high blocks and maintain cardiovascular stability, the "Oxford" has been developed.[86] Here, the mother is placed in the full left lateral position with an inflatable bag under her shoulder and three pillows under her head. Following spinal injection she is turned to the full right lateral and only placed in the wedged supine position immediately before surgery.

Although good conditions are usually achieved with bupivacaine alone, the addition of subarachnoid fentanyl 6.25–15 µg or sufentanil 2.5 µg reduces the risk of maternal intraoperative nausea or pain and improves early postoperative analgesia. Studies conflict as to whether morphine acts rapidly enough to improve intraoperative analgesia and the combination of fentanyl and morphine is popular. Intrathecal diamorphine 300 µg both improves intraoperative conditions and decreases postoperative opioid requirements. Although the addition of opioid or adrenaline alters the baricity of the solution, the clinical impact is unimportant. Spinal anaesthesia regresses more rapidly than epidural and a variety of options for postoperative analgesia are available.

Combined spinal-epidural anaesthesia

Combined spinal-epidural anaesthesia for CS was described by Brownridge in 1981,[87] and, with the advent of new equipment and refinement of techniques, has become a popular approach for elective CS in many units. It combines the advantages of spinal anaesthesia for surgery with the flexibility afforded by epidural catheterisation.[85] The technique is more reliable than epidural block alone, with minimal risk of perioperative conversion to general anaesthesia due to inadequate anaesthesia.

After conventional spinal anaesthesia, the epidural catheter is employed if required to extend anaesthesia cephalad, but principally dosed for postoperative pain relief. Either epidural saline or LA 10 ml injected within 10 minutes of the spinal causes a significant rise in the sensory level by a volume effect, although after that the effect of LA is greater.[88] A less commonly used approach is to establish low spinal block (for example, with 5 mg hyperbaric 0.5% bupivacaine) and to achieve surgical anaesthesia by incremental epidural dosing. This has the advantage of better haemodynamic stability, fewer adverse effects, and faster recovery at the expense of a longer preparation time for surgery. Failure to identify cerebrospinal fluid occurs in about 4–5% of cases and identification of subarachnoid placement is more rapid if the patient is sitting. In up to 10% of patients undergoing combined spinal-epidural anaesthesia a small amount of cerebrospinal fluid is visible in the epidural needle hub, following backflow along the spinal needle, and should not be interpreted as evidence of accidental dural puncture.

The single intervertebral segment needle-through-needle technique is the most popular approach. Compared to a double-space technique (inserting the epidural catheter first), it is faster and less painful and only disadvantaged in that epidural catheter position testing may be unreliable until postoperative regression of the block and in that a limited block may result if the catheter proves difficult to insert. Large series attest to the safety of CSE and concerns such as catheter penetration through the dural hole and transfer of epidural solution to the subarachnoid space rarely present as clinical events.[85]

Continuous spinal anaesthesia

While the efficacy compares favourably with alternatives, continuous spinal anaesthesia (using small incremental boluses of LA via a subarachnoid catheter), like spinal analgesia, is reserved for special situations in obstetrics because of both PDPH (especially when epidural equipment is used) and a higher incidence of neurological complications.[73,89] Despite the withdrawal of purpose-designed spinal microcatheters in many countries in the late 1980s, some 27 and 28 gauge subarachnoid catheters are again available and may be very useful in patients in whom conventional epidural or spinal techniques are unsuitable or inappropriate. Examples include parturients with severe musculoskeletal deformities of the lower spine (for example, untreated idiopathic scoliosis, Klippel–Feil syndrome, previous laminectomy or rod instrumentation) where epidural or spinal insertion is impossible, of high risk or unreliable. Haemodynamic stability is better than single-dose spinal anaesthesia, although technical problems and maldistribution of LA result in a failure rate of 5–10%. Continuous spinal analgesia in labouring parturients can also be readily converted to anaesthesia for instrumental delivery, CS or postpartum surgical procedures using incremental doses of hyperbaric or isobaric bupivacaine 5–10 mg.

Regional anaesthesia for emergency caesarean section

Overview

For non-elective surgery the factor of greatest relevance from an anaesthetic perspective is the urgency of delivery, which may range from immediate to many hours. In the absence of contraindications to regional anaesthesia, the time available may determine which method is used. Every effort should be made to avoid general anaesthesia, because it is in this setting that maternal morbidity and mortality are greatest. In addition, with urgent CS, fetal outcome is more likely to improve under regional anaesthesia compared with general anaesthesia. A better classification is urgent (non-life threatening maternal or fetal compromise) or emergency (life-threatening to mother or fetus). In each individual case the anaesthetist should communicate with the obstetrician to ascertain the current maternal and fetal condition, to determine if therapy to improve fetal condition before surgery is being instituted (for example, tocolytic drugs to stop uterine activity), and to obtain an exact timeframe for delivery (see Chapter 7). The American College and the Royal College of Obstetricians and Gynaecologists recommend that delivery should occur within 30 minutes of making the decision to perform CS for fetal distress.

Choice of technique

Although maternal factors (for example, uncontrolled antepartum haemorrhage or severe pre-eclampsia) are sometimes relevant, it is frequently the degree of urgency of delivery, the expertise of the anaesthetist, and the quality and expeditious use of available resources, personnel, and facilities that determine which method of anaesthesia is chosen. In a series of 360 consecutive emergency CS, 70% involved parturients with effective epidural analgesia who were safely extended to anaesthesia.[90] Ideally, the epidural catheter should have been tested and bilateral block obtained, because dosing a catheter which has been unsatisfactory for epidural analgesia in labour due to unilateral or asymmetric block may lead to delays and eventual general anaesthesia. Concern has been expressed with respect to combined spinal-epidural analgesia in parturients at high risk of CS, in whom the epidural catheter has not yet been tested, but a recent prospective series indicates that there is no greater likelihood of failure of epidural anaesthesia.[91]

Surgical anaesthesia can be readily achieved within five minutes with alkalinised 1.5% lignocaine with adrenaline (25 ml over two minutes)[92] or within 12 minutes, irrespective of the level of the established block, with 2% lignocaine with adrenaline 1:200 000 (20 ml over four minutes).[93] The addition of sodium bicarbonate 8.4% (1 ml per 10 ml of lignocaine with adrenaline) increases the non-ionised proportion of LA, thus hastening the onset and increasing the degree of motor block. 3% chloroprocaine, available in North America, is an attractive LA in this setting, featuring a rapid onset of action and low toxicity risk because of an elimination half-life of less than a minute secondary to plasma pseudocholinesterase metabolism. Previous concern about neurotoxicity appears to have been eliminated following reformulation of the preparation but postpartum backache and antagonism of epidural opioid analgesia remain problems.

Times to convert epidural analgesia to anaesthesia are similar to those required to provide general anaesthesia,[90] so only infrequently (for example, severe fetal distress or bleeding from vasa praevia where fetal demise is imminent) should it be impossible to use regional anaesthesia with sufficient expediency. In the above-mentioned survey, fetal distress was the indication for emergency CS in 38% of cases and in only 13% was this unheralded.[90] This emphasises the importance of early anaesthetic involvement and the use of epidural analgesia in labour for high-risk parturients (for example, pre-eclampsia, intrauterine growth retardation, oligohydramnios, meconium liquor, malpresentation or dystocia).

The rapid onset of spinal anaesthesia is ideal if epidural analgesia is assessed as inadequate or no epidural catheter is in place. A single-shot spinal in the lateral position in the operating room with immediate positioning in supine left tilt allows delivery to be affected within 10 minutes of arrival. Caution must be exercised when using spinal anaesthesia after failed epidurals, as high or total spinal block has been reported after normal doses (see "Immediate complications – local anaesthetic: total spinal").

Regional anaesthesia for retained placenta

Central neuraxis block from T7 to S5 produces excellent intraoperative conditions for removal of retained placental tissue.[94] For similar maternal reasons to those discussed above when considering CS, regional anaesthesia is preferable to general anaesthesia, providing intra- and postpartum blood loss has not been excessive and blood volume has been restored after obstetric haemorrhage. The case for regional block is even stronger now that effective tocolysis to assist with extraction of the placenta can be rapidly and safely obtained by the incremental administration of intravenous glyceryl trinitrate (50–100 µg boluses repeated minutely to a maximum 500 µg).

Epidural analgesia may be extended as for instrumental delivery or established *de novo*. It has been argued that bacteraemia represents a relative contraindication to regional blocks and that spinal anaesthesia should not be used if bacteraemia is suspected or the patient pyrexial. This argument would preclude spinal anaesthesia in all parturients, because bacteraemia after normal delivery is unpredictable (incidence 3.6–7.2%) and the incidence rises to 85% with manipulation of the uterus. The situation is analogous to that of chorioamnionitis during labour. In the absence of severe pyrexia or evidence of systemic sepsis and particularly if antibiotic therapy has commenced, the advantages of regional anaesthesia appear to outweigh the risks.

For removal of retained placenta, spinal anaesthesia may be provided using 10 mg hyperbaric bupivacaine to which 10 µg fentanyl may be added. For both placental evacuation and instrumental delivery, the short duration of intrathecal hyperbaric lignocaine 40–60 mg is appealing. However, the clinical use of 5% hyperbaric lignocaine remains controversial, despite evidence that the incidence of pain and dysaesthesia (transient radicular irritation) is much lower in the obstetric population. In addition, this agent may be less predictable in its distribution. In one of the few studies evaluating its obstetric use, worrisome high blocks occurred in four of 30 parturients and a total spinal block has resulted from only 50 mg.[95] In the surgical population, lower concentrations of lignocaine have been advocated. However, when 80 mg of 2% hypobaric and 5% hyperbaric lignocaine were compared for postpartum tubal ligation, the former proved inadequate, despite similar dermatomal distribution.[96]

Postoperative analgesia after regional anaesthesia

Many methods of analgesia can be employed after regional block for CS but intraspinal opioid analgesia has several advantages over systemic techniques. Although both spinal and epidural opioids are widely used, few comparative data are available. With spinal anaesthesia, a multimodal approach using subarachnoid morphine, bupivacaine wound infiltration, and oral paracetamol gives better analgesia than intravenous patient-controlled morphine followed by oral paracetomol and codeine, while not decreasing bowel motility to the same degree. Epidural boluses of morphine may be used, although side-effects are common. I prefer PCEA, as it combines the quality of epidural opioids with the flexibility of patient-controlled delivery.

Adjuncts or alternatives to regional analgesia

Wound infiltration and nerve blocks

Regional techniques involving wound infiltration or nerve block are clearly appropriate after general anaesthesia and are particularly useful in association with regional blocks if a postoperative epidural or intraspinal opioid management service is unavailable. The rationale for infiltration of LA into wounds is sound, but the results of clinical trials disappointing. After CS, subcutaneous wound infiltration alone is of no benefit, although repeated injection of 0.25% bupivacaine beneath the rectus sheath via a multiholed catheter or drainage tube after spinal anaesthesia reduces morphine requirements by 25% and both nausea and early sedation. Abdominal field block by subcutaneous infiltration covering T10–L1 bilaterally, plus bilateral rectus sheath block (deposition of LA after penetrating the anterior rectus sheath), are reported to be more effective than intramuscular opioid after general anaesthesia, but have not been adequately evaluated. A Pfannenstiel incision is innervated by the ilioinguinal and iliohypogastric nerves and in open studies bilateral blocks with 10 ml 0.25–0.5% bupivacaine reduce opioid requirement and possibly early postoperative pain after general anaesthesia. However, in association with spinal anaesthesia, a well-performed trial found no benefit from these blocks whether performed before or after CS.[97]

Non-steroidal anti-inflammatory drugs (NSAIDs)

Rectal, parenteral, and oral NSAIDs are now very popular for post-CS analgesia, mainly as adjuncts to intraspinal opioids. Although intramuscu-

147

lar ketorolac 30 mg produces analgesia equivalent to pethidine 75 mg, as a sole agent the quality of analgesia is unsatisfactory. NSAIDs have a dose-sparing effect on parenteral opioid and may reduce uterine contraction pain in the early postpartum period, but without significant improvement in overall pain scores. Epidural morphine 3–5 mg produces good analgesia in 70–85% of patients, but the addition of NSAIDs to 3 mg optimises both efficacy and the side-effect profile. The regular perioperative administration of indomethacin with subarachnoid morphine 250–300 µg reduces pain with movement on the first postoperative day and increases the median duration of effect from nine to 40 hours. Rectal diclofenac or paracetamol also significantly, but more modestly, increase subarachnoid opioid duration, for example from a mean of 14 to 19 hours after morphine 200 µg.[98] Parenteral diclofenac may reduce the minimum effective dose of subarachnoid morphine.

NSAID-induced inhibition of uterine activity does not increase postpartum bleeding and NSAIDs are contraindicated in only a small proportion of the obstetric population (history of peptic ulceration or gastrointestinal haemorrhage, aspirin-induced asthma, renal disease, and severe pre-eclampsia). NSAIDs are safe during lactation and breastfeeding, although drugs such as diclofenac, naproxen, ibuprofen, and ketorolac have a better side-effect profile than indomethacin, which occasionally causes headache and uncommonly depression, psychosis, and hallucinations.

Patient-controlled intravenous analgesia (PCIA)

PCIA is a popular technique after general anaesthesia, but is also used in some centres after regional block as the principal method or to supplement subarachnoid morphine. PCIA is more effective than intramuscular opioid and produces fewer side-effects than intraspinal morphine, although pain relief is less satisfactory and bowel function impaired. Compared with intermittent epidural diamorphine, PCIA with diamorphine causes more sedation but similar pain relief and higher satisfaction.[99] Studies vary when describing satisfaction from PCIA compared to intermittent epidural morphine. A comparison of intravenous with epidural routes using patient-controlled delivery with pethidine demonstrated that the latter produced significant dose sparing, better analgesia at rest and with movement, less sedation, and was preferred by over 90% of patients.

Fentanyl PCIA necessitates frequent supplementation or readjustment of variables. Efficacy during movement is reported to be better with morphine than pethidine PCIA but sedation and itch are greater. Morphine is the preferred opioid for PCIA because it avoids potential norpethidine toxicity, especially in those with renal dysfunction in the postpartum period, and it has no neonatal effects in breastfed infants (pethidine is associated with subtle changes in tone, alertness, and sucking on the third postoperative day).

Subarachnoid analgesia

Although subarachnoid fentanyl added to spinal bupivacaine improves intraoperative conditions and early postoperative analgesia, its duration is too short to be clinically useful. Diamorphine is a lipophilic opioid of rapid onset, which also reduces intraoperative supplementation and produces dose-dependent analgesia for up to six hours. Side-effects are also dose dependent, so although subarachnoid doses of 0.25–0.375 mg are safe, many patients require antiemetics and almost all experience mild pruritus.[100]

Morphine has been widely used since the early 1980s to provide prolonged postoperative analgesia after single-shot spinal block. Studies conflict as to whether it reduces intraoperative pain (which probably reflects its slow onset over 45–60 minutes) and thus whether subarachnoid fentanyl should also be added. Doses used in the 1980s (0.5–20 mg) are now known to be excessive and are associated with an unacceptable risk of delayed severe respiratory depression. Based on pharmacokinetic studies quantifying the proportion of epidural opioid transferred to the cerebrospinal fluid, "mini-dose" intrathecal morphine (200–250 µg) became popular in North America for post-CS analgesia. Large prospective series confirm its efficacy and an acceptable incidence of clinically detectable mild respiratory changes (approximately 1%).[101] Recent dose-finding studies suggest a ceiling analgesic effect, or optimum efficacy to side-effect profile, with 100–150 µg.[102] The majority of patients get prolonged analgesia but the time to first request for further analgesia is very variable, ranging from an average of nine to 28 hours. Thus, some patients require no other analgesics for over 24 hours, yet up to 20% request supplementation within 6–8 hours and 30–40% by 12 hours. Some units then provide supplementary PCIA (in one study 13% of patients used more than 40 mg of intravenous morphine in 24 hours),[103] while others offer NSAIDs, paracetamol, opioid or other suppository or oral analgesia and parenteral opioid if necessary. Side-effects, although dose dependent, are prominent after intraspinal morphine and both their frequency and severity may necessitate numerous staff interventions.

Two new spinal analgesics, the α_2-adrenergic agonist clonidine,[104] and the anticholinergic drug neostigmine, are safe to use in obstetrics. As a sole analgesic after CS conducted under general anaesthesia, subarachnoid clonidine 300–450 µg produces analgesia, which begins within five minutes, peaks at 20 minutes and lasts 9–14 hours. Despite central activity leading to a reduction in sympathetic activity, relative haemodynamic stability results from the direct peripheral vasopressor effect of high circulating levels of systemic clonidine. Sedation is the major side-effect, with many patients being undesirably drowsy from 30 minutes to eight hours after injection. Hypotension may also occur. Thus, while intrathecal clonidine alone appears unsuitable because of its side-effects, dose reduction through combination with opioid warrants investigation. Intrathecal neostigmine inhibits the metabolism of spinally released acetylcholine and its analgesic effects are potentiated by systemic opioid. Onset of action is 30–60 minutes and doses of 10, 30, and 100 µg do not change fetal heart rate, uterine contractility or Apgar scores, but are associated with an unacceptable incidence of nausea and vomiting. Unfortunately, recent work suggests 10 µg is not potent enough to reduce intravenous morphine requirements.

Epidural analgesia (bolus or infusion)

Epidural opioids provide excellent postoperative analgesia. The lipophilic opioids are characterised by rapid onset but brief duration so are less than ideal for intermittent bolus administration. Epidural sufentanil 20–30 µg, with or without adrenaline, is associated with a maximum duration of 3–5 hours, a high incidence of mild pruritus (up to 80%) and frequent drowsiness, which may interfere with maternal-infant bonding. Epidural fentanyl 100–200 µg is of even shorter duration. Epidural pethidine 50 mg is more effective than 100 mg intramuscularly and is preferred to intramuscular pethidine and epidural bupivacaine. It has an excellent side-effect profile (mild or moderate pruritus in 15%) and the optimum bolus of 25 mg relieves pain within 10–25 minutes but lasts only 2–3 hours. Epidural diamorphine (2.5–5 mg) is only available in the UK, takes effect in 10–30 minutes but provides a significantly longer duration of action, with 80% of patients having more than 6–8 hours of effective analgesia. Drowsiness and respiratory depression are infrequent and although pruritus is common (40–65%), it is mild and rarely requires treatment. In the USA, hydromorphone 0.6–1 mg provides a mean duration of 13–19 hours but up to 50% of patients request treatment for pruritus and nausea is common. It confers no advantage over morphine. Methadone, buprenorphine, and butorphanol have also been evaluated. Lipophilic opioids should be administered diluted to at least 5–10 ml in normal saline, because this increases onset and duration.

The alternative method of delivery is continuous infusion. Although combinations of opioid and LA are highly effective, the addition of LA does not appear to improve analgesia and introduces problems including impairment of ambulation (from lower limb motor or sensory loss) and heel pressure blisters. In clinical practice, epidural infusions are not popular after CS with either patients (dislike of intrusive infusion devices) or staff (labour intensive).

Epidural morphine is popular in North America. Extensive clinical experience supports its safe use on general wards, providing staff training, observational clinical monitoring by nursing staff, and management protocols are observed.[105] Neonatal transfer via breast milk is negligible after total doses up to 10 mg over 48 hours. The onset of analgesia is slow (peak effect 45–90 minutes), so initial administration should pre-empt the onset of pain. A blinded comparison of epidural morphine 3 mg and subarachnoid morphine 200 µg found that the epidural dose produced marginally better analgesia which was more likely to last 24 hours, at the expense of more nausea and pruritus. Although about 10% of women do not require any other postoperative analgesia after a single dose of epidural morphine,[105] variability is similar to subarachnoid morphine, with times to further analgesia of 6–26 hours. This reflects both pharmacokinetic and pharmacodynamic variability, in addition to trial methodological and population differences. Recent dose-response data indicate the minimum effective dose is 2.5 mg, with a ceiling effect above 3.75 mg, which is consistent with a potency ratio of intrathecal to epidural morphine of about 40:1. Comparative studies show better analgesia after epidural compared with parenteral morphine, at the expense of more side-effects, which may impinge on patient satisfaction.

Bothersome side-effects (see "Immediate complications – opioids" later) are the major disadvantage of intraspinal morphine analgesia and in the dose range up to 3.75 mg, do not appear to be dose related. Pruritus occurs in 60–90% and after a 3 mg dose, one-third of patients consider this an important problem. Nausea occurs in 20–40% and reactivation of herpes simplex labialis has been reported.

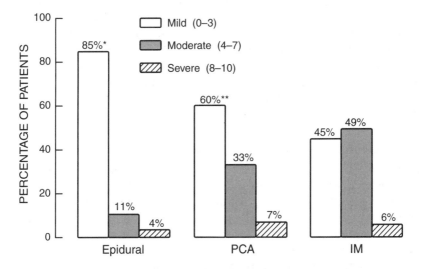

Fig 4.4 Epidural narcotic and patient-controlled analgesia for post-caesarean section pain relief. The percentage of patients in each group reporting mild (VAS 0–3), moderate (VAS 4–7) or severe (VAS 8–10) pain during the 24 h study period. * P <0.05 denotes epidural versus PCA and IM. ** P = NS denotes PCA versus IM (from Harrison DM, Sinatra R, Morgese L, Chung JH. *Anesthesiology* 1988;**68**:455, with permission)

Table 4.2   Subarachnoid and epidural opioid bolus for perioperative regional anaesthesia and analgesia

Drug	Preoperative dose		Postoperative epidural dose	Onset	Duration
	Spinal	Epidural			
Fentanyl	6.25–15 μg	25–100 μg	100–200 μg	5–10 min	1–3 h
Sufentanil	2.5 μg	–	20–30 μg	5–10 min	3–5 h
Diamorphine	0.25 mg	–	2.5–5 mg	5–20 min	6–8 h
Pethidine	–	–	25–50 mg	5–20 min	2–4 h
Morphine	100–200 μg	–	3–4 mg	45–75 min	6–24 h
Clonidine	75–300 μg	75–150 μg	150–600 μg	10–30 min	2–10 h

Epidural clonidine 75 μg administered before CS has no effect on maternal and fetal haemodynamics, but large postdelivery doses (400 μg) are of short duration (4–6 hours). A dose of 150 μg combined with subarachnoid morphine 250 μg increases the mean duration of morphine slightly and fewer patients require additional analgesia, but some nevertheless need supplementary opioids. Epidural clonidine is probably best suited to continuous infusion or PCEA and an infusion rate of 10–20 μg/h reduces supplemental PCIA morphine. When clonidine or adrenaline are added to sufentanil in postoperative PCEA system, each is equally effective in reducing sufentanil use. Unfortunately, although epidural clonidine is effective, particular as an adjunct to intraspinal opioid, its clinical utility is limited by potentiation of motor and sensory LA block (which may delay recovery room discharge) and unwanted sedation, which may be profound in the first few hours after bolus administration.[104] Although hypotension requiring treatment is very infrequent, a small study using Holter monitoring identified cardiac arrhythmias in two of 30 healthy patients given a 150 μg epidural bolus and the future of intraspinal clonidine in this setting remains uncertain.

Epidural analgesia (patient controlled)

PCEA is an attractive alternative approach to single or repeated staff-administered epidural boluses. It is ideal after regional block for CS because patients are generally healthy, well motivated and desire good pain relief, without bothersome side-effects or encumbrance of mobility, in order to optimise mother-infant interaction. PCEA significantly reduces drug consumption and sedation when compared to PCIA.[106] An open randomised trial demonstrated improved outcome and shorter postoperative stay with PCEA compared with PCIA after CS and when compared to a single bolus of epidural morphine, fentanyl or pethidine, PCEA causes fewer side-effects. Although many opioids can be used, morphine and hydromorphone have a slow onset and frequent side-effects, sufentanil is expensive and produces more light-headedness, nausea and pruritus than fentanyl, and diamorphine, apart from a relatively high incidence of pruritus, appears suitable but has not been evaluated. With the caveat that possible effects on the breastfed infant have not been investigated, pethidine PCEA using a patient demand bolus technique (5 mg/ml, 4–5 ml bolus of 20–25 mg, 20–30-minute lockout) is recommended. The addition of a background infusion increases drug usage without any analgesic benefit. With PCEA pethidine, median pain scores during coughing are 20 or less (0–100 scale), patient satisfaction high, and mean drug consumption 15–17 mg/h.[106] Three comparative studies of fentanyl versus pethidine, some with crossover design, show that pethidine has fewer side-effects (pruritus in 7% and nausea requiring antiemetic treatment over 48 hours less than 10%) and is preferred by patients. The addition of LA confers no benefit and apart from a small dose-sparing effect, neither clonidine nor adrenaline offers any significant advantages.

Large prospective series confirm the safety of postoperative PCEA in surgical patients and epidural pethidine has an exceptional clinical safety record that is supported by recent prospective audit.[51] Pump selection is critical and ambulatory style or disposable purpose-designed devices are essential. Although it is unlikely there are patient benefits with respect to surgical outcome, and cost analysis compared to alternative analgesic approaches has not been performed, pethidine PCEA after CS provides excellent analgesia without the need for intervention, supplementation, and treatment of side-effects.

Immediate complications of local anaesthetic

Total spinal block

Features and prevention

The classic symptoms of total spinal block, namely rapidly ascending sensory change, paralysis, apnoea, hypotension, and unconsciousness, are well recognised and the principles of resuscitation, based on airway, breathing, and circulation, familiar to all anaesthetists.[107,108] Avoidance of aortocaval compression and early protection of the airway to avoid aspiration must not be forgotten. Circulatory support with vasopressor therapy is likely and maternal and fetal monitoring should be intensive. High blocks which compromise swallowing, phonation, and respiration are less dramatic but can be difficult to distinguish from epidural or subdural block and may also require intervention to prevent aspiration or hypoxia. The consequences of accidental subarachnoid injection of LA are partly dose dependent and bupivacaine 12.5–15 mg, even in a high volume of diluent, is unlikely to produce adverse clinical effects, although a "total spinal" has been reported after only 15 mg. Medical and nursing staff should be aware that symptomatology may arise immediately, over minutes or occasionally very late (for example, 30 minutes postinjection with a change of patient position). A good prognosis follows early resuscitation, ventilation, and circulatory support, accompanied by anaesthesia or sedation until block regression to safe levels (usually 1–3 hours). One unit found urgent intubation was necessary in one in 5000 obstetric epidural blocks,[51] and maternal death due to substandard management of total spinal block is now very uncommon. Nevertheless, after no such deaths in the Confidential Enquiries between 1985 and 1993, the sole maternal death directly attributable to anaesthesia in the 1994–96 Report followed a combined spinal-epidural anaesthetic.

While sensitivity appears low, epidural catheter aspiration looking for cerebrospinal fluid is a simple preventive measure. A variety of tests to distinguish CSF from saline or LA have been suggested, including temperature, glucose, pH and protein tests, and the thiopentone precipitation test (acidic LA precipitates in alkaline thiopentone up to a dilution of 1 in 4). The appropriateness of a test dose remains controversial and in many case reports a false-negative test dose is described. The ideal test dose would have high sensitivity and specificity for both subarachnoid and intravenous injection but not cause high block. No single agent meets these criteria and an understanding of the value and limitations of various agents is essential. To detect subarachnoid injection, lignocaine 50 mg and bupivacaine 10 mg appear reasonably safe, but spinal block may not be evident for several minutes and sensory loss in sacral dermatomes is a more specific test than degree of lower limb strength. A sensation of warmth occurs earlier than after epidural injection, but may pass unnoticed. When accidental subarachnoid injection is recognised immediately, aspiration of at least 20–30 ml of LA-contaminated cerebrospinal fluid may recover up to 50% of the drug, although the feasibility and effectiveness of this manoeuvre are unknown. As opioids are also often administered, opioid-induced respiratory depression may contribute to hypoventilation and early administration of intravenous naloxone is advisable.

Clinical situations requiring caution

Life-threatening high block may be due to excessive and unpredictable spread of spinal anaesthesia, accidental subarachnoid injection of epidural solution, subarachnoid injection in a previously normally functioning epidural catheter or deliberate spinal anaesthesia after failed epidural block.[108] Total spinal block may occur unexpectedly despite failure to aspirate cerebrospinal fluid, a negative test dose, and a previously normal epidural response. Other mechanisms include failure to recognise initial subarachnoid or subdural catheter placement (with subsequent disruption of the arachnoid mater permitting entry of solution into the subarachnoid space), and multicompartment location of a multiholed catheter (with differential flow favouring the distal orifice with more forceful injection).

Anatomical studies suggest that penetration of the intact dura and arachnoid by a correctly placed epidural catheter is very unlikely in the absence of a dural tear by the needle.

After accidental dural puncture, subdural or subarachnoid drug passage from a resited epidural catheter can be demonstrated, with the size of the dural hole an important determinant of the proportion transferred. One option is to resite a catheter above the level of the dural puncture and to allow anaesthetic staff only to administer all drug doses cautiously and incrementally, looking for abnormal or high spread. Alarmingly, one series reports three total spinal blocks associated with 31 resited catheters dosed with three-quarters of the usual dose during labour.[109] Other larger series have failed to reproduce these figures. On the basis of better control and safety, however, deliberate subarachnoid placement or retention of the epidural catheter for continuous spinal analgesia or anaesthesia is a valuable alternative. Nevertheless, up to 30% of accidental dural punctures go unrecognised initially and these cases continue to pose a significant risk of subsequent high block.[110]

High block is also a concern where spinal anaesthesia for urgent CS is initiated several hours after accidental dural puncture and abandoned epidural analgesia in labour. This may be due to a relatively depleted cerebrospinal fluid volume and compression of the lumbar intrathecal sac, making a normal spinal dose a relative overdose. In addition, since 1989, a series of high or total spinal blocks have been described after deliberate spinal anaesthesia for CS in the situation where epidural analgesia was not, or could not be, converted to epidural anaesthesia. The mechanism appears to be principally a mass effect, with cephalad displacement of cerebrospinal fluid from a lumbar sac compressed by an epidural space containing large volumes of epidural fluid. As this event may not be uncommon but is unpredictable, some consider spinal anaesthesia contraindicated, although no excessively high blocks occurred in a series of 61 epidurals converted to spinal anaesthesia.[111] Whenever possible, epidural analgesia should be topped up and if it proves difficult to extend the block cephalad, rapid T4 block is often achieved with no or minimal addition of LA by siting a second, low thoracic, epidural catheter. Alternatively, a CSE technique with a reduced dose of hyperbaric bupivacaine (5–7.5 mg) and careful attention to patient positioning should increase safety, while permitting rapid extension if necessary by injection of epidural solution. Single-shot SA with 10–12.5 mg of bupivacaine remains safe, provided meticulous attention is paid to patient positioning to accentuate the thoracic curve (by elevation of the upper thorax, shoulders, and head in the "Oxford" position), thus restricting spread of hyperbaric solution beyond the midthoracic segments. General anaesthesia (with awake intubation) can then be reserved for the rare setting of an absolute contraindication to regional block in a patient with evidence of a potentially difficult airway.

Subdural block

Anatomy and diagnosis

The subdural space is said to contain a minute quantity of serous fluid and to lie between the dura mater and the arachnoid mater, although this anatomical description has been challenged and an interarachnoid space described. The subdural space is present throughout the spinal meninges and, unlike the epidural space, also extends intracranially. Deliberate subdural entry is difficult, although techniques for cervical injection and endoscopic examination have been described and a 7% incidence of inadvertent injection of contrast occurs during myelography. One pain clinic series reported an incidence of subdural injection of almost 1%, based on clinical diagnosis. Accidental subdural catheterisation and injection (either delayed or at the time of insertion) often involves obstetric patients and since the first documented case report in 1975, has become well recognised, although the incidence remains uncertain. Based on clinical diagnosis, it varies from almost 1% (chronic pain patients) to one in 1400 in the obstetric population.[51]

Subdural injection is often inferred from the clinical features, but atypical presentations and multicompartment blocks with multiholed catheters create confusion and ideally the diagnosis should be supported by epidurogram or other imaging.[112] A radiographic "railroad track" appearance after injection of contrast medium is typical, but a mixed picture with amorphous and lateral intervertebral spread within the epidural space is common, although it may not be possible to reliably discern the extra-arachnoid location of contrast. Identification of catheter location will permit patient counselling and advice about the risk of future recurrence.

Clinical features

A variety of potential consequences arise.[107,108] Subdural entry is usually indistinguishable from uneventful epidural location, although occasionally prominent backflow of solution or immediate headache (possibly from intrathecal sac compression and transmitted pressure) is noted. Subdural LA typically blocks nerve function with a similar latency to epidural injection and recovery rate is similar, but spread is greater than expected for the volume administered. The duration of subdural opioids may be prolonged. Common features of subdural block are high cephalad extension with volumes of only 2–10 ml (frequently involving cervical or cranial nerves, including trigeminal nerve block and Horner's syndrome) and markedly asymmetric or patchy distribution, with sacral sparing. Hypotension tends to be moderate and motor block variable in density. These characteristics are attributed to the wider subdural space around the dorsal nerve roots, favouring pooling in this area. Interesting atypical presentations have included limitation of cephalad extension and complete absence of lower limb motor block, despite excellent sensory anaesthesia for CS.

Subdural block thus shows a spectrum of clinical presentations, from early or delayed high sensory block with minimal systemic disturbance through to immediate life-threatening apnoea and hypotension. Ventilation and intubation may be required if consciousness, respiration or swallowing is impaired. Although successful continuous postoperative analgesia and anaesthesia for surgery have been described, catheter removal is more prudent, because of the risks of subsequent arachnoid rupture leading to total spinal anaesthesia.

Intravenous injection

Background and prevention

During pregnancy the engorgement of the epidural venous plexus and relatively low venous pressure (and hence tendency to collapse) predispose to an increased risk of venous catheterisation (incidence 3–20%, reduced if at least 10 ml of normal saline is injected before placement or if soft, flexible-tipped catheters are used) and more false-negative aspirations. LA toxicity (seizures, respiratory and cardiac arrest), usually after unintentional intravascular bupivacaine injection, has caused several maternal mortalities in North America and Australasia. Occasional deaths are still reported, although an apparent decline in the incidence of serious toxicity[75] has been attributed to greater awareness and better prevention of accidental intravenous injection (routine catheter aspiration, test doses, slow injection, incremental dosing, and the reduction of therapeutic doses for epidural analgesia in labour).[78] Other reasons may be the decline of single-shot epidural and caudal injection through a misplaced needle, the increasing use of spinal techniques and the greater safety margin of LAs such as lignocaine with adrenaline, chloroprocaine, and the single enantiomers. In older obstetric audits, convulsions occurred in one in 500–1500 epidural blocks, whereas a recent prospective series documented no cases in almost 11 000.[51] Caudal anaesthesia, albeit rarely used today, is a high-risk procedure, possibly because of the vascularity and tendency of veins to collapse with aspiration. In general surgical patients at a tertiary centre, the incidence of convulsions was one in 100, which contrasted markedly with one in 9000 for lumbar epidural techniques.[113]

Prevention of intravascular injection underpins safe practice. Although the sensitivity of an aspiration test for blood with uniport catheters is only about 70%, it appears to be close to 100% with multihole catheters. This test is easy and harmless and should be routine practice. The value of incremental test dosing has not been substantiated in prospective series and it may also fail to detect about 25% of intravascular catheters but is nevertheless recommended on the basis of reduced peak drug levels from slower injection times and potential detection of toxicity before serious events. Case reports suggest convulsions are unlikely when individual boluses are restricted to bupivacaine 20–25 mg or lignocaine 100 mg. All intravenous test doses have limitations. Air 1–2 ml has the highest specificity and sensitivity but is limited by the requirement for Doppler monitoring. LA alone is unreliable and risky and although almost all labouring women are able to distinguish intravenous from epidural fentanyl 100 μg, side-effects are common. Of various vasoactive drugs, the most popular and readily available is adrenaline but its efficacy, safety, and value are debatable. Pregnancy reduces sensitivity to chronotropes and vasopressors and labour pain and epidural injection produce tachycardia, which creates confusion and alters the positive heart rate response criteria for intravenous adrenaline. Intravascular adrenaline may provoke a hypertensive crisis in pre-eclamptic parturients and can significantly reduce uterine blood flow, which might compromise the sick fetus.[78]

Ropivacaine and levo-bupivacaine (the S-enantiomer) have greater safety margins than bupivacaine and appear safer should serious toxicity arise. These drugs may prove to be therapeutic advances as alternatives to racemic bupivacaine for epidural anaesthesia. Prevention of LA toxicity thus requires sound selection of technique, drug and drug dose, awareness of modifying influences including patient factors, pathophysiological disturbances and concurrent drug therapy, good technical skills and vigilance, and the thoughtful application of several strategies, rather than a single panacea. Although one centre using routine test dosing in labouring parturients reported a convulsion rate of one in 170,[114] this contrasts with our unit where intravenous test doses are not routine, yet no seizures have occurred in 10 995 prospectively audited obstetric epidural blocks.[51]

Features and management

The pathophysiology of central nervous system and cardiac LA toxicity has been reviewed.[115] Staff must recognise signs and symptoms of toxicity, particularly early central nervous system effects such as tinnitus, visual disturbance, oral and perioral tingling and numbness, metallic taste, drowsiness, and slurring of speech. Unfortunately, symptoms are unreliable, in that they may be masked by sedative drugs or be absent prior to the sudden onset of convulsions or cardiac arrest. All obstetric medical and nursing staff should be capable of managing serious toxicity, based on principles such as summoning of help, clearing the airway, ventilation with 100% oxygen, monitoring and support of the circulation (including early intubation and hyperventilation, uterine displacement, ECG monitoring and treatment of ventricular arrhythmias). Termination of convulsions with intravenous benzodiazepines or thiopentone followed by suxamethonium and intubation may be necessary (although most stop spontaneously) and the welfare of the fetus must be considered.[116]

Hypotension

Blood pressure changes and aortocaval compression

In healthy parturients, modest blood pressure (BP) reduction is anticipated with sympatholysis, although the magnitude varies with factors such as the circulating blood volume, vascular tone and the compensatory responses, patient position, speed of onset and extent of block, and drug interactions. Large falls in BP may reflect reduction in cardiac output and possible reduction of vital organ perfusion. Reduced uteroplacental flow may manifest as fetal heart rate and acid-base changes and reduced maternal cerebral flow as nausea, dizziness or syncope.

In the supine position in late pregnancy, partial or complete inferior vena caval compression and aortic occlusion near its bifurcation is likely in about 90% of parturients and prevention of aortocaval compression is pivotal to the safe management of regional blocks. The full left lateral or left lateral tilt position should be assumed until surgery commences, after which uterine displacement is achieved by either table tilt or wedging under the right hip and buttock. Occasionally, manual left uterine displacement or (despite the inferior vena cava's right midline anatomical position) right uterine tilt is more effective in reducing caval compression.

Perfusion pressure and vascular resistance (in both uterine arteries and the intervillous space) determine uteroplacental flow. Perfusion is stabilised by maintaining maternal cardiac output and various strategies can be employed to counteract the effects of sympathectomy and peripheral venous pooling associated with regional anaesthesia. Aortocaval compression may occur in the presence of normal arm BP measurement and impairment of maternofetal gas exchange not be apparent until signs of fetal acidaemia or hypoxia manifest (see above "Regional anaesthesia for caesarean section: fetal outcome").

Hypotension is the most common immediate complication of regional anaesthesia, although because definitions vary, comparisons between techniques, drugs, and management policies are problematic. Measurement variability is also a pitfall, with diastolic BP readings from automated devices about 10 mmHg lower than phase 4 Korotkoff sounds and even greater disparity in pre-eclampsia. Auscultated readings after epidural analgesia in parturients lying on their side yield falsely low results unless taken from the dependent arm. Clinically, maintenance of BP within 20% of baseline appears a reasonable target. Decreases of 20–30% from baseline or systolic BP of less than 90–100 mmHg are well tolerated by healthy women but because placental flow is perfusion pressure dependent and not autoregulated and adverse events are late features of underperfusion, these values serve as markers for intervention.

159

Hypotension associated with regional anaesthesia for caesarean section

Pathophysiology

Hypotension associated with regional anaesthesia for CS is more likely in elective surgery than in labouring parturients. After spinal anaesthesia, blood pressure falls more rapidly, usually within 3–10 minutes, and the 10° head-down position does not reduce the incidence. Ambulation before induction of regional block may reduce hypotension, as may injection in the lateral rather than the sitting position, though the latter may depend on sitting prior to recumbency. Bradycardia is uncommon (2%), but associated nausea frequent (up to one-third of patients). With epidural anaesthesia, absorbed LA potentially depresses vascular tone and myocardial function, but if sympathectomy occurs slowly, compensatory modification of cardiovacular effects limits haemodynamic change. Nevertheless, even if aortocaval compression is minimised, without vasopressor therapy, 60–85% of patients become hypotensive when receiving regional anaesthesia.

Intravenous fluid preloading

Previously considered mandatory, intravenous fluid preloading with crystalloid appears of only minor benefit and its preventive role is in doubt.[117] Because of rapid extracellular redistribution, crystalloid increases blood volume by only about 20% of volume administered and after the infusion of more than 3 l the incidence of mild or moderate hypotension is still 75%. Atrial natriuretic peptide levels rise in response to fluid loading and subsequent vasodilation may even be counterproductive. Aggressive rapid volume loading also significantly increases central venous pressure, reduces colloid osmotic pressure and haematocrit. This may be hazardous in parturients with cardiac disease or severe pre-eclampsia. In an urgent setting, spinal anaesthesia should not be delayed to permit preloading.

The maximum benefit is achieved with a crystalloid volume of about 10 ml/kg. Dextrose-containing fluid should be avoided because maternal hyperglycaemia and hyperinsulinaemia predispose to subsequent neonatal hypoglycaemia. Some studies (for example, comparing 500 ml hydroxyethyl starch with 1 litre of lactated Ringer's solution) suggest colloid, which has a longer intravascular half-life and more effectively expands blood volume, is more effective. Others show no advantage and disadvantages include cost and occasional anaphylactoid reactions.

Vasopressors

Several approaches to the prevention and management of hypotension are possible. The legs should not be in a dependent position although leg wrapping to prevent venous pooling is neither consistently useful nor popular.

Vasopressors are widely used and prophylactic administration is more effective than preloading,[118] although they should not be used alone as this may result in fetal acidosis. When accompanied by frequent monitoring, modest crystalloid preloading and prophylactic intravenous ephedrine (10 mg initially and a titrated infusion of, for example, 30 mg in 500 ml of crystalloid) reduce nausea and the incidence of hypotension during spinal anaesthesia for CS to 20–30%. Patients may respond to further vasopressor therapy, with ephedrine (5–10 mg IV) usually the drug of choice, because its predominantly β- and mild α-sympathomimetic action does not increase uterine artery resistance. Although animal work shows that direct α-sympathomimetics are more likely to increase vascular resistance and reduce uteroplacental flow, clinical studies indicate that small titrated doses are also safe. Phenylephrine (50–100 µg IV) slightly increases uterine artery resistance (as estimated by Doppler flow velocimetry), without significant clinical effect on the healthy fetus. This drug is useful in patients unresponsive to ephedrine or in whom the inotropic or chronotropic effects of ephedrine may be detrimental (for example, severe valvular stenosis or hypertrophic obstructive cardiomyopathy).

Hypotension associated with regional analgesia in labour

Hypotension may occur after regional analgesia secondary to LA-induced sympathectomy, reduction in sympathetic and catecholamine activity, and possibly from opioid-induced effects on sympathetic tone. The incidence depends on parturient factors (for example, the state of maternal hydration or coexisting disease), the technique and drugs used. In general, both epidural and CSE analgesia produce similar decreases in BP and clinically significant hypotension occurs in about 5%. Both continuous infusions and PCEA provide better haemodynamic stability than intermittent top-ups. The self-administration of small doses of epidural solution using PCEA appears safer in parturients who are upright compared with lying in the lateral position.

The routine use of intravenous fluid preloading is also controversial in this setting. A randomised study, which found a significant reduction in hypotension and fetal heart rate abnormalities after 1 l crystalloid did not show adequate protection against aortocaval compression. A 500 ml crystalloid bolus has no impact on haemodynamic changes after epidural analgesia, and 1 l is no more effective than 500 ml.[119] Routine infusion of 1 l of fluid reduces the frequency of uterine contractions[27] and omission of intravenous fluid before subarachnoid fentanyl has no haemodynamic sequelae when compared with administration of 500 ml of crystalloid. On the basis of this tocolytic effect of preloading, the danger of maternal overhydration during labour, the low frequency of hypotension and the ease of treatment with vasopressor, routine preloading in this setting is not recommended.

161

Motor block

Motor block associated with regional anaesthesia and analgesia

Motor block is an inevitable consequence of conventional epidural and spinal anaesthesia. Spinal anaesthesia produces more profound block[82] and subarachnoid hyperbaric bupivacaine has a longer postoperative duration before full regression compared with epidural lignocaine, though not bupivacaine. Some postoperative patients find this period of immobility an inconvenience, but loss of strength in the lower limbs and abdominal musculature is mainly an issue in the setting of regional analgesia in labour.

The intensity of motor block depends on factors such as LA dose and the duration (and possibly nature) of neural exposure. Comparative studies of epidural bupivacaine 0.25 and 0.5% (20–50 mg) show that lower limb weakness is greater with higher doses of LA, but following several boluses motor block is similar and a minimum of impaired hip flexion is almost universal. After an initial dose of 15 ml bupivacaine 0.04% (6 mg) with adrenaline and fentanyl, 17% have impaired hip flexion weakness and the addition of epidural adrenaline increases the intensity of motor block.[120]

An appropriate selection of epidural solutions is essential if lower limb and abdominal muscle weakness are to be minimised. When equianalgesic solutions are used for continuous infusion, bupivacaine 0.0625% and opioid for up to 10 hours leaves 70% of parturients with full lower limb strength, compared with less than 10% of those who receive 0.125% bupivacaine.[121] With a PCEA, the odds ratio for motor block versus no detectable block is 3.3 (95% CI 1.7–6.6) for bupivacaine 0.25% compared with bupivacaine 0.0625%, fentanyl, and adrenaline.

Motor block tends to increase with increasing duration of epidural analgesia, and its intensity may be less if nerve fibres have periods of partial recovery. Bupivacaine 0.125% infused at about 15 mg/h results in demonstrable lower limb weakness in at least 20% of parturients after a couple of hours but this is halved, despite similar analgesia, when opioid plus bupivacaine 0.0625% is infused (at less than 10 mg/h). With continuous infusion, the frequency and intensity of clinically detectable weakness increase with time. In contrast, PCEA with bupivacaine 0.0625% and opioid is associated with an unchanged or diminishing incidence of dense block after the first few hours.

Effects of motor block in labour

Increasing severity of motor block is associated with a reduction in spontaneous deliveries. Intermittent epidural boluses of 0.5% bupivacaine increase the number of instrumental deliveries when compared with 0.25% bupivacaine. Further reduction in bupivacaine concentration (by the addition of opioid) reduces the need for intervention.[63] Continuous epidural infusion using plain local anaesthetic produces low spontaneous delivery rates, but reduction in bupivacaine concentration below 0.125% has not significantly decreased the number of instrumental deliveries.[121]

Dense motor block precludes ambulation (see below) and reduces maternal satisfaction with regional techniques. Most women do not wish to ambulate freely once in established labour but avoiding motor block is nevertheless important. In a comparison of bupivacaine 0.25% and a bupivacaine-fentanyl mixture which reduced the delivered LA dose and leg weakness, parturients receiving the latter solution reported less unpleasant sensory and motor block and higher satisfaction scores.[122] In one recent survey, over 40% of parturients receiving epidural analgesia strongly agreed or agreed with the statement "Being able to move easily and possibly walk during labour was important to me".[123]

Reports that increased motor block is associated with more long-term backache after delivery are unfounded (see Chapter 8).

Ambulation during regional analgesia

The potential for full weight bearing and ambulation is best achieved with combined spinal-epidural analgesia, using initial subarachnoid opioid, alone or combined with bupivacaine. Although about 90% of parturients receiving spinal opioid combined with bupivacaine 2.5 mg have no demonstrable motor block,[69] even more have normal power, assessed clinically, after equally effective doses of 1–1.5 mg. Although 70% of parturients are ambulant during low-dose continuous infusion with bupivacaine 0.04%, opioid and adrenaline,[120] a PCEA technique after subarachnoid analgesia is arguably the optimum approach to ambulatory analgesia in labour.[66] During self-administration of bupivacaine 0.0625%, opioid and adrenaline, up to 80% of women are able to walk and the safety of small demand boluses, in terms of lack of postural hypotension, has been demonstrated.

The issue of safe ambulation in labour is not fully resolved, although recent investigation suggests that effects on proprioception are LA dose dependent and not clinically significant after spinal analgesia and low-dose epidural techniques.[124] Thus, provided a policy is in place to evaluate leg strength, check for postural hypotension and supervise initial weight bearing and ambulation, I believe testing proprioceptive function or the ability to perform a deep knee-bend is unnecessary. Extensive clinical experience in several units with thousands of parturients indicates "walking epidurals" are safe and falls are extremely unlikely.

Although potential benefits of ambulation in labour, such as reduction in labour duration and fetal heart rate abnormalities and higher rates of spontaneous delivery, have not been confirmed by recent potential clinical trials, many parturients prefer to have this option.

163

Shivering and temperature regulation

Shivering

Maternal shivering increases oxygen consumption, interferes with monitoring and has been described by consumers as the most annoying aspect of regional anaesthesia for CS. The aetiology is multifactorial. Anxiety contributes, as some patients shiver before establishing the block and, unless preventive measures are taken, hypothermia may develop from infusion of intravenous fluid at room temperature, inadequate surface covering, skin and body cavity exposure and blood loss during surgery. Maternal thermoregulatory shivering or shaking is also a physiological effect of epidural analgesia and anaesthesia. During labour, epidurals appear to increase the risk of shivering from about 10–20% to 20–50% of parturients and without preventive measures at epidural anaesthesia for CS, shivering is seen in 60–100%.

During regional blocks, the loss of sympathetically mediated skin and peripheral vasoconstriction may result in heat loss but a more important factor is the redistribution of heat from the central core to the periphery, which results in a rapid fall in core temperature. Thus surface prewarming or forced-air warming during CS, both of which increase skin temperature and reduce the redistribution of heat from the central compartment, are effective in preventing shivering.[125] During spinal anaesthesia for CS, core temperature falls, but in contrast to epidural anaesthesia where shivering severity increases, shivering declines compared to before the block.[82] This suggests that a more rapid increase in skin temperature is more effective in blunting the hypothermic response. Although experimental evidence exists for thermosensitive epidural tissues, warming of epidural solutions alone is of modest benefit, possible reducing the severity of shivering. Opioids alter the response of the hypothalamic thermoregulatory centre to changes in body temperature and are effective in prevention and treatment. Epidural fentanyl 25 μg or more, especially if combined with other measures, reduces the proportion of parturients who shiver after epidural analgesia with bupivacaine for either labour or CS by up to two-thirds, from about 75% to 25–35%.[126] Epidural pethidine 25 mg and sufentanil 25 μg also act within 10–15 minutes, although recurrent shivering may occur. If treatment is desired, intravenous pethidine 50 mg is effective within two minutes but increases sedation and may be undesirable on fetal grounds. Clonidine (30 μg IV as required) is equally effective, stopping shivering in 75% of cases and reducing its severity in the remainder.[127]

Maternal hyperthermia

In contrast to shivering and hypothermia associated with, in particular, epidural anaesthesia for CS, labour epidural analgesia with LA alone is associated with maternal temperature rise, usually beginning after at least five hours.

The average rise is 1°C over 7–10 hours duration, although the speed of labour may influence the time course and only about 5% of parturients reach 38°. The site of measurement, environmental factors and shivering also influence the incidence, time course, and degree of maternal hyperthermia. Maternal temperature and fetal tachycardia show a mild correlation.

No causal relationship between epidural analgesia and maternal hyperthermia has been established and studies have been flawed by their retrospective nature or failure to control for rupture of membranes or other confounders. Speculative theories for why epidurals may play a causal role are mainly based on an imbalance of heat loss and production, including thermoregulatory resetting.[128] The addition of opioid to LA may prevent temperature rise and recent prospective series suggest low-dose bupivacaine-fentanyl epidurals have little or no effect on maternal temperature. An association with neonatal fever has also not been established, but as uterine temperature is higher than oral and fetal heat is dissipated through the placental circulation, maternal hyperthermia has the potential to cause deleterious fetal effects and may lead to intervention on the basis of suspected maternal or neonatal infection.

Although more investigation is necessary, the mild maternal temperature rises which are sometimes seen in parturients receiving epidurals in labour may be unrelated to the block and do not appear clinically important. Only severe maternal hyperthermia and fetal tachycardia warrant investigation, active reduction of temperature, and antibiotic therapy.

Immediate complications of opioids

Opioid receptor-mediated side-effects[129] are reversible with pure antagonists such as naloxone and oral naltrexone, which cross the placenta but do not cause neonatal morbidity. Pure antagonists may also diminish analgesia, which is better preserved by agonist-antagonists such as nalbuphine. Attempts to prevent side-effects with prophylactic administration of antagonists have had limited success and treatment is generally reserved for patients experiencing symptoms. Many drugs are of therapeutic value for specific side-effects.

Pruritus

Neurophysiology

The neurophysiology of pruritus (itch) is complex and only partly understood.[130] Substance P, an 11-amino acid neuropeptide, plays a role in the mediation of pruritus. Scratching, which relieves pruritus, stimulates large afferent fast-conducting A-fibres adjacent to those conducting pruritic sensation and, via inhibitory interneurons, also inhibits central C-fibres

165

involved in the conduction of pruritic stimuli. Pruritus may be a manifesta-
tion of opioid-mediated facilitation of protective reflexes, can be down-
modulated by the cerebral cortex and an opioid-sensitive scratch centre
may be present in the floor of the fourth ventricle. Drugs with inhibitory
action on the dorsal horn of the spinal cord may reduce pruritus. Systemic
mast cell release of histamine is not involved and a central enkephalinergic
mechanism for pruritus would account for localisation to areas such as the
nose and upper face which are supplied by the trigeminal nerve. The
trigeminal spinal nucleus is rich in opioid receptors and continuous with the
substantia gelatinosa and Lissauer tract at C3–4. A segmental distribution
of pruritus, spreading cephalad from the site of injection, fits with cerebrospinal fluid spread of opioid to the trigeminal area.

Management

Pruritus is a common, annoying side-effect that varies with the route of
opioid administration, occurring more frequently after intraspinal than parenteral injection. It is usually localised to the face, neck, and upper thorax
and is only partly dose related. Pregnancy appears to increase susceptibility,
possibly secondary to altered opioid receptor binding due to competition by
oestrogens, higher endogenous opioid levels and greater cephalad spread.
Morphine and sufentanil are more pruritogenic than fentanyl and diamorphine, with pethidine and the κ-agonist, μ-antagonist butorphanol the least.
Intraspinal morphine results in an incidence of pruritus of 60–90% (onset
usually at 1–2 hours and the peak severity 2–4 hours) and over 50% of
patients request treatment.[131]

Pretreatment with antagonists is not effective in preventing intraspinal
morphine-induced pruritus and treatment is difficult. Simple treatments
including physical therapies (cooling, vibration, and transcutaneous electrical nerve stimulation), antihistamines and sedative drugs such as droperidol
show poor efficacy and opioid antagonists are more effective.[131] Naloxone
has a short elimination half-life and requires repeated injection (0.1–0.2 mg
IV or IM hourly) or infusion (0.1 mg/h). The failure rate is at least 25% and
pain relief is reduced. Nalmephene (0.5 µg/kg IV), a new long-acting
methylated antagonist with an elimination half-life of over 10 hours,
reduces the severity of pruritus and is as effective as a naloxone bolus and
infusion regimen, cost-effective, but more emetogenic. The long-acting oral
antagonist naltrexone (3 mg) is more cost effective than IV naloxone infusion and a good alternative is nalbuphine (5–10 mg IV). This mixed antag-
onist-agonist, which reduces the severity of pruritus, is more effective than
naloxone and diphenhydramine, does not reverse analgesia, and only occasionally causes mild sedation.[131] Pretreatment with epidural buprenorphine
and IV nalbuphine 15 µg/kg/h are also effective remedies for epidural morphine pruritus.

Propofol, in subhypnotic doses (10–20 mg IV bolus, with or without infusion at 30 mg per 24 hours), relieves epidural morphine-induced pruritus in surgical patients but appears ineffective in obstetric patients receiving either subarachnoid morphine after CS or spinal pethidine postpartum.

Nausea and vomiting

Opioid-induced nausea and nausea during labour

Nausea and vomiting are common, partly dose-related symptoms induced by all intraspinal opioids, although being of multifactorial aetiology, their incidence and severity vary considerably with the clinical setting. Nausea may occur through either or both gastrointestinal mechanisms (delayed gastric emptying) or central effects (sensitisation of the vestibular system to motion and opioid interaction in the brainstem vomiting centre). After epidural opioid, rapid systemic absorption into the dilated azygous venous plexus may produce symptoms and after subarachnoid administration particularly, distribution within the cerebrospinal fluid by bulk flow, or subsequent CSF circulation, may lead to opioid activity in the area postrema. The central pharmacokinetics of morphine predisposes to a high incidence compared to lipophilic opioids, with symptom severity peaking 2–4 hours after administration.

In labour, nausea and vomiting are common irrespective of pain relief and occur secondary to gastrointestinal stasis, the physiological stimulus of intense pain and the effect of systemic opioid or nitrous oxide. Regional analgesia incorporating opioids does not appear to increase the risk, although this has not been investigated under controlled conditions. Surveys suggest parturients using epidurals (with or without opioid), nitrous oxide or intramuscular pethidine are equally likely to complain of nausea and vomiting and nausea is infrequent (1–2.4%) and mild (median scores less than 10 on a scale of 0–100) with both combined spinal-epidural and epidural analgesia. Drug selection is nevertheless important, as subarachnoid pethidine increases nausea and vomiting almost 10-fold compared with sufentanil.

Nausea associated with caesarean section

Nausea is the second most common complication of regional anaesthesia for CS (after hypotension) and is mulitfactorial in aetiology. Metoclopramide 10 mg IV preoperatively reduces intraoperative nausea. Postoperative nausea occurs in up to 50% of patients receiving epidural morphine and prophylaxis with ondansetron is more effective than with metoclopramide. The lipophilic epidural opioids are less emetogenic and pethidine has the best side-effect profile in obstetric populations. Although 30% of patients report nausea at some time, it is of very mild degree with median VAS scores of zero.[131] In a comparison of PCEA pethidine with epidural morphine, the 24-hour incidence of nausea was 16% (4% requiring treatment) compared with over 52% (24% treated) respectively. P6 acupoint acupressure is also effective after epidural morphine.

Urinary retention and bladder dysfunction

Urinary retention in labour

Urinary retention in labour and postoperatively is of multifactorial origin and influenced by both LAs and opioids. The former may block sacral sympathetic and parasympathetic activity, resulting in bladder detrusor and sphincter paralysis. After CS under epidural analgesia, almost 50% of patients experience acute urinary retention and thus urinary catheterisation, at least until resolution of anaesthesia, is routine practice. After vaginal delivery, urinary retention is also a relatively common complication (2–18%) and occurs more frequently in parturients who have received an epidural during labour. As applies with operative delivery, a causal relationship is possible (dense epidural analgesia results in hypotonic bladder detrusor activity) but without matching of risk factors and randomisation, outcome data are confounded by selection bias. Although a high residual urine volume is likely in parturients who have had instrumental delivery under epidural block, two ultrasonographic studies of residual bladder volumes on the first two postpartum days after vaginal delivery found the epidural had no significant influence. A prolonged second stage of labour was the only factor to increase the odds of urinary volumes exceeding 50 or 100 ml.

Postoperative urinary retention

Urinary retention in the postoperative period is more common after intraspinal than systemic opioid administration, is not dose related and involves opioid-modulated control of bladder function in the sacral spinal cord. Inhibition of parasympathetic activity leads to detrusor muscle relaxation, increase in bladder capacity and retention. After epidural morphine these effects last from 15 minutes to 16 hours and are naloxone reversible.[129]

Irrespective of the aetiology, clinical staff must be vigilant because a single episode of bladder overdistension can produce irreversible detrusor damage and long-term bladder dysfunction. Good labour and postnatal nursing care, including surveillance, avoidance of traumatic instrumental delivery and early catheterisation have been important changes which appear to have reduced the incidence of this childbirth complication.

Respiratory depression

Respiratory depression may occur after any intraspinal opioid and although there are associated risk factors such as respiratory disease and the concurrent use of sedative drugs, the pregnant woman belongs to a low-risk group of mainly healthy patients who may be protected by the respiratory stimulant effects of progesterone. Nevertheless, rare cases of severe depression occur and all staff need to be prepared.

Respiratory depression may present within minutes, from rapid cephalad spread to the brainstem or early systemic absorption into blood after injection of lipophilic opioids. Alternatively, it may develop slowly or be delayed by many hours, secondary to intrathecal morphine circulating in cerebrospinal fluid from the lumbar to the cervical region and ventral medulla. Nevertheless, with the benefit of a better understanding of spinal opioid pharmacokinetics, rationalisation of drug doses and extensive clinical experience, respiratory depression is no longer the feared life-threatening complication seen after the introduction of intraspinal opioids. Mild depression occurs no more frequently than with alternative routes of opioid administration.[132]

Respiratory depression in labour

Hypoxaemic episodes occur in healthy women experiencing painful labour, particularly if they are obese. Desaturation most commonly occurs between contractions, due to hypoventilation after pain-induced hyperventilation, and during apnoeic periods in the expulsion phase of labour. Such episodes are most effectively avoided with epidural analgesia and are exacerbated by depression from systemic opioids and sedatives. The addition of fentanyl (total dose 50–350 µg) to epidural bupivacaine infusion increases the incidence of desaturation.[133,134] However, when compared to both no analgesia and systemic pethidine plus nitrous oxide, epidural LA/opioid analgesia still results in a lower incidence of minor desaturation.[133] Fetal oxygenation may fall during hypoxaemia but because this is well tolerated, the clinical impact is variable and only likely to be of significance in the compromised fetus. Clinically significant maternal respiratory depression from intraspinal pethidine or fentanyl, administered in labour or perioperatively, is rare.[51] Recently, several cases of rapid depression (some within a minute) after subarachnoid sufentanil in labour have been reported, suggesting rapid cisternal drug spread. Thus, although the risk of such an event is estimated to occur in only approximately one in 5000 cases (and probably fewer for fentanyl and pethidine), preparation and close supervision are mandatory.[135]

Postoperative respiratory depression

Severe respiratory depression is rare in the absence of drug errors. Epidural pethidine does not cause depression in bolus doses of 50 mg or less and is even safer if used as PCEA. Demand bolus doses of 20–25 mg are unlikely to cause serious depression if accidentally injected intravenously or intrathecally. Delayed depression is described very rarely after single dose, repeat boluses or continuous infusion of lipophilic opioids.[132]

After CS, subarachnoid morphine in doses of 0.1–0.25 mg does not depress ventilatory response to carbon dioxide, which contrasts with the effects of epidural morphine 5 mg, sufentanil 50 µg, and fentanyl 200 µg. The peak effect on respiration after epidural morphine occurs at between six and 10 hours, which coincides with most reports of severe delayed depression. Epidural morphine 4–5 mg results in mild but clinically evident respiratory depression in about one in 250–300 post-CS patients.[105]

The detection of respiratory depression may be difficult. Ventilatory response to carbon dioxide is reduced and hypercarbia may be present in the absence of obvious clinical changes such as bradypnoea. The most reliable indicator of respiratory depression is somnolence or sedation and most hospitals base monitoring protocols on assessment of level of conscious state, respiratory pattern, and rate. A common approach is to monitor intermittently (hourly) for up to six hours after lipophilic opioids and up to 24 hours for morphine, although protocols vary and occasionally pulse oximetry may be useful.[129,132]

Gastrointestinal function

The gastrointestinal effects of spinal opioids in pregnancy are usually undesirable. Delayed gastric emptying, biliary colic and constipation may be unpleasant, delay oral drug absorption and increase the risk of gastric regurgitation and aspiration. Aspiration is a rare but important event which still occurs after epidural analgesia in labour and in association with epidural anaesthesia (Report on Confidential Enquiries into Maternal Death in the United Kingdom 1991–1993). Epidural opioids may produce a systemic drug effect on gastrointestinal tract receptors but predominately have central effects in the spinal cord or cerebroventricular area of the brain. Naloxone is capable of reversing these effects but at doses which antagonise analgesia. Doses of opioid antagonists which reduce opioid-induced pruritus do not reduce nausea after CS. Selectively antagonising the unwanted peripheral gastrointestinal effects of opioids may be possible in future using the investigational drug N-methyl naltrexone, a permanently charged competitive antagonist that cannot cross the blood–brain barrier.

In labour, intramuscular pethidine and systemic, epidural and subarachnoid fentanyl may all delay gastric emptying in a dose-related manner. Epidural analgesia with LA alone has no effect but epidural fentanyl 50–100 µg or diamorphine 5 mg and subarachnoid fentanyl 25 µg, significantly delay emptying as estimated by paracetamol absorption studies.[136] When epidural fentanyl is infused at 20–30 µg/h, no significant effect occurs until at least 100 µg has been administered.[137] Although these effects on the gastric emptying of liquids should be considered, the profound effect of labour in delaying the gastric emptying of solids is well documented and the effect of systemic opioid is greater than that of intraspinal opioid. The role of prophylactic drugs and preventive strategies in avoiding gastric aspiration remains paramount irrespective of the drugs used for regional blocks.

When abdominal surgery is conducted under regional anaesthesia, bowel contraction results due to unopposed parasympathetic activity, but in the postoperative phase opioid analgesia depresses smooth muscle activity and may contribute to ileus. Nevertheless, the return of bowel function is more rapid if postoperative epidural analgesia is compared with systemic opioid analgesia and after CS, irrespective of the effect of intraspinal opioids, oral intake can usually be resumed within 12–24 hours.

Reactivation of herpes simplex virus (HSV)

The use of intraspinal morphine in obstetric patients and young adults has been associated with the reactivation of HSV, typically 2–5 days later. Single case reports describe HSV recurrence after epidural fentanyl and subarachnoid pethidine but both appear to have been coincidental. Lesions occur in the same area as the primary infection, usually in a trigeminal nerve distribution (herpes labialis). Recrudescence in the postpartum period places nearby infants at risk of neonatal infection, which carries significant morbidity and mortality. The mechanism of reactivation proposed is multifactorial, involving cerebrospinal fluid morphine activation of opioid receptors in the trigeminal nucleus where virus resides in latent form, reactivation by itching in facial areas, depression of cell-mediated immunity, and altered hormonal levels associated with pregnancy.[138]

The incidence of reactivation is controversial. Patients given epidural morphine after CS have a 3.5–10% incidence, although a small study reported 35%. Large prospective studies support a figure of 9% compared to 1% or less in controls.[139] Reactivation also occurs after subarachnoid morphine, although the risk has not been quantified. In a study of 816 patients randomised to parenteral or epidural morphine and followed for five days with clinical and microbiological diagnosis, epidural morphine, adjusted for history of HSV, conferred a 11.5 times greater risk of recurrent herpes labialis and no association with pruritus was identified [139].

A report of recurrent HSV blepharitis suggests it would be advisable to seek a history of HSV infection before prescribing intraspinal morphine, because of the potentially harmful consequences of ophthalmic and central nervous system infection.

References

1 Writer WDR. Breech presentation and multiple pregnancy: obstetrical aspects and anaesthetic management. *Clin Anaesthesiol* 1986;4:305–20.
2 Rolbin SH, Tey SS, Ananthanarayan C. Anaesthesia for preterm labour and delivery. *Curr Opin Anesthesiol* 1992;5:360–5.
3 Crawford JS. A prospective study of 200 consecutive twin deliveries. *Anaesthesia* 1987;42:33–43.

4 van Zundert A, Vaes L, Soetens M, et al. Are breech deliveries an indication for lumbar epidural analgesia? *Anesth Analg* 1991;**72**:399–403.

5 Chadwick HS, Easterling T. Anesthetic concerns in the patient with pre-eclampsia. *Semin Perinatol* 1991;**15**:397–404.

6 Santos AC. Spinal anesthesia in severely pre-eclamptic women: when is it safe? *Anesthesiology* 1999;**90**:1252–4.

7 Fisher M McD, Bowey CJ. Alleged allergy to local anaesthetics. *Anaesth Intens Care* 1997;**25**:611–14.

8 Goodman EJ, deHorta E, Tagiuam JM. Safety of spinal and epidural anesthesia in parturients with chorioamnionitis. *Reg Anesth* 1996;**21**:436–41.

9 Chestnut DH, Dewan DM, Redick LF, Caton D, Spielman FJ. Anesthetic management for obstetric hysterectomy: a multi-institutional study. *Anesthesiology* 1989;**70**:607–10.

10 Scott DB, Hibbard BM. Serious non-fatal complications associated with extradural block in obstetric practice. *Br J Anaesth* 1990;**64**:537–41.

11 Scott DB, Tunstall ME. Serious complications associated with epidural/spinal blockade in obstetrics: a two-year prospective study. *Int J Obstet Anesth* 1995;**4**:133–9.

12 Sage DJ. Epidurals, spinals and bleeding disorders in pregnancy: a review. *Anaesth Intens Care* 1990;**18**:319–26.

13 Katz J. The experts opine. The use of regional anesthesia in patients taking drugs which might alter the coagulation system remains a controversial subject. *Surv Anesthesiol* 1990;**4**:420–7.

14 Orlikowski CE, Rocke DA. The coagulopathic parturient. Anesthetic management. *Anesthesiol Clin North Am* 1998;**16**(2):349–73.

15 Bogod DG. Respiratory and cardiac problems in the peripartum period. *Curr Opin Anesthesiol* 1990;**3**:408–12.

16 Brighouse D. Anaesthesia for Caesarean section in patients with aortic stenosis: the case for regional anaesthesia. *Anaesthesia* 1998;**53**:107–8.

17 Whitfield A, Holdcroft A. Anaesthesia for Caesarean section in patients with aortic stenosis: the case for general anaesthesia. *Anaesthesia* 1998;**53**:109–12.

18 Stoddart P, O'Sullivan G. Eisenmenger's Syndrome in pregnancy: a case report and review. *Int J Obstet Anesth* 1993;**2**:159–68.

19 Reynolds F (ed). The effects on the baby of maternal analgesia and anaesthesia. London: WB Saunders, 1993.

20 Kinsella SM, Spencer JAD. Maternal and fetal cardiovascular effects of epidural analgesia during labour. *Contemp Rev Obstet Gynaecol* 1995;**7**:145–50.

21 Jouppila P, Jouppila R, Hollmen AI, et al. Lumbar epidural analgesia to improve intervillous blood flow during labor in severe pre-eclampsia. *Obstet Gynecol* 1982;**59**:158–61.

22 Marx GF, Elstein DI, Schuss M, et al. Effects of epidural block with lignocaine and lignocaine adrenaline on umbilical artery velocity wave ratios. *Br J Obstet Gynaecol* 1990;**97**:517–20.

23 Roberts SW, Leveno KJ, Sidawi JE, Lucas MJ, Kelly MA. Fetal acidemia associated with regional anesthesia for elective cesarean delivery. *Obstet Gynecol* 1995;**85**:79–83.

24 Marx GF, Luykx WM, Cohen S. Fetal-neonatal status following Caesarean section for fetal distress. *Br J Anaesth* 1984;**56**:1009–13.

25 Hirose M, Hara Y, Hosokawa T, Tanaka Y. The effect of postoperative analgesia with continuous epidural bupivacaine after cesarean section on the amount of breast feeding and infant weight gain. *Anesth Analg* 1996;**82**:1166–9.

26 Abboud TK, Shiek-al-Eslam A, Yanagi T, et al. Safety and efficacy of epinephrine added to bupivacaine for lumbar epidural analgesia in obstetrics. *Anesth Analg* 1985;**64**:585–91.

27 Cheek TG, Samuels P, Miller F, Tobin M, Gutsche BB. Normal saline iv fluid load decreases uterine activity in active labour. *Br J Anaesth* 1996;**77**:632–5.

28 Miller AC. The effects of epidural analgesia on uterine activity and labor. *Int J Obstet Anesth* 1997;**6**:2–18.

29 Halpern SH, Leighton BL, Ohlsson A, Barrett JFR, Rice A. Effect of epidural vs parenteral opioid analgesia on the progress of labor. A meta-analysis. *JAMA* 1998;**280**:2105–10.

30 Gambling DR, Sharma SK, Ramin SM, et al. A randomized study of combined spinal-epidural analgesia versus intravenous meperidine during labor. Impact on Cesarean delivery rate. *Anesthesiology* 1998;**89**:1336–44.

31 Clark A, Carr D, Loyd G, Cook V, Spinnato J. The influence of epidural analgesia on cesarean delivery rates: a randomized prospective clinical trial. *Am J Obstet Gynecol* 1998;**179**:1527–33.

32 Saunders NJStG, Spily H, Gilbert L, *et al*. Oxytocin infusion during the second stage of labour in primiparous women using epidural analgesia: a randomised double blind placebo controlled trial. *BMJ* 1989;**299**:1423–6.

33 Floberg J, Belfrage P, Ohlsen H. Influence of the pelvic outlet capacity on fetal head presentation at delivery. *Acta Obstet Gynaecol Scand* 1987;**66**:127–30.

34 Chestnut DH. Epidural analgesia and the incidence of cesarean section. *Anesthesiology* 1997;**87**:472–6.

35 Phillips KC, Thomas TA. Second stage of labour with or without extradural analgesia. *Anaesthesia* 1983;**38**:972–6.

36 Chestnut DH, Laszewski LJ, Pollack KL, *et al*. Continuous epidural infusion of 0.0625% bupivacaine–0.0002% fentanyl during the second stage of labor. *Anesthesiology* 1990;**72**:613–18.

37 Thorp JA, Hu DH, Albin RM, *et al*. The effect of intrapartum epidural analgesia on nulliparous labor: a randomized, controlled, prospective trial. *Am J Obstet Gynecol* 1993;**169**:851–8.

38 Ramin SM, Gambling DR, Lucus MJ, *et al*. Randomized trial of epidural versus intravenous analgesia during labor. *Obstet Gynecol* 1995;**86**:783–9.

39 Sharma SK, Sidawi JE, Ramin SM, *et al*. Cesarean delivery: a randomized trial of epidural versus patient-controlled meperidine analgesia during labour. *Anesthesiology* 1998;**89**:1336–44.

40 Bailey PW, Howard FA. Epidural analgesia and forceps delivery: laying a bogey. *Anaesthesia* 1983;**38**:282–5.

41 Neuhoff D, Burke MS, Porreco RP. Cesarean birth for failed progress in labor. *Obstet Gynecol* 1989;**73**:915–20.

42 Goyert GL, Bottoms SF, Treadwell MC, Nehra PC. The physician factor in cesarean birth rates. *N Engl J Med* 1989;**320**:706–9.

43 Bush DJ. Consent for obstetric anaesthesia and analgesia. In: Russell IF, Lyons G, eds. *Clinical problems in obstetric anaesthesia*. London: Chapman & Hall, 1997.

44 Waisel DB, Truog RD. Informed consent. *Anesthesiology* 1997;**87**:968–78.

45 Scott WE. Ethics in obstetric anaesthesia. *Anaesthesia* 1996;**51**:717–18.

46 Lonsdale M, Hutchinson GL. Patients' desire for information about anaesthesia. *Anaesthesia* 1991;**46**:410–12.

47 Farnill D, Inglis S. Patients' desire for information about anaesthesia: Australian attitudes. *Anaesthesia* 1993;**48**:162–4.

48 Garden AL, Merry AF, Holland RL, Petrie KJ. Anaesthesia information – what patients want to know. *Anaesth Intens Care* 1996;**24**:594–8.

49 Pattee C, Ballantyne M, Milne B. Epidural analgesia for labour and delivery: informed consent issues. *Can J Anaesth* 1997;**44**:918–23.

50 Swan HD, Borshoff DC. Informed consent – recall of risk information following epidural analgesia in labour. *Anaesth Intens Care* 1994;**22**:139–41.

51 Paech MJ, Godkin R, Webster S. Complications of obstetric epidural analgesia and anaesthesia: a prospective analysis of 10 995 cases. *Int J Obstet Anesth* 1998;**7**:5–11

52 Reynolds F. Epidural analgesia in obstetrics. Pros and cons for mother and baby. *BMJ* 1989;**299**:751–2.

53 Chamberlain G, Wraight A, Steer P. *Pain and its relief in childbirth*. Report of the 1990 NBT Survey. Edinburgh: Churchill Livingstone, 1993.

54 Groves PA, Oriol NE. How useful is intrapartum electronic fetal heart rate monitoring? *Int J Obstet Anesth* 1995;**4**:161–7.

55 Yentis SM. Time to abandon loss of resistance to air. *Anaesthesia* 1997;**52**:184.

56 McNeill MJ, Thorburn J. Cannulation of the epidural space. A comparison of 18- and 16-gauge needles. *Anaesthesia* 1988;**43**:154–5.

57 Brownridge P. Epidural analgesia in the first stage of labour. *Curr Anaesth Crit Care* 1991;**2**:92–100.

58 Reynolds F. Does the left hand know what the right hand is doing? An appraisal of single enantiomer local anaesthetics. *Int J Obstet Anesth* 1997;**6**:257–69.

59 Writer WDR, Stienstra R, Eddleston JM, et al. Neonatal outcome and mode of delivery after epidural analgesia for labour with ropivacaine and bupivacaine: a prospective meta-analysis. Br J Anaesth 1998;81:713–17.

60 Capogna G, Celleno D, Fusco P. Relative potencies of bupivacaine and ropivacaine for analgesia in labour. Br J Anaesth 1999;82:371–3.

61 Polley LS, Columb MO, Naughton NN, et al. Relative potencies of ropivacaine and bupivacaine for epidural analgesia in labor. Anesthesiology 1999;90:944–50.

62 Breen TW. Optimal labour analgesia 1996. Can J Anaesth 1996;43:327–32.

63 Olofsson C, Ekblom A, Ekman-Ordeberg G, Irestedt L. Obstetric outcome following epidural analgesia with bupivacaine-adrenaline 0.25% or bupivacaine 0.125% with sufentanil – a prospective randomized controlled study in 1000 patients. Acta Anaesthesiol Scand 1998;42:284–92.

64 Lyons G, Coumb M, Hawthorne L, Dresner M. Extradural pain relief in labour: bupivacaine sparing by extradural fentanyl is dose dependent. Br J Anaesth 1997;78:493–7.

65 Mercier FJ, Benhamou D. Promising non-narcotic analgesic techniques for labour. Bailliere's Clin Obstet Gynaecol 1998;12:397–407.

66 Paech MJ. New techniques for labour analgesia. Patient-controlled epidural analgesia and combined spinal-epidural analgesia. Bailliere's Clin Obstet Gynaecol 1998;12:377–96.

67 Elton CD, Ali P, Mushambi MC. "Walking extradurals" in labour: a step forward? Br J Anaesth 1997;79:551–4.

68 Vercauteren M. Intrathecal labour analgesia: a critical approach. Int Monitor Reg Anesth 1998;10:3–7.

69 Collis RE, Baxandall ML, Srikantharajah ID, et al. Combined spinal epidural (CSE) analgesia: technique, management and outcome of 300 mothers. Int J Obstet Anesth 1994;3:75–81.

70 Campbell DC, Banner R, Crone LA, et al. Addition of epinephrine to intrathecal bupivacaine and sufentanil for ambulatory labor analgesia. Anesthesiology 1997;86:525–31.

71 Gautier PE, de Kock H, Fanard L, et al. Intrathecal clonidine combined with sufentanil for labor analgesia. Anesthesiology 1998;88:651–6.

72 Gamlin FMC, Lyons G. Spinal analgesia in labour. Int J Obstet Anesth 1997;6:161–72.

73 Arkoosh VA. Continuous spinal analgesia and anesthesia in obstetrics. Reg Anesth 1993;18:402–5.

74 Swartz J, Biehl DR. Paracervical and pudendal nerve block for obstetric analgesia. Clin Anaesthesiol 1986;4:125–33.

75 Hawkins JL, Koonin LM, Palmer SK, Gibbs CP. Anesthesia-related deaths during obstetric delivery in the United States, 1979–1990. Anesthesiology 1997;86:277–84.

76 Morgan B. The use of regional anaesthesia in Caesarean section. Contemp Rev Obstet Gynaecol 1995;7:206–9.

77 Cooper MG, Feeney EM, Joseph M, McGuiness JJ. Local anaesthetic infiltration for Caesarean section. Anaesth Intens Care 1989;17:198–201.

78 Mulroy MF, Norris MC, Liu SS. Safety steps for epidural injection of local anesthetics: review of the literature and recommendations. Anesth Analg 1997;85:1346–56.

79 Capogna G, Celleno D. Improving epidural anaesthesia during cesarean section: causes of maternal discomfort or pain during surgery. Int J Obstet Anesth 1994;3:149–52.

80 Lussos SA, Datta S. Anesthesia for cesarean delivery. Part II: Epidural anesthesia. Intrathecal and epidural opioids. Venous air embolism. Int J Obstet Anesth 1992;1:208–21.

81 Russell IF. Levels of anaesthesia and intraoperative pain at caesarean section under regional block. Int J Obstet Anesth 1995;4:71–7.

82 Davies SJ, Paech MJ, Welch H, Evans SF, Pavy TJG. Maternal experience during epidural or combined spinal-epidural anesthesia for cesarean section: a prospective, randomized trial. Anesth Analg 1997;85:607–13.

83 Lussos SA, Datta S. Anesthesia for cesarean delivery. Part I: General considerations and spinal anesthesia. Int J Obstet Anesth 1992;1:79–91.

84 Morgan P. Spinal anaesthesia in obstetrics. Can J Anaesth 1995;42:1145–63.

85 Rawal N, van Zundert A, Holmstrom B, Crowhurst JA. Combined spinal-epidural technique. Reg Anesth 1997;22:406–23.

86 Carrie LES. Spinal and/or epidural blockade for Caesarean section. In: Reynolds F, ed. Epidural and spinal blockade in obstetrics. London: Baillière Tindall, 1990.

87 Brownridge P. Epidural and subarachnoid analgesia for elective caesarean section. *Anaesthesia* 1981;**36**:70.

88 Blumgart CH, Ryall D, Dennison B, Thompson Hill LM. Mechanism of extension of spinal anaesthesia by epidural injection of local anaesthetic. *Br J Anaesth* 1992;**69**:457–60.

89 Peyton PJ. Complications of continuous spinal anaesthesia. *Anaesth Intens Care* 1992;**20**:417–38.

90 Morgan BM, Magni V, Goroszenuik T. Anaesthesia for emergency caesarean section. *Br J Obstet Gynaecol* 1990;**97**:420–4.

91 Birnbach DJ, Stein DJ, Hartman JK, *et al.* Complications of combined spinal epidural (CSE) analgesia compared with lumbar epidural analgesia. *Anesthesiology* 1996;**85**:A860.

92 Gaiser RR, Cheek TG, HK Adams, Gutsche BB. Epidural lidocaine for cesarean delivery of the distressed fetus. *Int J Obstet Anesth* 1998;**7**:27–31.

93 Price ML, Reynolds F, Morgan BM. Extending epidural blockade for emergency caesarean section. *Int J Obstet Anesth* 1991;**1**:13–18.

94 Broadbent CR, Russell R. What height of block is needed for manual removal of placenta under spinal anaesthesia? *Int J Obstet Anesth* 1999;**8**:161–4.

95 Bembridge M, MacDonald R, Lyons G. Spinal anaesthesia with hyperbaric lignocaine for elective Caesarean section. *Anaesthesia* 1986;**41**:906–9.

96 Carter B, Wilson E, Pitkanen M, El-Tayeb H. 2% hyperbaric lidocaine is inadequate compared to 5% hyperbaric lidocaine spinal analgesia. *Anesthesiology* 1995;**83**:A955.

97 Huffnagle HJ, Norris MC, Leighton BL, Arkoosh VA. Ilioinguinal iliohypogastric nerve blocks – before or after cesarean delivery under spinal anesthesia. *Anesth Analg* 1996;**82**:8–12.

98 Dennis AR, Leeson-Payne CG, Hobbs GJ. Analgesia after caesarean section. The use of rectal diclofenac as an adjunct to spinal morphine. *Anaesthesia* 1995;**50**:297–9.

99 Stoddart PA, Cooper A, Russell R, Reynolds F. A comparison of epidural diamorphine with intravenous PCA using the Baxter Infusor following caesarean section. *Anaesthesia* 1993;**48**:1086–90.

100 Kelly MC, Carabine UA, Mirakhur RK. Intrathecal diamorphine for analgesia after caesarean section: a dose finding study and assessment of side-effects. *Anaesthesia* 1998;**53**:231–7.

101 Abouleish E, Rawal N, Rashad MN. The addition of 0.2 mg subarachnoid morphine to hyperbaric bupivacaine for cesarean delivery: a prospective study of 856 cases. *Reg Anesth* 1991;**16**:137–40.

102 Milner AR, Bogod DG, Harwood RJ. Intrathecal administration of morphine for elective Caesarean section. A comparison between 0.1 mg and 0.2 mg. *Anaesthesia* 1996;**51**:871–3.

103 Palmer CM, Emerson S, Volgoropolous D, Alves D. Dose response relationship of intrathecal morphine for postcesarean analgesia. *Anesthesiology* 1999;**90**:437–44.

104 Eisenach JC, de Kock M, Klimscha W. α_2-adrenergic agonists for regional anesthesia. A clinical review of clonidine (1984–1995). *Anesthesiology* 1996;**85**:655–74.

105 Fuller JG, McMorland GH, Douglas MJ, Palmer L. Epidural morphine for analgesia after Caesarean section: a report of 4880 patients. *Can J Anaesth* 1990;**37**:636–40.

106 Paech MJ, Moore JS, Evans SF. Meperidine for patient-controlled analgesia after cesarean section. Intravenous versus epidural administration. *Anesthesiology* 1994;**80**:1268–76.

107 Reynolds F, Speedy HM. The subdural space: the third place to go astray. *Anaesthesia* 1990;**45**:120–3.

108 Morgan B. Unexpectedly extensive conduction blocks in obstetric epidural analgesia. *Anaesthesia* 1990;**45**:148–52.

109 Hodgkinson R. Total spinal block after epidural injection into an interspace adjacent to an inadvertent dural perforation. *Anesthesiology* 1981;**55**:593–5.

110 Orkell RW, Sprigge JS. Unintentional dural puncture. A survey of recognition and management. *Anaesthesia* 1987;**42**:1110–13.

111 Adams TJ, Peter EA, Douglas MJ. Is spinal anesthesia contraindicated after failed epidural anesthesia? *Anesth Analg* 1995;**81**:659.

112 Collier CB. Accidental subdural block: four more cases and a radiological review. *Anaesth Intens Care* 1992;**20**:215–32.

113 Brown DL, Ransom DM, Hall JA, Leicht CH, Schroeder DR, Offord KP. Regional anesthesia and local anesthetic-induced systemic toxicity: seizure frequency and accompanying cardiovascular changes. *Anesth Analg* 1995;**81**:321–8.

114 Naulty JS, March MG, Leavitt KL, *et al.* Effect of changes in labor analgesic practice on the safety and efficacy of epidural anesthesia. *Anesthesiology* 1992;**77**:A983.

115 Hogan Q. Local anesthestic toxicity: an update. *Reg Anesth* 1996;**21**(6S):43–50.

116 Moore DC. Toxicity of local anaesthetics in obstetrics IV: management. *Clin Anaesthesiol* 1986;**4**:113–24.

117 Rocke DA, Rout CC. Volume preloading, spinal hypotension and Caesarean section. *Br J Anaesth* 1995;**75**:257–9.

118 Gajraj NM, Victory RA, Pace NA, van Elstraete AC, Wallace DH. Comparison of an ephedrine infusion with crystalloid administration for prevention of hypotension during spinal anesthesia. *Anesth Analg* 1993;**76**:1023–6.

119 Zamora JE, Roseag OP, Lindsay MP, Crossan ML. Haemodynamic consequences and uterine contractions following 0.5 or 1.0 litre crystalloid infusion before obstetric epidural analgesia. *Can J Anaesth* 1996;**43**:347–52.

120 Breen TW, Shapiro T, Glass B, Foster-Payne D, Oriol NE. Epidural anesthesia for labor in an ambulatory patient. *Anesth Analg* 1993;**77**:919–24.

121 Russell R, Reynolds F. Epidural infusion of low-dose bupivacaine and opioid in labour. Does reducing motor block increase the spontaneous delivery rate? *Anesthesia* 1996;**51**:266–73.

122 Murphy JD, Henderson K, Bowden MI, Lewis M, Cooper GM. Bupivacaine versus bupivacaine and fentanyl for epidural analgesia; effect on maternal satisfaction. *BMJ* 1991;**302**:564–7.

123 Paech MJ, Gurrin LC. A survey of parturients using epidural analgesia during labour. Considerations relevant to antenatal educators. *Aust NZ J Obstet Gynaecol* 1999;**39**:21–5.

124 Parry MG, Fernando R, Bawa GP, Poulton BB. Dorsal column function after epidural and spinal blockade: implications for the safety of walking following low dose regional analgesia for labour. *Anaesthesia* 1998;**53**:382–7.

125 Glosten B, Hynson J, Sessler DI, McGuire J. Preanesthetic skin-surface warming reduces redistribution hypothermia caused by epidural block. *Anesth Analg* 1993;**77**:488–93.

126 Shehabi Y, Gatt S, Buckman T, Isert P. Effect of adrenaline, fentanyl and warming of injectate on shivering following extradural analgesia in labour. *Anaesth Intens Care* 1990;**18**:31–7.

127 Capogna G, Celleno D. I.V. clonidine for post-extradural shivering in parturients: a preliminary study. *Br J Anaesth* 1993;**71**:294–5.

128 Mercier FJ, Benhamou D. Hyperthermia related to epidural analgesia during labor. *Int J Obstet Anesth* 1997;**6**:19–24.

129 Chaney MA. Side-effects of intrathecal and epidural opioids. *Can J Anaesth* 1995;**42**:891–903.

130 Ballantyne JC, Loach AB, Carr DB. Itching after epidural and spinal opiates. *Pain* 1988;**33**:149–60.

131 Alhashemi JA, Crosby ET, Grodecki W, Duffy PJ, Hull KA, Gallant C. Treatment of intrathecal morphine-induced pruritus following Caesarean section. *Can J Anaesth* 1997;**44**:1060–5.

132 Etches RC, Sandler AN, Daley MD. Respiratory depression and spinal opioids. *Can J Anaesth* 1989;**36**:165–85.

133 Griffin RP, Reynolds F. Maternal hypoxaemia during labour and delivery: the influence of analgesia and effect on neonatal outcome. *Anaesthesia* 1995;**50**:151–6.

134 Porter JS, Bonello E, Reynolds F. The effect of epidural opioids on maternal oxygenation during labour and delivery. *Anaesthesia* 1996;**51**:899–903.

135 Hughes SC. Respiratory depression following intraspinal narcotics: expect it! *Int J Obstet Anesth* 1997;**6**:145–6.

136 Kelly MC, Carabine UA, Hill DA, Mirakhur RJ. A comparison of the effect of intrathecal and extradural fentanyl on gastric emptying in laboring women. *Anesth Analg* 1997;**85**:834–8.

137 Porter JS, Bonello E, Reynolds F. The influence of epidural administration of fentanyl infusion on gastric emptying in labour. *Anaesthesia* 1997;**52**:1151–6.

138 Boyle RK. A review of anatomical and immunological links between epidural morphine and herpes simplex labialis in obstetric patients. *Anaesth Intens Care* 1995;**23**:425–32.

139 Boyle RK. Herpes simplex labialis after epidural or parenteral morphine: a randomized prospective trial in an Australian obstetric population. *Anaesth Intens Care* 1995;**23**:433–7.

5: General anaesthesia for obstetrics

RICHARD VANNER

With the increased use of regional blocks, general anaesthesia is no longer the preferred technique for either caesarean section or manual removal of placenta. The decline in the popularity of general anaesthesia has been supported by data published in the triennial reports on confidential enquiries into maternal deaths. These reports have consistently demonstrated anaesthetic-related mortality to be more likely when general rather than regional anaesthesia is performed, especially in the emergency situation. Although the percentage of caesarean sections performed under regional block is increasing, the dramatic rise in the number of operative deliveries means that a substantial number of general anaesthetics are still performed.[1] In England in 1994 there were approximately 604 000 deliveries of which 93 000 were performed by caesarean section. Of the caesarean deliveries, 55 000 were emergencies and 38 000 elective with general anaesthesia used in 34% and 29% of cases respectively.[2]

There are still many situations where general anaesthesia is indeed necessary. Regional blocks may be refused or contraindicated or have failed (see Chapter 4). Furthermore, in the true emergency, the speed and reliability of general anaesthesia may be considered beneficial.

Maternal mortality

Triennial reports on confidential enquiries into maternal deaths in England and Wales (UK since 1985) have been published since 1952. Recommendations from these reports have altered anaesthetic practice and have led to a gradual fall in maternal mortality from anaesthetic causes. Anaesthetic-related mortality is associated primarily with emergency caesarean section under general anaesthesia. Death is usually from hypoxia secondary to problems with tracheal intubation or from aspiration pneumonitis. Mortality from regional anaesthesia does occur as it does from elective caesarean section under general anaesthesia but these are fortunately rare events.[3-5] In the 1991–93 triennial report,[4] there were nine deaths from caesarean section under general anaesthesia, eight of them emergencies, and none from caesarean section under regional anaesthesia. By contrast only one anaesthetic death was documented in the 1994–96 report, following combined spinal-epidural anaesthesia for caesarean section.

Unfortunately, the reports on confidential enquiries into maternal deaths do not give the denominator of the total number of emergency caesareans under general anaesthesia. However, this can be extrapolated from a recent Department of Health statistical bulletin which recorded 18 000 emergency caesareans under general anaesthesia in England in 1994.[2] There were 1.28 times the number of maternities in the UK and therefore, assuming similar anaesthetic practice in the whole of the UK, there were 23 000 emergency caesareans under general anaesthesia in the UK in 1994. This provides a denominator to the 1991–1993 report[5] where there were eight anaesthetic-related deaths during emergency caesarean section under general anaesthesia in three years, a mortality of one in 8600.

However, of the general anaesthetic deaths in the 1991–93 report, in all nine caesareans regional anaesthesia was contraindicated; three refused regional anaesthesia, two had fetal distress, two had pulmonary hypertension, one had a placenta praevia which bled three litres and the other had septic shock. Thus there is a group of women who should have their caesarean section performed under general anaesthesia. This is a vulnerable group, not only because they are often the sickest and most high-risk obstetric patients but also because they need expertise in techniques that the obstetric anaesthetist practises less frequently.

Since the late 1970s there has been a gradual reduction in deaths from anaesthesia. It was thought that this was due to a reduction in caesarean sections performed under general anaesthesia and an increase in the number performed under regional anaesthesia. In a recent survey of maternity units in the UK,[1] 31 out of 226 units could provide figures for both 1982 and 1992. In those units 4983 emergency caesarean sections were performed under general anaesthesia in 1982 compared to 4900 in 1992. Therefore, the number of general anaesthetics has remained constant through the years. The increase in emergency caesarean sections performed under regional anaesthesia has been balanced by a 50% increase in the total number of emergency caesareans performed (5832 in 1982 to 9069 in 1992 in those 31 units). The reduction in deaths has mainly been in cases of unrecognised oesophageal intubation, probably due to the increased use of capnography in the 1980s. Improved antacid prophylaxis and the failed intubation drill as well as an increase in consultant anaesthetic sessions in maternity units have probably also helped.

Preparation of theatre and equipment

When starting their shift of duty, the obstetric anaesthetist should check all the anaesthetic machines and equipment in the delivery suite. Drugs for induction of general anaesthesia (thiopentone, suxamethonium, and atropine) should be drawn up, labelled, and placed in an unlocked refrigerator in theatre. These must be replaced every 24 hours. The intubation cart should also be checked: it should contain a variety of face masks, oral airways, four laryngoscopes (two normal Macintosh, one with a short handle, one half polio and one McCoy), a variety of tracheal tubes including those of both 6 and 7 mm internal diameter, Magill forceps and at least one 15 gauge gum elastic bougie. In case of a failed intubation both an unwrapped size 3 laryngeal mask airway and a cricothyrotomy kit (see below) must be available.

Monitoring in theatre should be of the same standard as the rest of the operating theatres in the hospital and should include pulse oximetry, capnography (always connected to the breathing circuit), non-invasive blood pressure, inspired oxygen analysis, anaesthetic agent analysis, ECG, airway pressure, expired tidal volume, ventilator disconnect alarm, nerve stimulator, temperature, and the capability for two invasive blood pressures. Ideally, the monitoring should be portable to allow transfer of the patient to the intensive care unit. A dedicated trained anaesthetic assistant should be readily available on a 24-hour basis.

Preparation of the patient

Preoperative assessment

First, the indication for general anaesthesia must be explored; it must be robust and should be recorded in the notes. It is important to assess the patient in a structured manner that can be repeated swiftly in the emergency situation. Ideally, the obstetrician or midwife should pick up potential anaesthetic problems and refer the woman for antenatal anaesthetic assessment. This allows previous notes or X-rays to be obtained, further investigations and a management plan devised. History must include obstetric details, previous anaesthetics with a review of previous anaesthetic charts if possible, medical health, recent drugs therapy including antacids, and known drug allergies. Examination must include airway assessment. The three best predictors of difficult intubation are inability to visualise the posterior pharyngeal wall when the mouth is opened wide and the tongue protruded,[6] a thyromental distance less than 7 cm with full head extension[7] and not being able to protrude the jaw so that the lower incisors fail to overlap the upper incisors.[8] Using the first two tests, Frerk[9] predicted that 14 out of 244 patients who were not pregnant could be a difficult intubation. When they were all intubated, 11 proved to be difficult (needing a bougie), nine of those having been predicted, therefore five cases (2%) were false positives (sensitivity) and two (1%) were missed (specificity). Assessment of mouth opening, neck movement, and body mass index may also help to predict possible difficulties with intubation.[10]

Unfortunately, failed intubation may still occur in a woman with a previous successful tracheal intubation before pregnancy.[11] Indeed, the Mallampati score can deteriorate during pregnancy[12] and even during labour.[13] If a difficult intubation is predicted either from examination of the airway or from a previous anaesthetic chart then regional anaesthesia must be reconsidered (see below) or awake fibreoptic intubation performed before inducing general anaesthesia.[14]

Antacid prophylaxis

The classic description of acid pulmonary aspiration by Mendelson in 1946[15] together with the early reports on confidential enquiries into maternal deaths in England and Wales have focused anaesthetists' attention on the gastrointestinal tract. Pregnancy itself does not prolong gastric emptying of solids or liquids but established labour may cause an unpredictable delay in gastric emptying which is markedly potentiated by opioid analgesia given by either the intramuscular or epidural routes.[16] Heartburn and regurgitation occur in 80% of pregnant women at term and even asymptomatic women have frequent gastro-oesophageal reflux.[17] All pregnant women at term can be regarded as having an incompetent lower oesophageal sphincter. Mortality from aspiration pneumonitis has been reduced since the late 1960s by the combination of antacid prophylaxis, preoxygenation, cricoid pressure, and tracheal intubation.[18]

Although severe aspiration pneumonitis may still occur in dogs after aspiration of gastric contents at pH 5.9,[19] it is now widely believed that a gastric pH of less than 3.5 is more harmful.[20] Therefore, in order to compare the effectiveness of different antacid regimens, high risk may be defined as those having a gastric pH of less than 3.5 with a volume of over 25 ml when aspirated with a Salem sump tube, It must be emphasised that others may also be at some risk of pneumonitis should they aspirate.

For elective caesarean section either ranitidine 150 mg or omeprazole 40 mg given orally the night before and again on the morning of surgery is effective at raising gastric pH. In one study comparing these antacids, six of 33 women who received ranitidine were at risk with a low pH compared to none of 32 in the omeprazole group, although all the women had gastric volumes of less than 25 ml.[20] If oral sodium citrate 30 ml of 0.3 M is given, this should be immediately before induction of general anaesthesia as it mixes effectively but only lasts for 30 minutes with normal gastric emptying.[16] In women at high risk of requiring an emergency caesarean delivery during labour, oral ranitidine 150 mg may be given six hourly with sodium citrate taken before induction of anaesthesia. Of 49 women treated this way only one (2%) was at risk, compared to eight (15%) of 53 women who had omeprazole 40 mg 12 hourly.[21] Omeprazole is enteric coated as it is destroyed by acid and may have an unpredictable effect after the first dose and is therefore not as effective as ranitidine as prophylaxis in labour. In a recent large study of 384 women undergoing emergency caesarean section under general anaesthesia, 120 received 30 ml of sodium citrate alone, of whom 28 (23%) were considered at risk of aspiration pneumonitis.[22] When intravenous metoclopramide was also given to 65 women there was no improvement as 15 (23%) were still considered to be at risk. However, significantly fewer women were at risk if, in addition to oral sodium citrate, they received ranitidine 50 mg intravenously immediately after the decision for surgery was made. With this antacid regimen, only four of 50 (8%) were at risk as defined by the above criteria.

Crossmatching blood

The blood transfusion service should receive blood with a request for group and screen for antibodies with the sample saved for all caesarean sections. Blood should be crossmatched if excessive bleeding is anticipated, if antibodies are present that would slow the crossmatch process and also if it is not possible to provide crossmatched blood within half an hour from request. There should be a blood refrigerator in all maternity units which always has two units of O Rh-negative blood available for use in emergencies (see Chapter 7). However, a safer alternative is to request group-specific blood before crossmatching as the group and antibody status are already known from antenatal testing. The crossmatch process can go ahead on a sample of this blood and a phone call to the delivery suite will confirm its compatibility by which time the blood will have been received by the anaesthetist.

Transfer of mother to the operating theatre

For emergency caesarean sections in labour the patient is normally transported to the operating theatre on her bed. She should be in the full left lateral position to prevent aortocaval compression and resulting fetal acidosis.[23] Supplemental oxygen should be given from a portable oxygen cylinder if there is evidence of fetal distress.[24] For elective surgery a woman may walk to the theatre area from the antenatal ward and, after going through the preoperative checklist, she may walk into theatre with the anaesthetic assistant. All mothers undergoing caesarean section must give consent and have identification bands secured around a wrist, although some maternity units allow women to labour without them.

General anaesthesia

General considerations (Box 5.1)

To neutralise stomach contents before induction of anaesthesia, the woman should drink 30 ml of 0.3 M sodium citrate. She is then positioned supine

---

Box 5.1   Checklist for general anaesthesia for caesarean section

- Consent and identification band
- Anaesthetic assessment, particularly the airway
- Intravenous infusion, blood for group and save or crossmatch
- Ranitidine 50 mg intravenously (unless given orally beforehand)
- Oral sodium citrate 30 ml 0.3 M
- Left uterine displacement on transfer and on operating table
- Monitoring, equipment check
- Anaesthetic assistant and surgeon present
- Preoxygenation for three minutes with calm reassurance to mother
- Apply cricoid pressure lightly while awake
- Intravenous induction and suxamethonium
- Intubate using a bougie if difficult, size 6 or 7 ID cuffed tube
- Ventilate with 50% nitrous oxide in oxygen with >1% isoflurane
- Non-depolarising muscle relaxant only after intubation confirmed
- After delivery: 66% nitrous oxide, 0.75% isoflurane, opioid
- Oxytocin
- Empty stomach with orogastric tube in emergencies
- Extubate on left side when awake and muscle relaxant reversed
- Adequate recovery facility with monitoring and one-to-one care

---

on the operating table with a 15° left lateral tilt. The supine position without tilt causes fetal acidosis at delivery.[25] All cases must have adequate uterine displacement in the supine position to reduce aortocaval compression and the abdomen should be uncovered briefly so that this may be checked. Compression of the inferior vena cava not only reduces cardiac output but also decreases uterine perfusion pressure by both a rise in uterine venous pressure and a fall in uterine artery pressure resulting from aortic compression. One plump pillow should be positioned under the head but not the shoulders. Slight head-up tilt may prevent air embolus and reduce the quantity of blood and amniotic fluid reaching the diaphragm via the paracolic gutters.

Peripheral intravenous access should be established, preferably with a 14 gauge cannula (and not smaller than 16 gauge) and an infusion of 0.9% saline or Hartmann's solution started.

Fluid preload is not required routinely before general anaesthesia. Blood loss at caesarean section under general anaesthesia may be up to one litre. Contraction of the uterus after delivery replaces about 500 ml of this loss. If placenta accreta is suspected (anterior placenta praevia and a previous caesarean section) then two 14 gauge cannulas, each with an infusion through a blood warmer, should be set up and crossmatched blood brought into theatre before surgery is started.

ECG, pulse oximetry, and non-invasive blood pressure monitoring should be attached and blood pressure checked. In cases of severe pre-eclampsia or with cardiac disease, invasive arterial and central venous pressure may be transduced. The capnograph should be switched on beforehand to allow calibration. The suction apparatus must be switched on and the Yankauer attachment positioned under the right-hand side of the pillow. An anaesthetic assistant, experienced in applying cricoid pressure, must be present. Ideally he or she should have recently practised the correct force on weighing scales (see below).

Depending on the degree of urgency of delivery, a urinary catheter may be inserted and the operating site cleaned and draped before induction of anaesthesia. On no account should the patient be anaesthetised before the surgeon is scrubbed and ready.

Preoxygenation can now commence and a note of the time made. For this, a Mapleson A breathing circuit (Magill) with 8 l/min oxygen flow may be used. The bag must distend and the expiratory valve pop open to ensure an adequate seal between the patient's face and the mask. Constant explanation and reassurance should be given during this time. The assistant now applies cricoid pressure lightly (10 N or 1 kg of force) with a single-handed technique. The position of the fingers should be checked and the mother asked to nod her head if cricoid pressure is comfortable.

Three minutes after the start of adequate preoxygenation anaesthesia is induced with 4–7 mg/kg of thiopentone given intravenously over about 20 seconds. Loss of consciousness is noted and suxamethonium 1.5 mg/kg given and flushed with the intravenous infusion. The cricoid pressure is increased to a firm pressure (30 N or 3 kg of force) with loss of consciousness. Laryngoscopy is not attempted for about 60 seconds or until suxamethonium fasciculations have stopped and full neuromuscular blockade has been achieved. Ventilation of the lungs should not be attempted during this time. Insertion of the laryngoscope may be awkward as the assistant's hand is applying cricoid pressure. This may be overcome by pointing the handle of the laryngoscope towards the patient's right shoulder during insertion of the blade. When the handle is then turned back to the midline it should rise above the assistant's hand and at the same time the tongue is pushed to the left. The half polio blade or short handle laryngoscope may be tried if insertion is difficult. If the assistant uses his or her left hand to apply cricoid pressure this is usually less of a problem.

After intubation and cuff inflation the tube position must be checked by observing chest expansion and auscultating for bilateral breath sounds. Correct placement is confirmed by the presence of a CO_2 trace on the capnograph. Cricoid pressure is then released and surgery may commence.

To minimise the possibility of maternal awareness, it is becoming increasingly popular to initially maintain anaesthesia with a high inspired concentration of volatile agent[26] (overpressure)(see below). An inspired oxygen concentration of 50%, together with nitrous oxide, until delivery is usual. Increased oxygen concentration may be of benefit in cases of fetal distress.[27] Ventilation should maintain the end-tidal CO_2 between 4 and 4.5 kPa to prevent maternal alkalosis and uterine artery vasoconstriction both of which reduce oxygen transfer to the fetus.

The pupils should be observed as immediately after induction they are often widely dilated and react briskly to light. After a few minutes of 2% isoflurane they reduce in size, at which point the inspired isoflurane may be reduced. Neuromuscular block is maintained with atracurium 0.3 mg/kg which may be given once tracheal intubation is confirmed. Failure to maintain adequate neuromuscular block may impede delivery. The blood pressure should be checked immediately after induction and at least every three minutes thereafter. Prolonged falls in systolic pressure of more than 20% must be avoided as reduced uterine perfusion leads to fetal acidosis.

Syntocinon 10 units is given intravenously at delivery to aid contraction of the uterus. This should be given slowly as Syntocinon is a vasodilator which may produce a marked tachycardia with hypotension. Syntocinon has a half-life of only four minutes and so 10–20 units may be added to the intravenous infusion. If the uterus does not contract, Syntocinon infusion can be increased to 10 units per hour for four hours through a separate intravenous infusion. Reduction of the inspired isoflurane concentration to 0.75% with an end-tidal concentration of 0.5% does not prevent uterine contraction.[28] Antibiotics may be given after delivery to reduce the incidence of postoperative infection. After delivery anaesthesia is maintained with 66% nitrous oxide in oxygen with the volatile agent continued until surgery is complete. Intravenous opioids such as morphine 0.2 mg/kg should be given. Towards the end of surgery the end-tidal CO_2 may be allowed to rise so that spontaneous ventilation returns.

In the emergency cases the stomach should be emptied with a large orogastric tube before extubation. A 20 gauge Salem sump tube with two lumens is suitable. A volume of over 100 ml is often obtained and this reduces the chance of aspiration during or immediately after extubation.[3] It is possible to measure gastric pH with test paper and to administer another dose of sodium citrate with a bladder syringe if the pH is less than 4.

When surgery is complete the mother is turned on to her left side. Neuromuscular block is reversed and checked with a nerve stimulator. Volatile agents and nitrous oxide are discontinued and ventilation with 100% oxygen continued until spontaneous breathing returns. The pharynx is cleared by gentle suction. When the mother is conscious the cuff of tracheal tube is deflated and the tube removed. Supplemental oxygen is given by face mask until the mother is fully awake. She should be awake before transfer to the recovery room and during transfer supplemental oxygen must be continued using a portable cylinder and she should remain in the lateral position.

Technique for elective caesarean section

It has been argued that women undergoing elective caesarean section under general anaesthesia are at much lower risk of aspiration pneumonitis and therefore do not require cricoid pressure during induction.[29] This is not current practice in the UK where all cases receive cricoid pressure.[30] General anaesthesia for elective caesarean section is much safer than in the emergency situation. Therefore, there is no reason to change current practice. Furthermore, the overriding advantage of using the same technique as in the emergency situation is that the technique can be practised as well as taught by consultant anaesthetists in a controlled environment.

Preoxygenation

Adequate preoxygenation is essential in obstetric patients. After preoxygenation, apnoea of one minute causes a much greater fall in arterial oxygen tension in pregnant compared with non-pregnant women.[31] This is thought to be due to the lower functional residual capacity (FRC) and a higher metabolic rate. The object of preoxygenation is to replace the alveolar nitrogen with oxygen to give a period of apnoea without hypoxaemia. Classically, preoxygenation in non-pregnant patients using a Mapleson A circuit with 8 l/minute oxygen flow takes three minutes with a normal minute volume. The time constant for this exponential process is given by dividing the FRC in litres by the alveolar ventilation in litres per minute and in three time constants there will be 95% denitrogenation.

A common problem with preoxygenation is failure to make an adequate seal between mask and face which allows room air to be inspired. It also prevents the reservoir bag from distending and therefore the expiratory valve fails to open, causing rebreathing of nitrogen. Preoxygenation using a rebreathing circuit such as a Mapleson D or a circle system may require a longer time or higher flows. Four deep breaths within 30 seconds of induction has been described as an alternative technique in a dire emergency.[32]

Cricoid pressure

The use of cricoid pressure to prevent regurgitation during induction of anaesthesia in patients at risk of pulmonary aspiration was first described by Sellick in 1961[33] but it was not adopted widely in the UK until the late 1960s. Although Sellick described cricoid pressure without a pillow, intubation is easiest with a pillow beneath the occiput and cricoid pressure is just as effective in this position.[34] Some also consider that support of the neck by a hand or neck support is required when the patient's head and neck are placed in the Magill position, as cricoid pressure may flex the head on the neck, making it more difficult to see the glottis at laryngoscopy.[35,36] Three recent studies have formally assessed this hypothesis[37,38,39] but their results are apparently contradictory. In one study,[37] the view of the glottis at laryngoscopy during cricoid pressure was slightly better when the neck was supported by hand than when it was not, concurring with the hypothesis. In contrast, in the other two studies,[38,39] there was no marked difference in the view at laryngoscopy, with and without support of the neck. Although the reason for the discrepancy between studies is not clear, one possibility is the difference in the pressure applied to the cricoid cartilage. In the first study,[37] a strong force (50–55 N) was applied to the cricoid cartilage whereas in the latter two, 40 N[38] or 30 N[39] was used. Therefore, it appears that cricoid pressure applied using an appropriate force does not worsen and may even improve[39] the view of the glottis at laryngoscopy. If too strong a force is used, however, cricoid pressure is more likely to flex the head and to make laryngoscopy more difficult, although it may be counteracted by providing neck support.

A study of 10 cadavers showed that 20 N of cricoid pressure prevented the regurgitation of oesophageal fluid with a pressure of 25 mmHg in all cases. A force of 30 N prevented regurgitation of oesophageal fluid with a pressure of 40 mmHg.[40] Gastric pressures over 25 mmHg are unlikely during emergency caesarean section under general anaesthesia.[41] Although suxamethonium can increase gastric pressure it rarely rises to over 25 mmHg. Therefore 20 N of cricoid pressure is probably enough and 30 N is more than enough to prevent passive regurgitation into the pharynx.

Normally the upper oesophageal sphincter prevents regurgitation into the pharynx; during intravenous induction of anaesthesia the sphincter relaxes just before loss of consciousness.[42] Cricoid pressure should therefore be applied to the awake patient before loss of consciousness. However, more than 20 N of force is uncomfortable and if this is exceeded, retching may occur[43] which could lead to oesophageal rupture.[40] Therefore light cricoid pressure should be applied to awake patients. Anaesthetic assistants can be trained to apply the correct force by practising on weighing scales.[44,45] Training can improve the performance and reduce errors to less than 5 N.[39] Therefore, a reasonable recommendation is to apply 10 N (1 kg) when the patient is awake and increase to 30 N (3 kg) with loss of consciousness.[45] The studies that have shown cricoid pressure to be potentially harmful have all applied excessive force. Forces of 40 N and over can cause airway obstruction,[43,46] difficulty in passing the tracheal tube,[47] oesophageal rupture[40] and impaired view at laryngoscopy without neck support.[37] Cricoid pressure itself has been shown to reduce lower oesophageal sphincter pressure in awake volunteers,[48] which is obviously undesirable in patients with a full stomach; however, it has not been shown to cause gastro-oesophageal reflux in similar subjects.[49]

Overpressure

It has become popular to increase the concentration of volatile anaesthetic initially to prevent awareness when the intravenous anaesthetic wears off (see below). This was not practised in the past because of fears of depression of the newborn and relaxation of the uterus. However, as it takes 10 minutes for the alveolar concentration of isoflurane to reach 60% of the inspired concentration, it is logical to use a higher concentration for a few minutes to speed up the rise in alveolar concentration to above MAC. Few studies have analysed the effects of this practice on mother and baby but one small study of 18 patients did not demonstrate any adverse effects.[26] However, this study did demonstrate low arterial blood concentrations of isoflurane in three control patients that did not receive the overpressure technique. Another study of 200 mothers receiving overpressure techniques with up to 1.8% isoflurane for the first five minutes reported acceptable Apgar scores.[27]

Maternal inspired oxygen concentration

The technique of fetal scalp blood sampling has demonstrated that fetal blood PaO_2 varies directly with maternal PaO_2. Although the increase in oxygen tension may be small, the increase in oxygen content is substantial because of the greater oxygen affinity of fetal haemoglobin (80% of fetal haemoglobin at term) and in emergency cases this may be even greater if it occurs on the steep part of the haemoglobin dissociation curve.[24] Piggott et al. studied 200 caesarean sections under general anaesthesia receiving either 100% oxygen with isoflurane or 50% oxygen with nitrous oxide and isoflurane. They showed higher umbilical vein oxygen tensions in the 100% group, particularly in the emergency cases, and also Apgar scores tended to be higher in this group.[27]

Effect on the newborn

The paediatrician should be present at all deliveries under general anaesthesia. They should be informed of any opioids given to the mother, so that when necessary, intramuscular naloxone 40 µg is given to the neonate. It was originally thought that prolonged induction to delivery times caused fetal acidosis at delivery. However, if maternal hypotension and aortocaval compression are avoided, this is not the case. Prolonged induction to delivery times do make the neonate more sleepy due to greater transfer of anaesthetic agents and if this time is over eight minutes there is a greater incidence of low one-minute Apgar scores. Uterine incision-delivery times of over three minutes are associated with an acidotic fetus and it is apparent that incision and manipulation of the uterus causes a reduction in uteroplacental blood flow.[50]

Anaesthetic agents

Induction agents

Intravenous induction agents for caesarean section must balance maternal unconsciousness with minimal neonatal depression and haemodynamic stability.[50] Thiopentone is still the agent of choice for caesarean section at a dose of 4–7 mg/kg. Peak umbilical vein concentrations (UV) occur after 1.5 minutes while peak umbilical artery concentrations (UA) occur after 3.5 minutes. There is a net fetal uptake of thiopentone for 10 minutes despite rapidly falling maternal vein (MV) concentrations. Despite Apgar scores of over 7 at one minute, neonates receiving thiopentone have mildly impaired neurobehavioural scores for 1–2 days. Ketamine provides good cardiovascular stability but causes unpleasant intraoperative dreaming in 6% and a dose of more than 1.5 mg/kg causes neonatal depression. Propofol 2.5 mg/kg has less increase in blood pressure after intubation than thiopentone; however, in a double-blinded study doses large enough to ensure maternal unconsciousness caused neonatal depression.[51] Etomidate gives good cardiovascular stability at a dose of 0.3 mg/kg, neonatal depression is not greater than thiopentone and the time to spontaneous breathing may be shorter; however, neonatal cortisol levels are lower.

Hypertension and tachycardia are frequently observed after laryngoscopy and intubation. This is undesirable in women with pre-eclampsia or heart disease and if regional anaesthesia is contraindicated, attempts should be made to blunt this hypertensive response. Various agents have been suggested. Alfentanil (10 µg/kg) is effective but may cause neonatal depression, although this is easily reversed with naloxone. Magnesium sulphate 40 mg/kg is an alternative but is painful to inject.[52] If not contraindicated, labetolol given by 10 mg increments may be useful. Intravenous boluses of lignocaine are not particularly effective. Should general anaesthesia be required in such patients, direct arterial pressure monitoring is helpful.

Inhalational agents

Nitrous oxide is taken up by the fetus and the UV/MV ratio is 0.83 after four minutes. Neonates do not seem unduly depressed by 50% concentrations in the mother as long as the induction delivery time is not prolonged.[50] All neonates should have oxygen for at least five minutes after delivery if the mother has had nitrous oxide to prevent diffusion hypoxia. Nitrous oxide does not relax the uterus which has a normal response to oxytocin. Volatile anaesthetic agents also cross the placenta and the UV/MV ratio is about 0.6 for both halothane and enflurane. Also fetal tissue uptake accounts for a steady UA/UV ratio of 0.5. It has been demonstrated that the combination of 0.5 MAC of nitrous oxide (50%) and 0.5 MAC of volatile agent (0.75% inspired isoflurane) causes negligible neonatal depression (with induction to delivery times of less than 11 minutes) and no more blood loss than with nitrous oxide alone.[28] More than 1 MAC of any volatile agent relaxes the uterus in a dose-dependent way and at 2 MAC the uterine response to oxytocics is blocked. Although these doses should usually be avoided as increased blood loss occurs, they can be used to therapeutically relax the uterus. Glyceryl trinitrate 800 µg by sublingual spray is also effective at relaxing the uterus. It may also be given by intravenous injection in 100 μg increments.

The use of the new volatile anaesthetic agents sevoflurane and desflurane for elective caesarean section has been investigated.[53,54] No significant differences in either maternal or neonatal outcome have been demonstrated when compared with isoflurane.

Neuromuscular blocking drugs

Suxamethonium gives rapid intubating conditions within 60 seconds and usually wears off in six minutes.[50] It is the agent of choice until a short-acting non-depolarising drug is developed. Plasma cholinesterase activity is 15% lower at term but its action is only occasionally prolonged. Magnesium sulphate does not prolong its action but prevents suxamethonium fasciculations.[55] In order to prevent fasciculations which may raise gastric pressure, it has been suggested that a small dose of non-depolarising relaxant be given before suxamethonium. This practice should be avoided, as the rise in gastric pressure has not been consistently demonstrated and neuromuscular block is not as complete when compared with suxamethonium alone.

The new non-depolarising muscle relaxant rocuronium has also been studied in elective caesarean section. A dose of 0.6 mg/kg usually provides good intubating conditions in less than 80 seconds and the block may be reversed 30 minutes after injection.[56] Rocuronium has not been shown to have any adverse effects on mother or baby and it has been suggested that it may gain widespread use as an alternative to suxamethonium. Although it would appear to be a reasonable choice when suxamethonium is contra-indicated, in the event of a failed intubation with failed ventilation the mother will not be saved by the return of spontaneous respiration.

As a result of their ionisation, non-depolarising neuromuscular blocking drugs cross the placenta extremely slowly. Evidence of muscle relaxation is therefore most unlikely. Either vecuronium 0.06 mg/kg or atracurium 0.3 mg/kg is suitable for caesarean section as they provide muscle relaxation for 30 minutes at which time the block can be safely reversed. Much smaller doses (half) should be used in women receiving magnesium sulphate as clinical effect is potentiated.[55]

Recovery

Lack of adequate postoperative care is an important cause of maternal mortality.[3] It is recommended that "midwifery staff deputised to look after post-operative patients should be specifically trained in monitoring, the care of the airway and resuscitative procedures and should be supervised by a defined anaesthetist at all times".[3] It is helpful to provide a written recovery protocol for management after general anaesthesia. This should include standards on the duration of one-to-one nursing care, appropriate monitoring, and discharge to postnatal wards. The anaesthetist must be readily available in the initial postoperative period. The recovery area must be close to the operating theatre and be equipped with suction, oxygen, appropriate monitoring equipment and ideally, an anaesthetic machine.

Prophylaxis against thromboembolic disease in the form of subcutaneous heparin 5000 units twice a day should be prescribed to those with known risk factors: age over 35 years, emergency surgery, obesity, gross varicose veins, high parity, pre-eclampsia, immobility of more than four days before surgery, concurrent illness, and previous or family thromboembolic history.

Postoperative analgesia

Without regional anaesthesia and spinal opioids, postoperative pain may be more difficult to treat. At the end of surgery bilateral ilioinguinal nerve block or infiltration of the wound with local anaesthetic may be helpful when regional blocks have not been used. In the postoperative period a combination of intramuscular morphine 0.2 mg/kg four hourly and non-steroidal anti-inflammatory drugs such as rectal diclofenac 150 mg/day may be adequate. If suppositories are to be given, patient consent should be obtained. Although repeated intramuscular injections may be undesirable for both patients and staff, they do allow mobility. Intravenous patient-controlled analgesia (PCA) has gained in popularity but must be portable. Good pain relief can be achieved with 1 mg boluses of morphine with a five-minute lockout period. Background infusion is not usually required. Nausea and vomiting are the most troublesome side-effects and an antiemetic may be added to the PCA syringe or alternatively given as required.

Oral or rectal analgesics should be prescribed and provide the mainstay of pain relief in the days following surgery. Delays in gastric emptying may affect drug absorption, although most women start eating and drinking within 24 hours of delivery.

Complications

Problems with intubation

Difficult intubation

A number of factors contribute to possible difficulty with intubation in the obstetric patient. Anatomically, there is an increase in total body water, enlargement of breast tissue and most likely a full set of teeth. With emergency anaesthesia induced often by a trainee anaesthetist with the patient tilted to the side and also receiving cricoid pressure, it is hardly surprising that intubation not infrequently proves difficult. To minimise the difficulty, the head and neck must be correctly positioned before induction and adequate time must be allowed for maximal neuromuscular block to develop before attempting laryngoscopy.

If there is a Cormack and Lehane grade 2 or 3 view at laryngoscopy a 15 gauge gum elastic bougie should be used immediately.[57] If this can be passed between the vocal cords a 7 mm tracheal tube may be railroaded into the correct position. If difficulty is encountered passing the tube, it should be rotated anticlockwise through 90° and if this manoeuvre should fail, a size 6 tube may be tried. No more than two attempts at intubation should be allowed, with a change of technique (repositioning or use of different laryngoscope) hopefully leading to correct placement of the tracheal tube.[10]

It is important to abandon attempts at intubation and make the diagnosis of a failed intubation at an early stage before hypoxaemia occurs. On no account must a second dose of suxamethonium be given. A grade 4 view at laryngoscopy should lead to immediate introduction of the failed intubation drill without attempt at intubation. It has recently been suggested that cricoid pressure is released in order to have another attempt at intubation,[58] but if cricoid pressure was applied correctly this would be unlikely to improve the view at laryngoscopy.[39]

Failed intubation (Fig 5.1)

Failed intubation occurs once in every 250 general anaesthetics in maternity.[11] Once it is established that intubation is impossible, the failed intubation drill must be implemented without delay. Senior anaesthetic assistance should be called and cricoid pressure maintained (see below). An oral airway should be inserted and manual ventilation of the lungs should be attempted using 100% oxygen via a face mask. In the failed intubation drill described by Tunstall in 1976, it was recommended that a woman should be turned to her left side.[59] This practice has now been questioned as not only is it difficult to turn a pregnant woman onto her side but also maintenance of cricoid pressure and manual ventilation are both made more challenging. Moreover, should surgery proceed, the woman then needs to be returned to the wedged supine position. Should bag and mask ventilation prove unsuccessful, the failed ventilation drill should be followed (see below).

Current recommendations are to maintain cricoid pressure during the failed intubation drill and certainly aspiration is more likely when there are problems with the airway.[60] However, 30 N force can only be maintained for four minutes.[61] Therefore the force applied may need to be reduced to a comfortable level. In a recent report of 23 failed intubations over a 17-year period in one maternity unit, all mothers survived.[11] Cricoid pressure was maintained during their failed intubation drill and 14 (60%) were not difficult to ventilate with a mask and oral airway, seven (30%) were difficult to

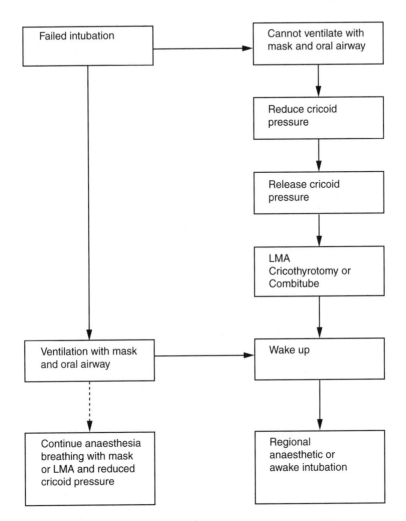

Fig 5.1   Failed intubation and failed ventilation drills

ventilate and in two (9%) it was impossible. In the 14 patients in whom mask ventilation was not difficult, maintaining cricoid pressure was not harmful and may well have prevented regurgitation and pulmonary aspiration.[62] Although some cases had laryngeal oedema, it is possible that cricoid pressure contributed to the difficulties in mask ventilation in the other nine cases.[46]

Failed ventilation (Fig 5.1)

The "can't intubate, can't ventilate" scenario is a life-threatening emergency. The amount of cricoid pressure applied may be reduced by half and ventilation tried again as excessive force may obstruct the airway. If ventilation is still impossible cricoid pressure should be released and ventilation tried again. Cricoid pressure should be released in the supine position while looking with a laryngoscope with suction in hand. If ventilation is still impossible the oral airway should be replaced with a laryngeal mask airway (LMA). (Nasal airways are best avoided as they may provoke excessive haemorrhage in the obstetric patient.) Although the LMA does not protect against aspiration of gastric contents and despite several case reports of successful insertion of the LMA in this situation with cricoid pressure maintained,[63] correct insertion of the LMA is more likely without cricoid pressure.[64] Cricoid pressure is still effective if reapplied after insertion of the LMA[65] although it may cause partial airway obstruction.[66]

Although blind tracheal intubation through the LMA has been described, it is not recommended in the failed intubation drill as laryngospasm may result.

If attempts at ventilation are still impossible the next step is to insert a cricothyrotomy cannula. Complications with this technique are not uncommon and so it should be practised regularly on mannequins or in the mortuary. Complications occur with insertion, ventilation with high-pressure oxygen or as a result of barotrauma from hyperinflation when exhalation through the upper airway is obstructed. A cricothyrotomy kit with a 4 mm ID cannula and a standard 15 mm connector (Quicktrach, VBM Medical) is better than an intravenous cannula as it allows ventilation with a normal breathing circuit, thus avoiding high-pressure circuits. It also allows exhalation through the cannula, thus avoiding barotrauma with upper airway obstruction.[67]

The final option in the failed ventilation drill is to perform a surgical tracheostomy. Even with an experienced surgeon, this takes more than three minutes. In the maternity unit with an inexperienced operator, this is likely to be prolonged and uncontrolled haemorrhage may result.

The Combitube is an alternative emergency airway. The leading tube nearly always enters the oesophagus and the other lumen gives a good airway provided there is no laryngospasm. The small adult 37 gauge tube should be used (the large 41 gauge should be obsolete). Insertion can be traumatic as blood on the cuff is often seen[68] which may be related to overdistension of the pharyngeal balloon. Oesophageal rupture has also been reported.[69]

Spontaneous ventilation returns as the effects of the suxamethonium wear off. At this point the decision must be made to either continue anaesthesia with an unprotected airway or to wake the patient up and perform another anaesthetic technique. In situations where the mother's life depends on immediate surgery (massive haemorrhage) a spontaneous breathing anaesthetic may be continued. Elective cases where there is no absolute contraindication to regional block should be allowed to wake up. In case of fetal distress there is often difficulty deciding which course to follow. A scoring system for urgency of delivery to aid in the management of failed intubation has been suggested.[10]

If general anaesthesia is to be maintained the woman is deepened with a volatile agent such as halothane or sevoflurane (as these are less irritant than isoflurane) before surgery is started. This avoids straining and possible gastro-oesophageal reflux in response to surgical stimulation. Nitrous oxide may be added provided oxygen saturation is satisfactory and this will allow the concentration of volatile agent to be reduced. High concentrations of volatile agents may result in uterine atony and increased blood loss. After delivery, Syntocinon by bolus and infusion is recommended although it may not be effective when more than 2x MAC of volatile agent is used. Emptying the stomach with an orogastric tube is not advisable in this situation as vomiting and laryngospasm may be precipitated.

It is imperative that all anaesthetists working in the maternity unit are familiar with the failed intubation and ventilation drill. Although many algorithms on how to manage this potentially lethal situation have been produced, the time to read them is not when difficulties with intubation are being encountered.

Anaesthesia for the known difficult airway

Regional anaesthesia is obviously preferred when airway problems are suspected or have occurred. Spinal block provides rapid operating conditions and avoids the risk of total spinal anaesthesia following misplacement of epidural solutions. An intrathecal catheter offers more flexibility than a single-shot spinal. Alternatively, a slow incremental epidural technique may be used if cardiovascular stability is crucial. If regional anaesthesia is contraindicated then awake intubation, usually with the aid of a fibreoptic bronchoscope, followed by general anaesthesia is the technique of choice.[14] However, this requires time, equipment, and expertise. If these are not available then caesarean section must be performed with the infiltration of local anaesthetic. A technique using 80 ml of 0.5% lignocaine with adrenaline has been described but is seldom practised.

Aspiration

Aspiration is the process by which material is carried from the pharynx to the lower respiratory tract. The clinical outcome depends on the volume and nature of the aspirate, its distribution, and the host defence mechanisms. The consequences can vary from relatively benign to fulminant acute respiratory failure and death.[70]

Retrospective work has estimated that the incidence of aspiration in women undergoing caesarean section is about one in 600.[60] More recent prospective analysis revealed no cases of clinical aspiration in 256 elective and 389 emergency caesarean sections under general anaesthesia.[71] Large-volume aspiration of acidic gastric contents may precipitate the appearance of acute lung injury within two hours. Dyspnoea and tachypnoea develop often with a cough productive of pink frothy sputum. Tachycardia and hypotension are observed. Localised or diffuse wheeze and crackles may be heard. Diffuse alveolar infiltrates, usually in the lower lobes, are apparent on the chest X-ray. Worsening hypoxaemia may develop and lead to the adult respiratory distress syndrome (ARDS).

If aspiration occurs, immediate pharyngeal suction of regurgitated material must be performed. The mother should be positioned on her side to prevent further aspiration. If the mother is unconscious, intubation and tracheal suction may be appropriate. Aspiration of food particles may cause airway obstruction at the level of the larynx, trachea or bronchi and laryngoscopy or bronchoscopy may be required to remove solid material. Bronchial lavage is not helpful and may disseminate the aspirated material. If the mother is awake, however, coughing is effective at expelling small fragments of particulate material. Following aspiration, the mother must be nursed on either a high-dependency or intensive care unit. Bronchodilators may sometimes be helpful, but corticosteroids are of no proven benefit and may predispose to infection. Antibiotic treatment is usually not started unless infection is identified. Cardiovascular support may be needed initially with the sudden extravasation of fluid into the lung. Mechanical ventilation may be needed with worsening hypoxaemia in which case further lung injury from hyperoxia and barotrauma must be minimised. Mortality may be as high as 50% if ARDS develops.

Awareness

The last 30 years have fortunately seen a reduction in the incidence of awareness during general anaesthesia for caesarean section. The spectrum of awareness ranges from dreaming through recall of events to being fully conscious and in pain.[72] Light levels of anaesthesia during caesarean section were at one time considered desirable to minimise neonatal depression. This fatuous belief is no longer held as it is now realised that not only is painful awareness a real possibility but that endogenous release of maternal catecholamines decreases uterine perfusion, producing fetal acidosis. Although adequate maternal anaesthesia does increase the amount of drug reaching the baby and causes some neonatal depression, this is an entirely reversible process.

Various methods for detecting maternal awareness have been described. Neither spectral EEG analysis nor lower oesophageal contractility monitoring is widely used. The isolated forearm technique, where an arterial tourniquet is inflated before neuromuscular blockade, is popular with some but may lack sufficient sensitivity.[72]

Awareness is likely to occur if inadequate doses of induction agents are used in addition to little or no inspired volatile agent. If volatile anaesthetic agents are not used the incidence of awareness is as high as 25%.[28] Fortunately such techniques have been abandoned although cases of awareness are still reported. To investigate the incidence of awareness a team at St James Hospital in Leeds, UK, questioned over 3000 patients following caesarean section under general anaesthesia. Before 1985 the protocol for general anaesthesia was induction with thiopentone 3–4 mg/kg maintained with halothane 0.5% in 50% oxygen with nitrous oxide up to delivery. At this time the halothane was switched off, the nitrous oxide increased to 70% and an intravenous opioid given. This technique produced an incidence of awareness of 1.3% with recall of dreaming during surgery of 7%. The protocol was changed in 1985. The induction dose of thiopentone was increased to 5–7 mg/kg and halothane replaced with isoflurane 1% which was continued after delivery at a lower concentration. This change reduced the incidence of awareness to 0.4% and dreaming to 4%. None of the 3000 patients reported being in pain and none could recall the whole operation.[73]

Unless patients are questioned specifically about awareness then underreporting occurs. During their consent to caesarean section under general anaesthesia women should be informed of an incidence of recall of part of the operation of one in 100 but that pain will not be part of the experience.[73] If painful awareness occurs, a psychiatric sequel, such as post-traumatic stress disorder, is a distinct possibility.

References

1 Brown GW, Russell IF. A survey of anaesthesia for Caesarean section. *Int J Obstet Anesth* 1995;4:214–18.

2 Department of Health. *NHS maternity statistics, England: 1989–90 to 1994–95.* Bulletin 1997/28, Tables 5 and 19. London: DoH, 1997.

3 Department of Health. *Report on confidential enquiries into maternal deaths in the UK 1988–1990.* London: HMSO, 1994.

4 Department of Health. *Report on confidential enquiries into maternal deaths in the UK 1991–1993.* London: HMSO, 1997.

5 Department of Health. *Report on confidential enquiries into maternal deaths in the UK 1994–1996.* London: HMSO, 1997.

6 Mallampati SR, Gatt SP, Gugino SP, *et al.* A clinical sign to predict difficult tracheal intubation: a prospective study. *Can Anaesth Soc J* 1985;32:429–34.

7 Patil VU, Stehling LC, Zaunder HL. *Fibreoptic endoscopy in anesthesia.* Chicago: Year Book Medical Publishers, 1983.

8 Calder I, Calder J, Crockard HA. Difficult direct laryngoscopy in patients with cervical spine disease. *Anaesthesia* 1995;50:756–63.

9 Frerk CM. Predicting difficult intubation. *Anaesthesia* 1991;46:1005–8.

10 Harmer M. Difficult and failed intubation in obstetrics. *Int J Obstet Anesth* 1997;6:25–31.

11 Hawthorne L, Wilson R, Lyons G, Dresner M. Failed intubation revisited: 17-yr experience in a teaching maternity unit. *Br J Anaesth* 1996;76:680–4.

12 Pilkington S, Carli F, Dakin MJ, *et al.* Increase in Mallampati score during pregnancy. *Br J Anaesth* 1995;**74**:638–42.

13 Dresner M. Increased Mallampati score during labour. Proceedings of the Obstetric Anaesthetic Association Meeting, Glasgow, 1996.

14 Broomhead CJ, Davies W, Higgins D. Awake oral fibreoptic intubation for Caesarean section. *Int J Obstet Anesth* 1995;**4**:172–4.

15 Mendleson CL. The aspiration of stomach contents into the lungs in obstetric anesthesia. *Am J Obstet Gynecol* 1946;**52**:191.

16 O'Sullivan G. Gastric emptying during pregnancy and the puerperium. *Int J Obstet Anesth* 1993;**2**:216–24.

17 Vanner RG, Goodman NW. Gastro-oesophageal reflux in pregnancy at term and after delivery. *Anaesthesia* 1989;**44**:808–11.

18 Benhamou D, Vanner RG. Controversies in obstetric anaesthesia: cricoid pressure is unnecessary in obstetric general anaesthesia. *Int J Obstet Anesth* 1995;**4**:30–3.

19 Schwartz DJ, Wynne JW, Gibbs CP, Hood CI, Kuck EJ. The pulmonary consequences of aspiration of gastric contents at pH values greater than 2.5. *Am Rev Respir Dis* 1980;**121**:119–26.

20 Ewart MC, Yau G, Gin T, Kotur CF, Oh TE. A comparison of the effects of omeprazole and ranitidine on gastric secretion in women undergoing elective Caesarean section. *Anaesthesia* 1990;**45**:527–30.

21 Yau G, Kan AF, Gin T, Oh TE. A comparison of omeprazole and ranitidine for prophylaxis against aspiration pneumonitis in emergency Caesarean section. *Anaesthesia* 1992;**47**:101–4.

22 Stuart JC, Kan AF, Rowbottom SJ, Yau G, Oh TE. Acid aspiration prophylaxis for emergency Caesarean section. *Anaesthesia* 1996;**51**:415–21.

23 Crawford JS, Burton M, Davies P. Anaesthesia for section: further refinement of technique. *Br J Anaesth* 1973;**45**:726–32.

24 Bassell GM, Marx GF. Optimization of fetal oxygenation. *Int J Obstet Anesth* 1995;**4**:238–43.

25 Crawford JS, Burton M, Davies P. Time and lateral tilt at Caesarean section. *Br J Anaesth* 1972;**44**:447–84.

26 McCrirrick A, Evans GH, Thomas T. Overpressure isoflurane at Caesarean section: a study of arterial isoflurane concentrations. *Br J Anaesth* 1994;**72**:122–4.

27 Piggott SE, Bogod DG, Rosen M, Rees GAD, Harmer M. Isoflurane with either 100% oxygen or 50% nitrous oxide in oxygen for Caesarean section. *Br J Anaesth* 1990;**65**:325–9.

28 Warren T, Datta S, Ostheimer GW, Naulty JS, Weiss JB, Morrison JA. Comparison of the maternal and neonatal effects of halothane, enflurane and isoflurane for cesarean delivery. *Anesth Analg* 1983;**62**:516–20.

29 Jordan MJ, Brighouse D. Controversies in obstetric anaesthesia – modern pre-medication renders rapid sequence induction obsolete in general anaesthesia for elective Caesarean section. *Int J Obstet Anesth* 1993;**2**:106–9.

30 Cook TM, McCrirrick A. A survey of airway management during induction of general anaesthesia in obstetrics: are the recommendations in the Confidential Enquiries into Maternal Deaths being implemented? *Int J Obstet Anesth* 1994;**3**:143–5.

31 Archer GW, Marx GF. Arterial oxygen tension during apnoea in the parturient woman. *Br J Anaesth* 1974;**46**:358–60.

32 Norris MC, Dewan DM. Pre-oxygenation for Caesarean section: a comparison of two techniques. *Anesthesiology* 1985;**62**:827–9.

33 Sellick BA. Cricoid pressure to control regurgitation of stomach contents during induction of anaesthesia. *Lancet* 1961, 2:404–6.

34 Vanner RG, O'Dwyer JP, Pryle BJ, Reynolds F. Upper oesophageal sphincter pressure and the effect of cricoid pressure. *Anaesthesia* 1992;**47**:95–100.

35 Crawford JS. *Principles and practice of obstetric anaesthesia*, 5th edn. Oxford: Blackwell Scientific Publications, 1984.

36 Crawford JS. The 'contracricoid' cuboid aid to tracheal intubation (letter). *Anaesthesia* 1982;**37**:345.

37 Yentis SM. The effects of single-handed and bimanual cricoid pressure on the view at laryngoscopy. *Anaesthesia* 1997;**52**:332–5.

38 Cook TM. Cricoid pressure: are two hands better than one? *Anaesthesia* 1996;**51**:365–8.
39 Vanner RG, Clarke P, Moore WJ, Raftery S. The effect of cricoid pressure and neck support on the view at laryngoscopy. *Anaesthesia* 1997;**52**:896–900.
40 Vanner RG, Pryle BJ. Regurgitation and oesophageal rupture with cricoid pressure: a cadaver study. *Anaesthesia* 1992;**47**:732–5.
41 Hartsilver EL, Vanner RG, Bewely J, Clayton T. Gastric pressure during emergency Caesarean section under general anaesthesia. *Br J Anaesth* 1999;**82**:752–4.
42 Vanner RG, Pryle BJ, O'Dwyer JP, Reynolds F. Upper oesophageal sphincter pressure and the intravenous induction of anaesthesia. *Anaesthesia* 1992;**47**:371–5.
43 Vanner RG. Tolerance of cricoid pressure by conscious volunteers. *Int J Obstet Anesth* 1992;**1**:195–8.
44 Herman NL, Carter B, van Decar TK. Cricoid pressure: teaching the recommended level. *Anesth Analg* 1996;**83**:859–63.
45 Vanner RG, Asai T. Safe use of cricoid pressure (editorial). *Anaesthesia* 1999;**54**:1–3.
46 Allman KG. The effect of cricoid pressure application on airway patency. *J Clin Anesth.* 1995;**7**:197–9.
47 Lawes EG, Duncan PW, Bland B, Gemmel L, Downing JW. The cricoid yoke – a device for providing consistent and reproducible cricoid pressure. *Br J Anaesth* 1986;**58**:925–31.
48 Tournadre JP, Chassard D, Berrada KR, Bouletreau P. Cricoid cartilage pressure decreases lower esophageal sphincter tone. *Anesthesiology* 1997;**86**:7–9.
49 Skinner H, Girling K, Bedforth N, Mahajan R. Effect of cricoid pressure on gastro-oesophageal reflux. *Br J Anaesth* 1998;**80**:A163.
50 Lussos SA, Datta S. Anesthesia for cesarean delivery. Part III: General anesthesia. *Int J Obstet Anesth* 1993;**2**:109–23.
51 Capogna G, Celleno D, Sebastiani M, *et al.* Propofol and thiopentone for Caesarean section revisited: maternal effects and neonatal outcome. *Int J Obstet Anesth* 1991;**1**:19–23.
52 Allen RW, James MFM, Uys PC. Attenuation of the pressor response to tracheal intubation in hypertensive proteinuric pregnant patients by lignocaine, alfentanil and magnesium sulphate. *Br J Anaesth* 1991;**66**:216–23.
53 Gambling DR, Sharma SK, White PF, van Beveren T, Bala AS, Gouldson R. Use of sevoflurane during elective cesarean birth: a comparison with isoflurane and spinal anesthesia. *Anesth Analg* 1995;**81**:90–5.
54 Abboud TK, Zhu J, Richardson M, Peres da Silva E, Donovan M. Desflurane: a new volatile anesthetic for cesarean section. Maternal and neonatal effects. *Acta Anaesthesiol Scand* 1995;**39**:723–6.
55 James MFM. Magnesium in obstetric anaesthesia. *Int J Obstet Anesth* 1998;**8**:115–23.
56 Abouleish E, Abboud T, Lechevalier T, Zhu J, Chalian A, Alford K. Rocuronium (Org 9426) for caesarean section. *Br J Anaesth* 1994;**73**:336–41.
57 Cormack RS, Lehane J. Difficult tracheal intubation in obstetrics. *Anaesthesia* 1984;**39**:1105–11.
58 Brimacombe JR, Berry AM. Cricoid pressure in chaos. *Anaesthesia* 1997;**52**:924–6.
59 Tunstall ME. Failed intubation drill. *Anaesthesia* 1976;**31**:850.
60 Olsson GL, Hallen B, Hambraeus-Jonzon K. Aspiration during anaesthesia: a computer-aided study of 185 358 anaesthetics. *Acta Anaesthesiol Scand* 1986;**30**:84–92.
61 Meek T, Vincent A, Duggan JE. Cricoid pressure: can protective force be sustained? *Br J Anaesth* 1998;**80**:672–4.
62 O'Mullane EJ. Vomiting and regurgitation during anaesthesia. *Lancet* 1954;**1**:1209–12.
63 Brimacombe JR, Berry AM. The laryngeal mask airway for obstetric anesthesia and neonatal resuscitation. *Int J Obstet Anesth* 1994;**3**:211–18.
64 Asai T, Barclay K, Power I, Vaughan RS. Cricoid pressure impedes the placement of the laryngeal mask airway. *Br J Anaesth* 1995;**74**:521–5.
65 Strang TI. Does the laryngeal mask airway compromise cricoid pressure. *Anaesthesia* 1992;**47**:829–31.
66 Asai T, Barclay K, McBeth C Vaughan RS. Cricoid pressure applied after placement of the laryngeal mask prevents gastric insufflation but inhibits ventilation. *Br J Anaesth* 1996;**76**:772–6.
67 Dworkin R, Benumof JL, Benumof R, Karagianes TG. The effective tracheal diameter that causes air trapping during jet ventilation. *J Cardiothorac Anesth* 1990;**4**:731–6.

68 Mercer MH, Gabbot DA. Influence of neck position on ventilation using the Combitube airway. *Anaesthesia* 1998;**53**:146–50.

69 Klein H, Williamson M, Sue-Ling HM, *et al.* Esophageal rupture associated with the use of the Combitube. *Anesth Analg* 1997;**85**:937–9.

70 Lykens MG, Bowton DL. Aspiration and acute lung injury. *Int J Obstet Anesth* 1993;**2**:236–40.

71 Warner MA, Warner ME, Weber JG. Clinical significance of pulmonary aspiration during the perioperative period. *Anesthesiology* 1993;**78**:56–62.

72 Bogod DG, Orton JK, Yau HM, OH TE. Detecting awareness during general anaesthetic Caesarean section. *Anaesthesia* 1990;**45**:279–84.

73 Lyons G, MacDonald R. Awareness during Caesarean section. *Anaesthesia* 1991;**46**:62–4.

6: The parturient with co-existing disease

PHILIPPA GROVES, MICHAEL AVIDAN

Introduction

Anaesthetists can make an important contribution to the management of the pregnant woman with coexisting disease. Cooperation between obstetrician, physician, anaesthetist, and neonatologist from early pregnancy gives the best chance of successful outcome for both mother and baby. This chapter does not attempt to cover all diseases that may occur in pregnancy but focuses on the more important conditions that may be encountered by the obstetric anaesthetist. The aim is therefore to emphasise key aspects of certain diseases, especially when the disease, or its management, is significantly altered by pregnancy or when there are particular anaesthetic implications.

Pre-eclampsia

Hypertensive disorders in pregnancy affect more than 10% of women. Preeclampsia (or pregnancy-induced hypertension) may be defined as the development of hypertension with proteinuria, hyperuricaemia, and oedema, usually after 20 weeks gestation unless associated with a hydatidiform mole. Oedema is not essential for the diagnosis as it is a frequent symptom in normal pregnancy. Chronic hypertension is that which predates pregnancy or develops before the 20th week. Pregnant women with chronic hypertension are at increased risk of superimposed pre-eclampsia and placental abruption, whilst perinatal morbidity and mortality are both increased.

To diagnose pre-eclampsia, the diastolic blood pressure (usually Korotkov IV) must be greater than 90 mmHg on two separate readings fours hours apart or greater than 110 mmHg on a single reading. Proteinuria more than 0.3 g/l in a 24-hour collection or 1 g/l in two random samples is significant.

Aetiology

The precise mechanism by which pre-eclampsia develops remains unclear. Failure of trophoblastic invasion and arterial occlusion with fibrin, platelets, and macrophages are known to occur. This reduces uteroplacental blood flow, leading to placental ischaemia. Widespread endothelial damage follows possibly resulting from the release of a humoral factor from the placenta (Fig 6.1).[1] Plasma cellular fibronectin (a marker of endothelial cell activation and damage) concentrations are significantly higher in pregnancies complicated by pre-eclampsia.

Cardiovascular adaptation seen in normal pregnancy is impaired in the pre-eclamptic patient. Sensitivity to angiotensin II is usually lost but in pre-eclampsia sensitivity is increased. Furthermore, cardiac output and plasma volume are reduced, whilst systemic vascular resistance is increased. In pre-eclampsia there is also an imbalance favouring thromboxane A_2, a vasoconstrictor and promoter of platelet aggregation, over prostacyclin which opposes these actions. The use of aspirin is therefore an attractive theoreti-

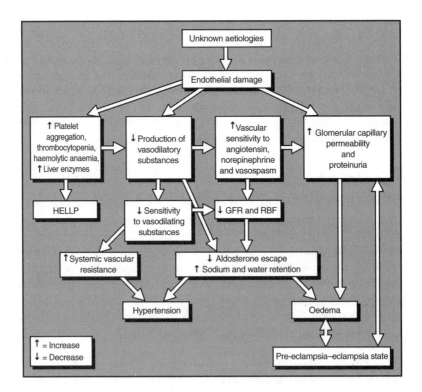

Fig 6.1 Hypothesis of mechanism by which endothelial damage leads to preeclampsia and eclampsia (from Boxer and Malinow[1] with permission). HELLP: haemolysis, elevated liver enzymes, low platelets

cal treatment for this condition. However, the Collaborative Low-dose Aspirin in Pregnancy (CLASP) Study suggests that low-dose aspirin may only be of benefit in those at high risk of early-onset pre-eclampsia.[2]

Risk Factors

Several risk factors associated with the development of pre-eclampsia have been identified (Box 6.1). Pre-eclampsia is primarily a disease of first pregnancy; should this pregnancy proceed normally, development of pre-eclampsia in a subsequent pregnancy is unlikely. Conversely, a history of pre-eclampsia increases risk for future pregnancies. Pre-eclampsia is more likely to develop where there is a family history of the condition. The risk is also greater in those with pre-existing hypertension and other medical conditions such as diabetes, obesity, and renal disease. There is also a strong association between pre-eclampsia and multiple pregnancy and hydatidiform mole, suggesting that excessive placental tissue increases risk. It appears likely that the development of pre-eclampsia has an immunological basis.

Box 6.1   Risk factors for pre-eclampsia

- Nulliparity
- Past history of pre-eclampsia
- Family history of pre-eclampsia
- Past history of hypertension
- Extremes of maternal age
- Hydatidiform mole
- Coexisting disease:
    renal disease
    obesity
    diabetes
    antiphospholipid syndrome
- Multiple pregnancy

Clinical features

Although most commonly diagnosed on routine blood pressure check, the widespread endothelial damage seen in pre-eclampsia produces a multisystem disorder.

Cardiovascular

Endothelial damage leads to altered production of humoral mediators of smooth muscle reactivity. This produces increased systemic vascular resistance, hypertension, decreased circulating volume, and increased left ventricular work. Central venous pressure (CVP) correlates poorly with left ventricular end-diastolic volume in pre-eclampsia. Therefore overreliance on CVP values when managing intravenous fluid replacement may potentially precipitate pulmonary oedema despite relative hypovolaemia (see below).

Respiratory

Excessive urinary loss of plasma proteins reduces colloid osmotic pressure. This, combined with endothelial damage in pulmonary vasculature, increases the risk of pulmonary oedema in the pre-eclamptic patient, especially if injudicious fluid loading is performed.

Renal

Renal blood flow and glomerular filtration rate are reduced with associated increases in renin, angiotensin atrial natriuretic factor, and catecholamines. Endothelial damage, rather than hypovolaemia, is the major cause of poor urine output. Progression to renal failure is possible should haemorrhage or hypoxia occur. Decreased urate clearance produces the well-recognised increase in serum levels.

CNS

The major neurological features of pre-eclampsia, namely headache, visual disturbance, eclamptic fits, and intracerebral bleeding, are thought to be the result of altered cerebral blood flow. Although originally attributed to changes similar to those of hypertensive encephalopathy, symptoms are more likely caused by cerebrovasospasm severe enough to cause focal ischaemia. Indeed, 20% of women with eclampsia have little or no evidence of hypertension.

Hepatic

Serum transaminase levels may be raised secondary to vasospasm and ischaemia. Subcapsular swelling produces right upper quadrant pain and may herald haematoma or even rupture. Elevated liver enzymes form part of the HELLP syndrome. The HELLP (Haemolysis, Elevated Liver enzymes, Low Platelets) syndrome is not uncommon in severe pre-eclampsia. Patients may present with malaise, epigastric pain or nausea and vomiting. Haemolysis results from red cell trauma by damaged endothelium and fibrin mesh deposits. Elevated liver enzymes are caused by hepatic necrosis with disseminated intravascular coagulation (DIC) responsible for a reduction in platelet number.

Haematology

The hypercoagulable state of pregnancy and endothelial damage with sluggish peripheral flow increase the risk of venous thrombosis. Consumptive coagulopathy may develop, producing an increase in fibrin degradation products (FDP). Platelet numbers fall due to increased aggregation and destruction and when their number fall below $100 \times 10^9/l$, other parameters of coagulation should be checked before performing a regional block.

Management (see Chapter 7)

The ultimate cure for pre-eclampsia is termination of pregnancy or delivery. Management should focus on control of blood pressure, preventing fits, and appropriate fluid management. For the anaesthetist, there are concerns over the safety of certain regional techniques and the problems associated with general anaesthesia.

Hypertension

Controlling blood pressure reduces both maternal and neonatal morbidity. Treatment should aim to keep the blood pressure at or below 140/90 mmHg. Aggressive reductions in blood pressure should be avoided as placental perfusion may be compromised.

Methyldopa is one of the most commonly used antihypertensive agents in the UK. Its lack of adverse effects on the baby is well established although larger doses may cause maternal sedation and depression. For this latter reason, treatment is usually changed after delivery. β-Blockers may be effective in controlling blood pressure but there is a suggestion that atenolol is associated with intrauterine growth retardation. Similar adverse effect does not appear to be associated with the mixed α- and β-blocker labetalol. Nifedipine has been used when treatment with methyldopa is either inadequate or contraindicated. Care should be taken if calcium channel blockers are used in conjunction with magnesium as significant hypotension and respiratory weakness may result.

When acute control of blood pressure is required nifedipine, hydralazine or labetalol may be used. The use of hydralazine, a direct arterial vasodilator, is limited to the emergency situation, as tachyphylaxis develops. Angiotensin-converting enzyme inhibitors are contraindicated in pregnancy as they may cause renal failure in the developing fetus.

Convulsions

It has now been established that magnesium sulphate is more effective at preventing further fits in the eclamptic patient than either phenytoin or diazepam.[3] However, there is still debate about the indications for magnesium in pre-eclampsia as it is often difficult to predict who may go on to develop eclampsia. Furthermore, there have been suggestions that in some situations, magnesium may have adverse effects on the baby. Further studies are required to determine the place of magnesium in the treatment of pre-eclampsia.

205

Fluid Management

Relative hypovolaemia and poor urine output are often seen in severe pre-eclampsia. Should the urine output fall below 0.4 ml/kg/min, CVP monitoring is advisable.[4] In those with impaired coagulation, it is prudent to use a long line inserted through a peripheral vein. Aggressive fluid replacement or attempts to maintain a predetermined CVP should be avoided as pulmonary oedema may be precipitated. Indications for pulmonary artery catheterisation continue to be debated. Its use is not without complications and placement has not been demonstrated to improve outcome. It may, however, provide useful information in patients with pulmonary oedema or renal failure.

Anaesthetic management

Regional analgesia and anaesthesia and coagulation

Abnormalities in coagulation may potentially contraindicate regional analgesia and anaesthesia in the pre-eclamptic patient. Blocks may usually be sited with a platelet count of greater than 75×10^9 /l provided clotting studies are normal. There is little evidence to support the usefulness of the bleeding time as a diagnostic test before embarking upon regional anaesthesia.[5] The thromboelastograph has been used to evaluate clotting in women with PET.[6] However, it has yet to become an established tool in pre-eclampsia management. The use of low-dose aspirin and prophylactic subcutaneous heparin does not contraindicate epidural or spinal blocks.[7] In the presence of severe coagulopathy, regional blocks should be avoided.

Epidural or spinal anaesthesia for caesarean section

Controversy surrounds the safety of spinal anaesthesia in severe pre-eclampsia. It has been argued that precipitous falls in blood pressure may follow induction of spinal anaesthesia,[8] although evidence to support this comes from poorly controlled studies. Several small studies now point to the safety of spinal anaesthesia in severe pre-eclampsia. For this issue to be resolved, the results of large prospective randomised studies are awaited. Whichever method of anaesthesia is chosen, fluid loading should be performed with care and vasopressors used judiciously.

General anaesthesia

General anaesthesia may be required for caesarean section when there is a severe coagulopathy, maternal hypovolaemia or depressed level of consciousness. Efforts should be made to obtund the hypertensive response to tracheal intubation as this may potentially increase the risk of cerebral haemorrhage. This may be done with a combination of magnesium (30–40 mg/kg) and alfentanil (5–10 µg/kg).[9] Magnesium increases sensitivity to non-depolarising muscle relaxants and may mask fasciculations after suxemethonium. The β-blocker esmolol produces fetal bradycardia and should be avoided predelivery but may be valuable in preventing a rise in blood pressure on extubation.

Although there is a possibility of airway oedema in the pre-eclamptic patient, its significance in relation to difficulty with intubation has in the view of some been overstated.[4] Whether or not this is true, it may be wise to deflate the cuff of the tracheal tube before extubation and occlude the lumen whilst checking that the woman can breathe, to ensure that the upper airway is not too oedematous.

Postpartum management

High-dependency or intensive care may be necessary after delivery when strict attention to fluid balance is vital. Magnesium therapy is usually continued for 24 hours after which calcium channel blockers may be started. Antihypertensive regimens may be reviewed and methyldopa replaced by β-blockers.

Cardiac disease

Cardiac disease remains a leading non-obstetric cause of maternal death although the pattern of disease is changing. The incidence of cardiac disease in pregnancy has fallen over the last 25 years and it is now estimated to complicate 1.5–2% of pregnancies.[10] This fall is due to the decline in rheumatic heart disease which in the past has accounted for the majority of cases. However, because of improved medical and surgical treatment of congenital heart disease, increasing numbers of women born with these defects are now reaching childbearing age. Maternal mortality for women with heart disease varies depending on severity . Those in New York Heart Association (NYHA) symptomatic classes I and II (Box 6.2) generally do well with mortalities of <1%.[11] However, those in NYHA classes III and IV have a 75–90% risk of maternal mortality and a high incidence of fetal loss. Certain specific conditions also carry a high mortality (Boxes 6.3 and 6.4).

Cardiac disease and pregnancy

Box 6.2 New York Heart Association functional classification
Class I — Asymptomatic
Class II — Slight limitation of physical activities; comfortable at rest
Class III — Marked limitation with less than ordinary activity causing fatigue, palpitation, dyspnoea or angina; remains comfortable at rest
Class IV — Symptomatic at rest

Box 6.3   Circumstances in which successful pregnancy outcome is likely

New York Heart Association class I or II symptoms before pregnancy
Absence of pulmonary hypertension
Able to increase stroke volume or tolerate tachycardia
Simple acyanotic congenital defects
Regurgitant valve disease

Box 6.4   High-risk conditions

Mitral stenosis
Left ventricular outflow tract obstruction
Pulmonary hypertension
Peripartum cardiomyopathy
Complicated coarctation of the aorta

It has been suggested that the key to a good outcome for those with cardiac disease in pregnancy is accurate diagnosis, allowing the best estimate of the impact of cardiovascular changes of pregnancy and the recognition of a high-risk situation. The Confidential Enquiries into Maternal Deaths stress the importance of thorough investigation of any woman with symptoms suggestive of heart disease.[12,13] Therefore, early referral to a cardiologist for assessment is appropriate if cardiac disease is suspected. There should be no hesitation in obtaining a chest X-ray as screening can be provided to make the risk to the fetus negligible.[14]

The physiological adaptation to pregnancy (see Chapter 1) may not be tolerated by the woman with cardiac disease. Cardiac output increases by 30–50% as a result of increases in both stroke volume and heart rate. These changes start early in the first trimester and are approaching maximum by 24 weeks gestation.[15] Cardiac output increases again in labour and is maximal in the third stage with placental expulsion, uterine contraction with associated autotransfusion and the cessation of aortocaval compression. During the first few hours of the puerperium, cardiac output remains elevated.

Antibiotic prophylaxis should be administered to women with structural cardiac disease undergoing operative delivery and for those with prosthetic heart valves, surgical shunts or a history of bacterial endocarditis. In other cases antibiotic prophylaxis is discretionary.

Anaesthetic considerations

A multidisciplinary approach to antenatal care is vital for any pregnant woman with heart disease. This should include a senior obstetrician, cardiologist, and anaesthetist. Delivery should take place in a unit accustomed to the care of pregnant cardiac patients. There must be a clear plan for delivery and, where necessary, emergency intervention. Anaesthetic management should be documented well in advance of delivery. There is no place for initial assessment of a pregnant patient with cardiac disease in labour unless absolutely unavoidable.

Acyanotic congenital heart disease

Most patients with asymptomatic acyanotic congenital heart disease have a successful outcome to pregnancy (Box 6.3).

Atrial septal defect (ASD)

This is one of the most common congenital heart defects in adults. The secundum defect may be diagnosed for the first time in pregnancy. The complications of the defect – arrhythmias, pulmonary hypertension, and right ventricular failure – are not commonly seen until the fourth and fifth decades and most women tolerate pregnancy well. Supraventricular arrhythmias are poorly tolerated as they may increase left-to-right shunting and the acute onset of these should be treated promptly. Cardioversion may be required if right ventricular failure or systemic hypotension occur. Women with ASDs do not tolerate rapid blood loss well and diversion of blood through the defect may result in an abrupt fall in cardiac output. Epidural analgesia in labour is beneficial as increases in systemic vascular resistance with contractions are avoided.

Ventricular septal defect (VSD)

This occurs in less than 10% of adults with congenital heart disease. Outcome depends on the size of the defect and degree of pulmonary hypertension. Most large VSDs are corrected in childhood and thus in adult patients, the defect is usually small and pregnancy is well tolerated. In the asymptomatic patient special monitoring and management in labour are not required. However, with larger VSDs, epidural analgesia in labour may be beneficial in avoiding the increases in systemic vascular resistance associated with painful contractions. For caesarean section, either regional or general anaesthesia may be used; epidural may be preferable to subarachnoid block because the changes in systemic resistance are slower and more time for compensation is available.

Congenital aortic stenosis

This not uncommon congenital cardiac condition in adults is usually the result of a bicuspid valve. It may be asymptomatic despite a loud systolic murmur and these patients usually have uncomplicated pregnancies. Complications are heralded by the onset of dyspnoea, angina or resting tachycardia and such patients require hospital admission. Echocardiography should be performed to assess peak aortic velocity, ventricular function, and valve area which at the onset of new symptoms may be reduced to less than 0.75 cm^2.

As patients with aortic stenosis have a fixed cardiac output they are unable to compensate for decreases in systemic vascular resistance except by increasing their heart rate. However, at rates greater than 140, diastolic filling is reduced together with cardiac output. Atrial fibrillation causes reduced ventricular filling and should be treated promptly.

Epidural analgesia and anaesthesia should be used with caution, gradually administering local anaesthetic to extend block height slowly; single-shot spinal anaesthesia is best avoided. General anaesthesia should also be administered cautiously, again because of the possibility of dropping systemic vascular resistance. Controversy surrounds the choice of anaesthesia for caesarean section in women with aortic stenosis.[16,17] It has been suggested that the choice of anaesthetic may be less important than the care with which it is given; women with symptomatic aortic stenosis need a highly experienced anaesthetist and full monitored care.[18]

Persistent patent ductus arteriosus

Although this condition constitutes a significant proportion of congenital heart disease, surgical correction of large defects early in life means that important lesions rarely present in pregnancy. Anaesthetic considerations are similar to those for VSD and ASD when epidural analgesia in labour is recommended.

Coarctation of the aorta

Coarctation is usually corrected in infancy although occasionally it may be diagnosed in pregnancy. Even those with uncorrected coarctation tolerate pregnancy well, although there is a risk of aortic dissection, rupture of a berry aneurysm, infective endocarditis, and heart failure.

Cyanotic congenital heart disease

Tetralogy of Fallot

Patients with uncorrected defects have an increased morbidity and mortality in pregnancy, especially if they have a history of syncope, polycythaemia, right ventricular failure, and oxygen saturations of <80%. The decrease in systemic vascular resistance during pregnancy increases the right-to-left shunt, producing maternal cyanosis, poor fetal growth and increased fetal loss.

210

Further reduction in systemic vascular resistance, venous return, and blood volume are poorly tolerated because they increase right-to-left shunt. Hence, for labour and vaginal delivery it has frequently been suggested that these patients are probably most safely managed with systemic medication, inhalational analgesia or pudendal block, although the quality of these methods of pain relief may be poor. Regional techniques should only be used with extreme caution and general anaesthesia is probably the technique of choice for caesarean section.

Eisenmenger's syndrome

This refers to congenital heart disease (usually ASD, VSD, patent pulmonary ductus) in which increased pulmonary vascular resistance leads to a reversed shunt (right to left). These patients have a poor life expectancy (survival beyond age 40 is rare) and are at severe risk in pregnancy (maternal mortality around 30%). It has been recommended that such women should not get pregnant or should have a therapeutic abortion in early pregnancy. Clearly, the final decision is with the woman and if pregnancy continues she will require admission to a specialist centre and her progress must be closely monitored, particularly her oxygen saturation and fetal growth. Prophylactic subcutaneous heparin is often administered. Delivery by caesarean section under general anaesthesia with full invasive monitoring has been recommended. Anaesthetic considerations are similar to those for tetralogy of Fallot. Decreases in systemic vascular resistance and venous return and increases in pulmonary vascular resistance, resulting from hypercarbia, acidosis, and hypoxia, should be avoided. Regional blocks are normally avoided and general anaesthesia should only be administered with extreme caution.

Rheumatic valve disease

Although the incidence of rheumatic heart disease has declined dramatically in the British population, cases may still present in young immigrants.

Mitral stenosis

The mitral valve is most commonly affected by rheumatic fever and symptoms usually appear in the second or third decade if the initial streptococcal infection occurred in childhood. The natural history of the condition is for symptoms to proceed rapidly towards total incapacity within a few years if surgical correction does not occur. Flow through the stenotic valve is reduced, increasing left atrial pressure and eventually leading to pulmonary oedema. Secondary pulmonary hypertension may develop culminating in right ventricular failure. During pregnancy the increase in heart rate reduces diastolic filling time and increases left atrial pressure. Should atrial fibrillation develop, left atrial pressure rises, further hastening the onset of pulmonary oedema. Patients are usually managed with β-blockers and additional diuretics. If medical treatment fails, balloon valvotomy may be performed. Anticoagulants are often used to minimise the risk of mural thrombus formation.

For women not receiving anticoagulants, epidural analgesia for labour using low-dose local anaesthetics is recommended. Rapid ventricular rates associated with painful contractions are avoided and increases in central blood volume minimised. For caesarean section epidural block may again be suitable but levels should be increased cautiously to avoid sudden decreases in systemic vascular resistance.

Aortic stenosis

This is relatively rare in pregnancy as there is usually a 35–40-year latent period between acute rheumatic fever and symptoms of severe stenosis. Anaesthetic considerations are dealt with above under congenital aortic stenosis.

Valvular insufficiencies

Regurgitant valve disease is well tolerated in pregnancy because the physiological vasodilation and slight increase in heart rate tend to reduce regurgitation. Thus, epidural analgesia is recommended for labour and delivery. However patients who also have Marfan's syndrome are at risk of aortic dissection or rupture in pregnancy and are usually maintained on β-blockade.

Valvular prostheses

These women usually have adequate cardiac reserve for pregnancy but in those with mechanical prosthesis, meticulous attention to anticoagulant therapy is required because of the induced hypercoagulable state. Although maternal mortality is low, morbidity is increased as are fetal mortality and congenital malformations, more so after mitral valve replacement. Bioprostheses should not increase the risks for mother or baby but have a limited life and may deteriorate at an increased rate during pregnancy.

Other heart diseases

Cardiomyopathies

Hypertrophic cardiomyopathy

This condition is usually well tolerated in pregnancy. Although restricted, stroke volume does increase through pregnancy. Women may become symptomatic during pregnancy, reporting dyspnoea, chest pain, and palpitations. β-Blockers are usually the first line of treatment. The risk of sudden death does not appear to be increased. Sudden reductions in afterload are not well tolerated and regional blocks should be used with care.

Peripartum cardiomyopathy

This term is used when dilation of all cardiac chambers and cardiac failure occur during pregnancy or in the first six months postpartum with no other obvious cause. The condition is rare (one in 3000–4000 deliveries) and it is unclear whether it is caused by pregnancy or whether pregnancy exacerbates a pre-existing latent myocardial disorder. At presentation, women may require full cardiac support and may go on to require transplantation. Long-term prognosis is variable with mortality between 15% and 60%. Some women make a good recovery although this may take many months. Recurrence in subsequent pregnancies is not inevitable but is more likely if heart size has not returned to normal within six months of the first episode.

Myocardial infarction

This is a rare event, occurring only in about one in 10 000 pregnancies. However, the incidence may increase as women delay childbearing until they are older. Roth and Elkayam reported that infarction usually occurs in the third trimester in women older than 33 years.[20] The maternal mortality rate is about 20% with a fetal loss in 13%. Most fetal deaths are associated with maternal deaths. Coronary atherosclerosis is the commonest cause but is only present in about 50% of cases where coronary anatomy has been investigated. Coronary thrombosis with normal coronary anatomy has been explained by transient coronary spasm with a background of the hypercoagulable state of pregnancy.

Diagnosis can be difficult as the index of suspicion is low. Furthermore, the creatinine kinase MB isoenzyme is produced by the myometrium and so other methods of confirming the diagnosis are required. Management should follow the usual principles of care, but plans should be made for prompt rescue of a viable fetus should the mother's condition deteriorate suddenly. In the case of cardiac arrest left uterine displacement should not be forgotten and early evacuation of the uterus (within 4–5 minutes) is important.[21] This action may save both mother and baby by relieving aortocaval compression and allowing effective cardiac massage. The use of thrombolytic therapy in pregnancy is relatively contraindicated because of the risks of teratogenicity (although streptokinase and t-PA do not cross the placenta in animals) and haemorrhage (especially if administered at the time of delivery).

For those surviving the initial event, delivery should normally be postponed if possible for 2–3 weeks after infarction to allow some healing to occur. The mode of delivery should be determined on an individual basis; advantages of elective caesarean section include control of the time of delivery and the avoidance of a long and stressful labour, whereas vaginal delivery avoids some of the risks of anaesthesia and a major surgical procedure.[22] Epidural block and elective instrumental delivery reduce cardiac workload and oxygen demands, but obviously extreme caution should be observed to avoid fluctuations in preload and afterload.

Primary pulmonary hypertension

This is a rare disorder that occurs most often in young women.[23] The natural history is usually death within two years of the onset of symptoms. Mortality in pregnancy is in the region of 50%. The pulmonary vasculature becomes increasingly non-reactive and produces a high resistance to right ventricular work, resulting in hypertrophy. Eventually left ventricular output falls because of the failing right ventricle. As for Eisenmenger's syndrome, regional blocks are usually avoided although their successful use for both labour and caesarean section has been reported.[24]

Diabetes mellitus

Diabetes mellitus is one of the more common metabolic disorders. It results from either a decrease in insulin secretion (type 1 or insulin dependent) or from increased resistance to insulin in target tissues (type 2 or non-insulin dependent). Gestational diabetes refers to diabetes that is first diagnosed during pregnancy.

Diabetes and pregnancy

Hypoglycaemia is not uncommon in the first half of diabetic pregnancy as maternal glucose levels fall. The second half of pregnancy is associated with an increase in insulin requirements as hormonal changes result in peripheral insulin resistance.

The changing metabolic demands of pregnancy can result in poor diabetic control. Hypoglycaemic episodes, especially in those on insulin therapy, are not unusual in early pregnancy. Diabetic ketoacidosis, which usually occurs only in insulin dependent diabetes, may be precipitated by infection or trauma. Hyperosmolar non-ketotic coma (diabetic coma) is more common in non-insulin dependent diabetics. Of the chronic complications of diabetes, pregnancy may accelerate the development of proliferative retinopathy. Women with diabetes are more likely to develop pre-eclampsia and polyhydramnios.

In 1954 Pederson suggested that glucose crosses the placenta but insulin does not; maternal hyperglycaemia therefore stimulates the fetal pancreas to produce excess insulin and the resulting anabolic effect produces macrosomia.[25] The increased size of the baby makes operative and instrumental delivery more probable and increases the risk of shoulder dystocia.

Elevated levels of both insulin and glucose lead to increased oxygen requirements, increasing the potential for fetal hypoxia. Increased levels of glycosolated haemoglobin result in a further reduction in fetal oxygenation

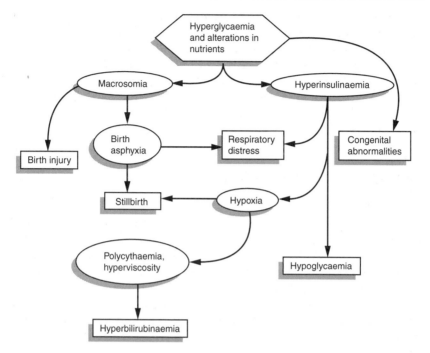

Fig 6.2   The relationship between hyperglycaemia in the mother and problems of the infant (from Steel and Johnstone[26] with permission)

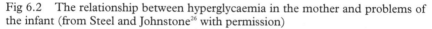

as the ability of maternal haemoglobin to release oxygen in the placental circulation is impaired. Congenital malformations and intrauterine death are therefore not surprisingly increased in diabetes.

High insulin levels also inhibit the enzymes involved in surfactant production. The incidence of respiratory distress syndrome is increased in babies born to poorly controlled diabetic mothers. Neonatal hypoglycaemia and hyperbilirubinaemia are also more common (Fig 6.2), as is the development of diabetes itself.

Anaesthetic Considerations

Diabetic women are more likely to undergo instrumental or operative delivery. Regional analgesia in labour is therefore preferred as the risks of general anaesthesia are avoided. Regional block also attenuates the stress response to labour, thereby decreasing catecholamine and cortisol levels and improving glycaemic control and uteroplacental flow. Furthermore, the mother is more able to recognise the symptoms of hypoglycaemia. During labour, glucose and insulin infusions may be required and blood sugar monitored regularly especially in the period immediately following delivery when insulin requirements may fall dramatically.

215

For elective caesarean section, regional block is again preferred. Fluid preload should not contain either lactate or glucose. The latter has been associated with impairment of umbilical cord gases. The complications of maternal diabetes, namely large and small vessel disease, autonomic neuropathy with gastroparesis, and the stiff joint syndrome, all make general anaesthesia potentially more hazardous. For postoperative pain relief, NSAIDs should be used with caution in those with renal impairment.

Coagulation disorders (Fig 6.3)

Thrombophilia

Venous thromboembolic disease is one of the most common medical disorders complicating pregnancy. The term "thrombophilia" has been applied by the British Society for Haematology to those familial or acquired disorders of haemostasis likely to increase the risk of thrombosis.[27] Congenital thrombophilias are significantly more common than inherited bleeding diatheses and include deficiencies or abnormalities of antithrombin III (ATIII), protein C, protein S, activated protein C resistance (factor V Leiden), and elevated levels of factor VIII. Resistance to activated protein C, the most common genetic risk factor for venous thrombosis, is found in 4% of the general population and 20% of those with diagnosed venous thromboses. Protein S deficiency poses a risk for arterial as well as venous thrombosis.

The most important acquired thrombophilic disorder is the antiphospholipid syndrome (see below). This may be associated with systemic lupus erythematosus and often presents as recurrent thromboses, early miscarriage, and thrombocytopenia.

Thrombophilia and pregnancy

Pregnancy is a physiological thrombophilic state in which levels of procoagulant proteins are increased and anticoagulant activity is reduced. The risk of thrombosis is increased by the gravid uterus compressing the inferior vena cava, causing venous stasis. Platelet activity and plasminogen activator inhibitors increase, both continuing into the postpartum period.

Pregnant women with significant risk factors for thromboembolic disease, especially ATIII deficiency (ATIII is the principal inhibitor of the enzymes of the coagulation network), should receive anticoagulant therapy throughout their pregnancy.[28] The use of warfarin in the first trimester is associated with increased fetal loss and congenital malformations.[29] Warfarin may cause skin necrosis when given to those with protein C or S deficiency and should only be introduced once fully heparinised.[30] As term approaches, heparin, with its shorter half-life and reliable reversibility with

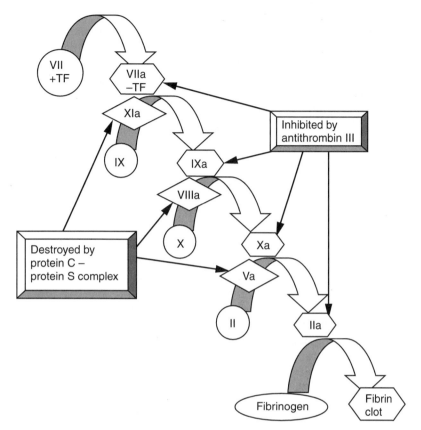

Fig 6.3   The roles played by protein C, protein S, and antithrombin III in opposing coagulation. The diagram shows their actions on various clotting factors

Box 6.5   Risks factors for thromboembolic disease

History of venous thrombosis
Thrombophilia
Caesarean section
Varicose veins
Increasing age
Increasing parity
Major concurrent illness
Pre-eclampsia
Antiphospholipid syndrome
Antepartum bed rest
Obesity

protamine, is considered safer. In women with ATIII deficiency, heparin may be given with ATIII replacement as its activity is dependent on adequate levels of ATIII. Women receiving heparin should be monitored for the development of osteopenia and thrombocytopenia.

Low molecular weight heparins (LMWH), such as enoxaparin and dalteparin, are now being increasingly used. Their pharmacokinetic profile offers more reliability and their longer duration of action allows once-daily administration.

Anaesthetic considerations

The choice of anaesthetic technique may be limited in the fully anticoagulated woman. Regional blocks are generally avoided for fear of producing an expanding haematoma, resulting in neuronal death. This is fortunately an extremely rare complication in the obstetric population. Should surgery be required, general anaesthesia may actually increase the risk of thrombosis as it predisposes to intravascular coagulation.[31]

Assessment of the risks and benefits of regional block should therefore be determined for individual patients. Platelet counts of greater than 100×10^9/ml are generally considered safe and values down to 75×10^9/ml are usually acceptable if clotting studies are normal. Prolongation of clotting time increases risk but it is not possible to state an absolute value at which the risk becomes unacceptable. Various authors have chosen figures which they consider acceptable although studies to validate such opinions are probably not possible. Prothrombin times in excess of 30% of normal range and prolongation of the aPTT by more than 10 seconds to many clinicians represent an unacceptable risk. Bleeding time has been shown to be of little value.[5] Thrombelastography is an interesting research tool but its place in clinical practice has yet to be determined.

It is generally considered safe to perform a regional block on women receiving aspirin and prophylactic doses of subcutaneous heparin (if in doubt the aPPT should be checked).[8] Where full doses of heparin are used, blocks are not usually performed for at least six hours after the last dose and the aPTT has been checked. For LMWH the picture is less clear. To determine the level of anticoagulation, anti-Xa levels are required which are neither easy or quick to perform. It has been stated that blocks are safe provided that at least 12 hours have elapsed after the last dose and that a further dose is not given for the next two hours.[32] However, there are several published cases (not in obstetrics) of spinal haematomas following large doses of enoxaparin.[33]

Von Willebrand's disease

Von Willebrand's disease (vWD) is the most common inherited abnormality of haemostasis, occurring in up to 1% of the population. The von Willebrand factor (vWF) is necessary for platelet adhesiveness and it serves as a carrier for factor VIII (FVIII). The disease may be classified according to severity into three groups. In group 1, accounting for 90% of sufferers, there is a decrease in FVIII:vWF activity. The more severe groups 2 (subdivided into A, B, M, and N) and 3 represent varying abnormalities of platelet-associated vWF. The most sensitive test for all types of vWD is ristocetin cofactor activity, which assesses the ability of vWF to bind with platelet membranes.

Cryoprecipitate has been used to treat vWD but carries a risk of infection. Rh-negative patients should be treated with Rh-negative cryoprecipitate. Other treatment options include recombinant factor VIII:C, fractionated factor VIII:C, fresh frozen plasma, and desmopressin (DDAVP). DDAVP probably leads to the release of platelet-activating factor from monocytes. The recommended dose of DDAVP is 0.3 mcg/kg diluted in 100 ml of isotonic saline infused over 30 minutes. Intranasal preparations are also available. In patients with type 2B vWD, DDAVP may cause a fall in platelet count and should therefore be avoided.[34] DDAVP may also cause water retention and hyponatraemia. If treatment with DDAVP is not efficacious, FVIII:vWF concentrates may be given. Commercial preparations of FVIII concentrates, which are used to treat haemophilia, remove ristocetin co-factor activity and are not useful in vWD. Immunisation against hepatitis (A and B) may be given to those not immune who may require blood products.

Von Willebrand's disease and pregnancy

Type I vWD disease is usually improved by pregnancy as FVIII and vWF concentrations are increased during pregnancy. Women with types II and III vWD, however, may still have a bleeding tendency. Maternal coagulation factors do not rise until the second trimester so women with type I vWD having surgery during the first trimester may bleed profusely.

Anaesthetic considerations

Early consultation with an experienced haematologist is helpful. Regular assessments of FVIII levels can predict which women may potentially develop problems at the time of delivery. For those women with significantly reduced levels of FVIII:vWF, vascular trauma during regional block may produce an expanding spinal or epidural haematoma with resultant neurological damage. Where factor VIII:vWF levels are less than 50%, prophylactic treatment may be given at the onset of labour. For those with vWD group 1 or 2A, DDAVP may be given, whilst in the more severe forms FVIII vWF concentrates are required. Delayed postpartum haemorrhage is a possibility and so levels should be checked in the postnatal period.

219

Sickle cell disease

Sickle cell disorders encompass a group of haemoglobinopathies that represent the most common inherited form of anaemia in pregnancy. Sickle cell anaemia is the result of a genetic point mutation resulting in a substitution of valine for glutamic acid at the sixth position of the β-chain of haemoglobin. Red cells of patients with sickle cell disease aggregate and sickle when the partial pressure of oxygen drops below 5.3 kPa. Sickling also occurs with vascular stasis, falls in body temperature, and acidaemia. As a consequence red cell lifespan is only about 17 days compared with normal values of 120 days.

Sickle cell disease and pregnancy

The physiological changes of pregnancy and labour may result in an exacerbation of sickle cell disease. Women have an increased risk of pneumonia, pyelonephritis, cholecystitis, pulmonary emboli, retinal haemorrhages, and thrombosis. Pre-eclampsia, abruption, placenta praevia, intrauterine growth restriction, and preterm labour are also more common. Such pregnancy complications have also been demonstrated in women with sickle cell trait.[35] It is estimated that 35% of women with sickle cell disease have crises during the antenatal period, with vaso-occlusive problems being the most common.[36] Blood transfusion may be given to maintain a haemoglobin level above 8 g/dl and an HbA value of greater than 40%. Sickle cell crises are less likely if the haemoglobin is kept above 10 g/dl.

The newborn is protected from sickling as fetal haemoglobin (HbF) contains γ rather than β-chains. Increased maternal levels of HbF may be beneficial in reducing adverse effects.[37] Hydroxyurea, in combination with recombinant erythropoietin, stimulates the production of HbF but its safety in pregnancy has not been established as it may reduce white cell and platelet counts.[38]

Anaesthetic considerations

Management is directed to avoiding conditions which predispose to sickling and so women should be kept warm, well oxygenated, hydrated, and pain free. Monitoring hydration may be aided by central venous and urinary catheterisation but the risk of infection may militate against their use. Analgesia is imperative and is most efficacious with regional block as tolerance to narcotics following long-term administration is not uncommon. Furthermore, the incidence of caesarean section is increased in women with sickle cell disease and a working epidural both reduces the need for general anaesthesia and may be used to provide excellent postoperative pain relief.

Left lateral tilt is particularly important in sickle cell patients to avoid stasis of blood and sickling in the lower limbs. The use of a pulse oximeter on a toe may provide useful information. Maternal morbidity may occur in the postpartum period if the mother becomes cold, dehydrated or if pain control is inadequate. With the risks of thrombosis and infection, postnatal antibiotics and thromboprophylaxis are advisable.

Obesity

The WHO definition of obesity is based on body mass index (BMI), which is calculated by dividing the weight in kg by the square of the height in metres. Values greater than 25 are classed as overweight. Classifications based purely on weight lack both sensitivity and specificity. The risks of obesity are presented in Table 6.1.

Table 6.1   Problems associated with obesity in pregnancy

Obstetric problems	Medical problems	Anaesthetic problems
• Diagnosis and dating of pregnancy • Gestational diabetes • Pre-eclampsia • Fetal macrosomia	• Pulmonary dysfunction • Hypertension • Coronary artery disease • Liver disease • Cholelithiasis	• Difficult IV access • Problems siting regional blocks • Unpredictable spread of epidural and spinal solutions • Increased incidence of failed intubation and pulmonary aspiration • Reduced pulmonary reserve and tendency to hypoxia • Excessive aortocaval compression from abdominal panniculus

Obesity and pregnancy

Obesity is a common problem observed in about 10% of pregnancies. It is associated with increased maternal morbidity and mortality as physiology is adversely affected. Oxygen consumption and CO_2 production are increased. However, functional residual capacity and expiratory reserve volume are reduced and closing volume is increased, all predisposing to hypoxaemia. Lung compliance is reduced and a history of sleep apnoea may be elicited. Increased diaphragmatic splinting may further limit respiratory reserve.

Blood volume, already elevated in obese patients, rises during pregnancy, increasing the possibility of left ventricular failure, especially where there is pre-existing hypertension or ischaemic heart disease. Varicose veins and deep vein thrombosis are also more likely, as is the development of pre-eclampsia. Hiatus hernia is more common in the obese, increasing the risks

221

of regurgitation and aspiration during general anaesthesia. Gestational diabetes is seen more often in obese women.

Obesity increases the incidence of obstetric intervention. Induction of labour is more likely because of hypertension and diabetes. Fetal macrosomia may potentially lead to shoulder dystocia.

Anaesthetic considerations

All obese parturients should be assessed by an anaesthetist during pregnancy. A thorough history and examination should identify particular anaesthetic risk factors. In severe cases respiratory function tests, arterial blood gases, and ECG may be performed. The degree of airways closure in different positions may be assessed by pulse oximetry.

Systemic opioids should be used with caution because their sedative effects can worsen existing hypoventilation and hypoxia. Epidural analgesia in labour is particularly beneficial in these women.[39] It offers excellent analgesia, decreases respiratory work and oxygen consumption and prevents increases in cardiac output. Furthermore, the block may be extended for operative delivery should this become necessary. There may, however, be technical difficulties in establishing an epidural block in a morbidly obese woman; epidural insertion should therefore be attempted early in labour.

Successful epidural analgesia may be aided by a long Tuohy needle, the use of the sitting position and threading the catheter at least 5 cm into the epidural space to avoid displacement. The volume of local anaesthetic required to provide adequate epidural analgesia is less in the obese parturient, therefore blocks should be established cautiously.[40] This may be because the epidural space has a decreased capacity due to adipose tissue and venous engorgement from severe aortocaval compression from the gravid uterus and excess abdominal fat. If dural puncture occurs during attempts at epidural insertion, it may be appropriate to consider threading an epidural catheter into the intrathecal space and using continuous spinal analgesia.

Regional block is preferred for operative delivery. Occasionally it may be impossible to measure non-invasive blood pressure successfully and an intra-arterial cannula may be required (this also enables serial blood gas sampling). Positioning to avoid aortocaval compression may be difficult but must not be overlooked as cardiovascular collapse has been reported in obese patients adopting the supine position. Both epidural and spinal anaesthesia have been used with success, although there may be excessive cephalad spread of solutions.[40] Difficult and prolonged surgery is to be expected and so a combined spinal-epidural technique may be preferable to single-shot spinal anaesthesia.

General anaesthesia presents significant risks of failed intubation and aspiration of stomach contents. Positioning is again important; if the shoulders are elevated the breasts tend to fall away from the chin which makes insertion of the laryngoscope into the mouth easier. Adequate pre-oxygenation is essential because oxygen saturation falls more rapidly during apnoea in obese patients.[41] The cricoid cartilage may be impossible to identify and cricoid pressure may not be applied correctly. Large tidal volumes may minimise airway closure but a high FiO_2 may be required to maintain adequate oxygenation. In such cases increased concentrations of volatile agent are necessary to ensure unconsciousness.

Respiratory insufficiency and hypoxaemia are likely following surgery and supplemental oxygen may be required for several days. The patient should be nursed sitting up and effective analgesia from a regional block (see Chapter 4) permits pain-free coughing and increased ventilatory excursion and encourages mobilisation. Wound infection and dehiscence are both possible. Deep vein thrombosis is a further risk for obese patients and women should be given thromboprophylaxis with subcutaneous heparin.

Neurological and neuromuscular disorders

Epilepsy

Epilepsy occurs in approximately 0.5% of the population. It is most commonly idiopathic and usually presents in the first two decades of life, occasionally presenting for the first time in pregnancy.

Epilepsy and pregnancy

In a study of 59 pregnant women with epilepsy, Knight and Rhind reported that 50% had no change in seizure frequency during pregnancy, whilst 45% had an increase in frequency and 5% improved.[41] Possible mechanisms for the increase in seizures are fluid retention, alkalosis, stress, and sleep deprivation. Maternal drug levels fall as a result of reduced protein binding and increased renal clearance. Furthermore, compliance with anticonvulsant medication may be altered.

Congenital malformations are 2–3 times more common in babies born to epileptic mothers. Although generally thought to be an effect of anticonvulsant medication, there may also be a genetic predisposition. Although stopping or reducing medication to the minimum effective dose before conception is a good idea theoretically, in practice this can be difficult or even dangerous. Maternal seizures are obviously undesirable whatever the gestation and so most women are advised to continue their normal medication in pregnancy and to have alterations made on therapeutic rather than theoretical grounds.

If status epilepticus occurs in pregnancy, it should be treated immediately with standard therapy. There should be awareness of the possibility of aspiration and the maintenance of oxygenation and acid-base balance.

Intubation and ventilation should therefore be performed early. Benzodiazepines and barbiturates can both be used to terminate seizures. Any deleterious effects of these drugs on the baby are of less significance than the effects of uncontrolled seizures.

Anaesthetic considerations

Hyperventilation associated with prolonged use of Entonox in labour produces maternal hypocarbia, lowering seizure threshold. Pethidine is also best avoided as its major metabolite, norpethidine, has convulsant activity. Although local anaesthetic toxicity may stimulate seizures, appropriate doses for epidural analgesia are safe and therefore recommended for pain relief in labour.

If general anaesthesia is required, drugs with epileptogenic potential such as ketamine and enflurane are probably best avoided. Ventilation should aim to keep carbon dioxide at normal levels. Babies born to mothers receiving anti-epileptic treatment should receive vitamin K as they may have reduced levels of clotting factors.

Myotonic disorders

These are a rare group of inherited disorders characterised by difficulty in initiating muscle movement and delayed muscle relaxation following contraction. Myotonic dystrophy is the most common myotonic disorder. It may be induced by hypothermia, shivering, surgery, and various anaesthetic agents. The anaesthetist should be informed about these patients early in pregnancy so that the degree of disability can be assessed and the potential for unusual responses to anaesthetic agents explored. There may be respiratory muscle weakness and cardiac involvement with conduction problems and arrhythmias. Cardiomyopathy is occasionally observed. Smooth muscle may also be affected.

Myotonic dystrophy and pregnancy

Although pregnancy is uncommon because of ovarian atrophy, symptoms may worsen as pregnancy advances. Muscle weakness may produce uterine inertia prolonging labour and increasing obstetric intervention. Retained placenta and postpartum haemorrhage are also more common.

Anaesthetic considerations

The degree of cardiac and respiratory impairment should be assessed antenatally. Respiratory depressants should be used with extreme caution because of their potential to cause apnoea. Regional blocks are recommended for labour especially where operative delivery is a possibility as general anaesthesia should be avoided. The addition of small doses of opioids to epidural solutions may be helpful to reduce the incidence of shivering. If caesarean section is required the block may be extended, but care should be taken in those with respiratory impairment. Regional anaesthesia does not prevent generalised contractures.

General anaesthesia may occasionally be necessary but should be avoided if at all possible. Suxamethonium should not be used. Non-depolarising muscle relaxants are safe but dosage should be reduced if mothers are receiving quinidine therapy. Efforts must be made to prevent intraoperative hypothermia. Reversal of neuromuscular blockade with neostigmine is thought to be safe. Postoperatively, women require high-dependency care and monitoring.

Multiple sclerosis

Multiple sclerosis is a demyelinating disease characterised by exacerbations and remissions, usually presenting in young adulthood. The interval between exacerbations is unpredictable and in the early stages there may be complete recovery from symptoms between attacks. However, over the years residual symptoms may lead to profound disability.

Multiple sclerosis and pregnancy

Infection, stress, injury, and surgery are all associated with relapses. Relapse rates during pregnancy are similar or slightly reduced when compared to non-pregnant controls. However, 40% of women suffer a relapse in the first six months after delivery. Multiple sclerosis does not affect fertility, pregnancy, labour or delivery.

Anaesthetic considerations

All pregnant women with multiple sclerosis should be seen by an anaesthetist antenatally. There is concern regarding the safety of regional blocks with suggestions that further damage may be done to demyelinated areas. There is, however, a lack of data implicating the use of regional blocks in the development of postnatal relapse. Epidural analgesia has been successfully used for labour and delivery, but in one report a woman experienced an anaesthetic area on the inner thigh after delivery.[42] This resolved in a matter of weeks and the authors concluded that epidural anaesthesia should not be contraindicated provided that the patient is aware of the risks and benefits and agrees to its use. Crawford et al. reported just one postoperative relapse among 37 patients receiving epidural anaesthesia.[43] More recently, Bader et al. demonstrated that relapse was no more common in women receiving regional blocks compared with those using other forms of pain relief.[44] They did, however, suggest that more concentrated local anaesthetic solutions may produce higher relapse rates, although this was based on a small number of patients.

Should general anaesthesia be required for patients with multiple sclerosis, there is no reason to deviate from a standard technique (see Chapter 5).

Myasthenia gravis

Myasthenia gravis is an autoimmune condition characterised by weakness and fatigability of skeletal muscles predominantly with ocular, bulbar, and respiratory involvement. It affects between one in 10–50 000, more commonly women, and usually presents in the third or fourth decade. In up to 90% of sufferers IgG antibodies against acetylcholine receptors may be isolated. Treatment is with anticholinesterases, such as pyridostigmine, immunosupressants, plasmapheresis, and thymectomy.

Deterioration in symptoms may result from myasthenic crisis, which represents a worsening of the condition, or from cholinergic crisis produced by excessive anticholinergic therapy. Patients with myasthenia may be particularly sensitive to drugs potentiating muscular weakness such as aminoglycoside antibiotics, magnesium, and β-mimetics.

Myasthenia and pregnancy

Myasthenia does not affect fertility but in about 40% of women symptoms may worsen during pregnancy, most commonly in the first trimester. Maternal risks are of respiratory failure and both myasthenic and cholinergic crises.

Premature labour is more common in myasthenic patients, possibly due to increased circulating levels of acetylcholine from anticholinesterase therapy.[45] During labour, when oral absorption of drugs is unpredictable, parenteral administration of anticholinesterase therapy may be required. As the uterus consists of non-striated muscle, the duration of labour should not be affected.

Neonatal myasthenia occurs in 10–30% of babies born to mysathenic mothers. This is a transient phenomenon caused by placental transfer of maternal antibodies. Presentation may occur at birth or be delayed for up to 48 hours and treatment is with respiratory support and anticholinesterase therapy. Postpartum deterioration may be expected in 30–50% of cases and so patients should be observed closely. Regular oral medication should be restarted as soon as possible.

Anaesthetic considerations

Antenatal anaesthetic assessment in these patients is extremely important. Respiratory and bulbar involvement must be sought. Serial vital capacity measurements can be a useful bedside guide of possible deterioration during pregnancy. An ECG is recommended because focal necrosis of the myocardium may occasionally occur.

Parenteral opioids and sedatives should be used with caution in myasthenic patients, particularly if there is respiratory or bulbar involvement. Regional analgesia is recommended for labour as it avoids the need for systemic medication and the block may be extended for instrumental or operative delivery.

For those with severe disease and respiratory muscle involvement, general anaesthesia may be required for operative delivery. These patients are very sensitive to muscle relaxants and intubation can be achieved with small doses of suxamethonium (30–50 mg) which may well suffice for the duration of surgery. Mivacurium, which is metabolised by pseudo-cholinesterase, is best avoided. If non-depolarising agents are required, reversal of neuromuscular blockade may be accomplished with incremental doses of neostigmine and glycopyrrolate. Monitoring the degree of neuro-muscular block with a nerve stimulator is mandatory. Provision for post-operative ventilatory support and chest physiotherapy should be made where necessary. As postpartum deterioration is not uncommon, women should initially be cared for on a high-dependency unit.

Back problems

Scoliosis

Minor degrees of scoliosis are common, occurring in up to 15% of the pregnant population. More severe forms are seen in about one in 10 000 people, predominantly women. These may be associated with respiratory and cardiac disease and patients may have undergone surgical correction (see below). A restrictive lung disorder may be present. Increased pulmonary vascular resistance from impaired lung development may lead to pulmonary hypertension and ultimately right heart failure. There may be associated neuromuscular disease and patients may also suffer from malignant hyperthermia.

During pregnancy the severity of the spinal curvature may be increased. There may be inability to increase the circumference of the thoracic cage and as the gravid uterus splints the diaphragm and reduces the functional residual capacity, increasing ventilation perfusion mismatch may produce maternal hypoxaemia.

The existence of pelvic deformity increases the need for caesarean section. Where possible, this may be performed under regional anaesthesia. Epidural anaesthesia may, however, be difficult to site and variable in spread. Such anatomical difficulties increase the incidence of accidental dural puncture. To aid location of epidural space, three-dimensional MRI scanning has been used. Should general anaesthesia be required, particular attention should be given to airway assessment as difficulty with intubation may occur.

Spinal Surgery

Surgery on the spinal column may be performed for scoliosis (see above), disc problems, spondylolisthesis or following trauma. As a result the anatomy of the lower back may be abnormal, increasing the risks of regional

227

block. Depending on the underlying problem, backache may be a particular problem during pregnancy. Anaesthetic referral should occur early in pregnancy so that details of surgery can be obtained before labour and delivery. Regional blocks may be difficult to site, the spread of solutions may be inadequate and there may be an increased risk of accidental dural puncture. Compared with epidural techniques, spinal block is usually more predictable. As with scoliosis, difficulties with intubation should be anticipated.

Ankylosing spondylitis

Ankylosing spondylitis is chronic inflammatory arthropathy producing fibrosis, ossification, and alkylosis, particularly affecting the sacroiliac, facet, and costovertebral joints. It is seen in about 0.05% of the female population and may be associated with aortic regurgitation and restrictive lung disease. The condition is not affected by pregnancy. Regional blocks may be technically difficult to perform but do not appear to cause increased complications. Tracheal intubation may be difficult if there is a fixed flexion deformity of the cervical spines or temporomandibular joint involvement. Awake fibreoptic intubation may be necessary if general anaesthesia is needed.

Spina bifida

Spina bifida occulta

This occurs when the two halves of the vertebral arch fail to fuse but without herniation of meninges or neural tissue. The overlying skin is intact but there may be a tuft of hair, cutaneous angioma, lipoma or skin dimple. The defect has a reported incidence of up to 35%, often only picked up as an incidental X-ray finding, as it rarely causes symptoms. It usually occurs at just one level, most commonly L5–S1.

It is uncommon for spina bifida occulta to increase complications of regional anaesthesia as it is usually below the level at which blocks are sited and the defect is frequently minor. More extensive defects may, however, lead to problems such as increased dural puncture and unpredictable spread of solutions.[46]

Spina bifida cystica

Here there is herniation of meninges (meningocoele) and neural tissue (meningomyelocoele). In the more severe myeloschisis the neural folds fail to meet and the neural plate remains open to air. These conditions are invariably associated with a neurological deficit below the level of the lesion and often accompanied with hydrocephalus. In some patients the spinal cord may be tethered and the conus may extend as far as the L2–3 interspace. Kyphoscoliosis often develops with age. Fortunately, spina bifida cystica is becoming rare with awareness of the benefit of dietary folate supplements and improved antenatal screening.

Patients with lesions above T11 may not experience pain in labour. For lower lesions the risks and benefits and regional blocks should be assessed. Respiratory function should be checked and the possibility of raised intracranial pressure considered. An MRI scan is helpful to confirm the anatomical defect and assess any tethering of nerve tissue. Although there are reports of regional blocks in these patients, the possibility of increased complications must be considered.

Chronic backache

Backache is one of the most commonly reported symptoms, with many different causes. It occurs in about 50% of all pregnancies and in up to 10% may be severe enough to prevent women from working.[47] For those suffering with chronic backache before pregnancy, symptoms often deteriorate as pregnancy advances. With recent suggestions that regional blocks may exacerbate backache (see Chapter 8), there has been concern over their safety. Studies of women reporting backache during pregnancy have failed to demonstrate any adverse effects of epidural analgesia in labour on the severity of subsequent symptoms.[48] Indeed, those choosing regional analgesia reported fewer postnatal problems. However, in some chronic back conditions, especially following surgery, there may be an increased failure rate for regional blocks.

Renal disease

Although there are many causes of maternal renal impairment, for the purposes of this chapter discussion will focus on women with pre-existing chronic renal disease. Nevertheless, acute renal failure may develop during pregnancy from ascending urinary tract infection, pre-eclampsia or severe haemorrhage. Improvements in the medical management of women of childbearing age who have undergone renal transplantation have led to many completing pregnancy successfully.

Renal disease and pregnancy

Regardless of the cause or degree of renal insufficiency, in recent years there have been significant advances in the expected outcome of pregnancy in women with chronic renal failure. It would appear that when pregnancy is well managed, fetal survival is now commonplace and that maternal renal function, although still at risk of deterioration, is not adversely affected in the majority of cases.[49]

Normotensive women with minimal renal dysfunction have about a 90% chance of a successful pregnancy with little or no deterioration of renal function; however, those with preconceptual hypertension and moderate renal dysfunction (baseline serum creatinine >125 μmol/l) have a 20% chance of renal function deterioration and 35% chance of severe problems with hypertension.[50] Renal insufficiency, secondary scleroderma, polyarteritis, and membranoproliferative glomerulonephritis have particularly bad prognoses in pregnancy.

Pregnancy in women with endstage renal failure is uncommon because fertility tends to be reduced. Successful outcome is estimated to occur in about 50% of women on haemodialysis. Management can be difficult, with meticulous attention being required to dialysis regimens, blood pressure control, and treatment of bleeding episodes. Successful pregnancy has also been reported in women treated with continuous ambulatory peritoneal dialysis (CAPD); this mode of dialysis, together with the use of erythropoietin, may help to improve pregnancy outcome for endstage renal patients.[51]

The severity of maternal disease determines fetal outcome. Significant renal impairment is associated with an increased risk of spontaneous abortion, premature labour, and intrauterine growth restriction.

Transplantation may offer the best chance of childbearing for these women and it appears that pregnancy does not have an adverse long-term effect on renal allograft function or survival.[52] However, problems may arise for both mother and baby. As with any chronic renal disease, there is an increased risk of premature labour and growth restriction together with the risks of exposure to drugs such as azathioprine, cyclosporine, and corticosteroids. For the mother there is an increased risk of pre-eclampsia, infection, and hypercalcaemia.

Anaesthetic considerations

There should be a thorough antenatal assessment to determine the extent of the disease. The degree of hypertension and current medication should be noted. Fluid balance and electrolytes may vary in those receiving dialysis or filtration. Anaemia is common and prolonged bleeding from platelet dysfunction may be observed. The presence of a peripheral neuropathy should be documented if regional blocks are to be used. Delayed gastric emptying may increase the risk of aspiration during general anaesthesia.

There is no absolute contraindication to regional blocks in women with renal insufficiency. However, care should be taken to maintain renal perfusion whilst not causing fluid overload. Particular vigilance is required in fluid balance of women with proteinuria. If anticoagulants have been used during haemodialysis, at least six hours should elapse before siting a regional block. It is wise to confirm that clotting is normal by checking the aPTT. When performing a block it is essential to use an aseptic technique.

Women with renal impairment are more likely to be delivered by caesarean section because of both growth retardation and maternal disease.

The choice of anaesthesia should be made on an individual basis but there is usually no absolute contraindication to regional anaesthesia. If fluid balance is likely to be a particular problem, central venous monitoring may be useful but invasive arterial monitoring should be considered carefully before potentially damaging an artery that may be used later to form an arteriovenous fistula. When positioning patients for surgery, care should be taken to protect shunts or fistulas. Steroid cover is indicated for those on long-term corticosteroid therapy. If a general anaesthetic is required, suxamethonium should be used with caution if the serum potassium level is already high as it may further increase the value by 0.5–1.0 mEq/l. Atracurium is probably the non-depolarising muscle relaxant of choice for maintenance of neuromuscular blockade as elimination is independent of renal function.

Acute fatty liver of pregnancy

Acute fatty liver of pregnancy affects approximately one in 10 000 deliveries. Its aetiology is not fully understood but depression of the enzyme glucose-6-phosphatase occurs, resulting in hypoglycaemia, impaired fat transport, and fat accumulation in the liver. It carries a significant risk of death to both mother and baby. The condition usually presents in the third trimester with malaise, abdominal pain, and jaundice. The differential diagnosis is between hepatitis, cholestasis, bile duct obstruction, and pre-eclampsia. Occasionally there may be rapid progression to hepatic failure. Diagnosis is made on blood results as ultrasound scanning may fail to detect fatty infiltration and liver biopsy may be contraindicated by coagulopathy. Bilirubin, ALT, and AST are all elevated and there may be a haemolytic anaemia, thrombocytopenia, and disseminated intravascular coagulopathy. Oliguria progressing to acute renal failure is a possibility.

Treatment is supportive and early delivery may be indicated to avoid intrauterine death. Indeed, resolution of the condition may take place following delivery. Caesarean section may therefore be required with anaesthetic technique dictated by the state of coagulation. If not impaired, regional anaesthesia is indicated and spinal block may be preferred to minimise vascular trauma. Where general anaesthesia is performed an appropriate technique for patients with liver dysfunction should be used.

Systemic lupus erythematosus

Systemic lupus erythematosus (SLE) is a multisystem disorder affecting approximately one in 2000 people. A disease of exacerbation and remission, SLE is nine times more common in women and is observed in one in 1500 pregnancies. Autoantibodies or immune complexes may damage almost any organ with the most common presentations being arthropathy, skin rash, fever, nephritis, hypertension, and neurological disorders. The diagnosis is usually confirmed by the presence of antinuclear autoantibodies, with double-stranded DNA autoantibodies being the most specific for SLE.

The mainstay of treatment for SLE is with corticosteroids to which azathioprine may also be added. Antihypertensive medication may be required to control blood pressure. Aspirin and other NSAIDs are used for arthropathy.

The antiphospholipid syndrome (APS) may be associated with SLE. This condition is characterised by autoantibodies, anticardiolipin, and lupus anticoagulant that bind to phospholipids.[53] Up to 50% of women with APS also have SLE. APS is associated with recurrent arterial and venous thrombosis leading to a high incidence of intrauterine growth restriction, placental thrombosis, premature labour, and intrauterine death. The term "lupus anticoagulant" is something of a misnomer as it has no anticoagulant activity *in vivo*. Indeed, many patients with this condition are receiving anticoagulants to prevent intravascular thrombosis.

SLE and pregnancy

There is debate as to whether pregnancy results in exacerbation of SLE, although it is generally accepted that it does not alter the long-term course of the disease. In those who conceive during the active phase of SLE, worsening of the condition is to be expected. It is not clear whether pre-eclampsia is more common in women with SLE as lupus nephritis may similarly present with hypertension, oedema, and proteinuria. Thrombocytopenia is also often observed in SLE patients.

Neonatal lupus erythematosus may be seen in up to a third of cases of maternal SLE, affected infants presenting most often with cardiac or cutaneous abnormalities.

Anaesthetic considerations

As SLE is a multisystem disorder various anaesthetic risk factors may be observed. A thorough history and complete examination should be performed. Assessment of myocardial and respiratory reserve should be made and where necessary echocardiography and respiratory function tests performed. Any neurological deficit should be documented. Temporomandibular function and neck mobility must be checked to predict ease of intubation should this be necessary.

The presence of coagulation disorders may contraindicate regional block. Prolonged prothrombin and activated partial thromboplastin times may be found and require further investigation. Thrombocytopenia is common especially in those who are lupus anticoagulant positive. Patients may also be receiving aspirin and heparin therapy to prevent thrombosis.

Individual assessment of the risks and benefits of regional blocks should be made.

HIV and AIDS

Human immunodeficiency virus (HIV) and the acquired immunodeficiency deficiency syndrome (AIDS) are becoming increasingly common in women of childbearing age. The prevalence of HIV-positive women in the UK is at present virtually impossible to calculate, although it is estimated to occur in up to 0.3% in certain urban populations. About 50% of those diagnosed as HIV positive will develop AIDS within 10 years. HIV is a retrovirus transmitted through sexual contact, intravenous drug abuse, transfusion of infected blood products or vertically during pregnancy and delivery. The receptor for HIV is the CD4 surface antigen on T-helper cells which, when triggered, leads to the latter's destruction.

Zidovudine (AZT), a viral reverse transcriptase inhibitor, has been shown to reduce dramatically the incidence of vertical transmission of HIV.[54] However, AZT monotherapy has limited long-term benefit and may encourage the emergence of resistant viral strains. Combination therapy with protease inhibitors and non-nucleoside reverse transcriptase inhibitors may be necessary. Furthermore, side-effects of AZT are troublesome and include bone marrow toxicity, anaemia, granulocytopenia, headache, nausea, myalgia, myopathy, hepatotoxicity, and lactic acidosis. Concurrent infection such as *Pneumocystis carinii* pneumonia (PCP), tuberculosis, herpes, and toxoplasmosis may also require treatment.

HIV and pregnancy

Data from the European Collaborative Study (ECS) have shown that only 14% of HIV-infected pregnant woman are severely immunocompromised.[55] There is to date little significant evidence to suggest that HIV increases the rate of complications in pregnancy or that pregnancy alters the course of HIV infection. There may, however, be a higher rate of growth restriction, premature labour, and stillbirth although these may be the result of associated factors such as drug abuse.

Vertical transmission of HIV may occur *in utero*. This is more common towards the end of pregnancy or during delivery and in mothers whose CD4 count is significantly reduced. To minimise the risk of vertical transmission, fetal blood sampling, scalp electrodes, and artificial rupture of membranes are best avoided.

Anaesthetic considerations

A number of studies indicate that general anaesthesia and opiates may have a negative effect on immune function. Although this immune-suppressive effect probably is of little clinical importance in healthy individuals, its implications for the HIV-infected patient are unknown. Both cellular and humoral immune functions are suppressed after surgery. Although the aetiology of postoperative immunosuppression is unclear, many known mediators of the stress response are potent immunosuppressants. Postoperative immunosuppression, which typically lasts for several days, may last longer in inherently immunosuppressed patients and may predispose to the development of postoperative infections or facilitate tumour growth or metastasis.[56] General anaesthesia cannot suppress the stress response and may exacerbate postoperative immunosuppression by suppression of cellular and humoral immune function. Immunosuppression resulting from general anaesthesia occurs within 15 minutes of induction and may persist for as long as 11 days.

It has been suggested that general anaesthesia be avoided when a regional technique is possible in AIDS patients, because of apparent depression of cell-mediated immunity after general anaesthesia.[57] The use of epidural anaesthesia followed by epidural analgesia with local anaesthetics may aid in preservation of perioperative immune function that persists beyond the duration of the block. This may be associated with a decreased incidence of postoperative infectious complications. In a study of HIV-positive parturients who received regional anaesthesia, there were no neurologic or infectious complications related to the anaesthetic or obstetric course. In the immediate postpartum period, the immune function measurements remained essentially unchanged, as did the severity of the disease.[57]

There have been fears that epidural block and lumbar puncture (LP) in HIV-positive patients may allow entry of the virus into the CNS. The natural history of HIV includes CNS involvement early in the clinical course and expression of this infection varies widely. However, it is conceivable that a small but significant number of HIV-infected individuals may not have CNS involvement. In these patients, neuraxial anaesthesia and LP may represent a risk. The safety of epidural blood patches for treatment of postdural puncture headache has been reported in HIV-positive patients.[58] However, the procedure is not without a small risk of introducing virus to the CNS.

Steps must be taken to avoid HIV transmission to health care workers. Education must stress the importance of transmission via blood, cerebrospinal fluid (CSF), vaginal secretions, and amniotic fluid. The use of two pairs of surgical gloves is recommended as it decreases the incidence of potential skin contamination from glove puncture from 11% to 2%.[59] Should needlestick injury occur, the risk of seroconversion for HIV is estimated to be 0.4%, whereas that for hepatitis B is about 30%. Should needlestick injury from an HIV-positive patient occur, current recommendations for postexposure prophylaxis for health care workers are four weeks of treatment with zidovudine, lamivudine (3TC), and indinavir.

Respiratory disease

Cystic fibrosis

Cystic fibrosis is an inherited autosomal recessive condition affecting about one in 2500 people. It presents in childhood with respiratory disease or occasionally malabsorption from pancreatic insufficiency. Repeated respiratory infection may lead to bronchiectasis and airway collapse, producing hypoxaemia. Diagnosis is confirmed by increased sodium chloride in sweat testing. The disease may also be detected by DNA testing which may be done *in utero* by chorionic villus sampling. Treatment of respiratory disease is with physiotherapy with aggressive antibiotic therapy for acute infection. Pancreatic supplements may also be required.

Cystic fibrosis and pregnancy

With advances in medical management, more women with the condition are becoming pregnant. Whilst pregnancy does not appear to affect the progress of cystic fibrosis, complications are more often seen in those with more severe disease.[60] The risk of premature labour is increased, as is perinatal mortality. Care should be taken to avoid prescribing antibiotics for the mother such as tetracyclines and sulphonamides which may have adverse effects on the baby.

During labour, women with cystic fibrosis should be kept well hydrated to aid in sputum production. If oxygen therapy is required this must be humidified. Elective instrumental delivery may reduce the possibility of pneumothorax during the active phase of the second stage of labour.

Anaesthetic Considerations

For labour analgesia, regional block is recommended as it provides effective pain relief and abolishes increased ventilatory demands.[61] Furthermore, if instrumental or operative delivery is required the block can be extended, eliminating the need for general anaesthesia. Care should be taken to avoid too high a block as this may impair the woman's ability to cough, potentially leading to sputum retention.

General anaesthesia is usually well tolerated and has the advantage that ventilation and tracheal suction may easily be performed via the tracheal tube. However, there is a risk of bronchospasm and pneumothorax. Postoperative high-dependency care may be required and humidification of supplemental oxygen is necessary.

Asthma

Asthma is a chronic disease characterised by reversible airway obstruction, inflammation of the airways and hyperresponsiveness to various stimuli. It is seen in about 1% of pregnancies.

Asthma and pregnancy

Asthma may improve, worsen or remain static during pregnancy. Improvement may result from increased progesterone levels. There have been reports of an increased incidence of pre-eclampsia, growth restriction and premature labour in asthmatic patients. For those taking steroids, gestational diabetes is more likely.

Prostaglandins may precipitate bronchospasm and should be used with care for either induction of labour or control of postpartum haemorrhage. Similar risks apply to ergometrine. In pre-eclampsia β-blockers are best avoided as they too may cause bronchospasm.

Anaesthetic considerations

Regional analgesia in labour is recommended as it decreases respiratory work and reduces maternal stress and hyperventilation which may cause bronchospasm. The block may be extended for operative delivery and general anaesthesia may therefore be avoided. A history of intolerance to NSAIDs should be obtained as these may produce bronchospasm in some asthmatics. When general anaesthesia is required, a rapid-sequence induction should be used to prevent aspiration although bronchospasm may result. Volatile agents are beneficial as they bronchodilate. Although deep extubation reduces the risk of bronchospasm, it is advisable to allow the patient to regain consciousness before removing the tracheal tube to minimise the chance of aspiration.

References

1 Boxer LM, Malinow AM. Pre-eclampsia and eclampsia. *Curr Opin Anesthesiol* 1997;**10**:188–98.
2 CLASP. A randomised trial of low-dose aspirin for the prevention and treatment of pre-eclampsia among 9364 pregnant women. *Lancet* 1994;**343**:619–29.
3 Eclampsia Trial Collaborative Group. Which anticonvulsant for women with eclampsia? Evidence from the Collaborative Eclampsia Trial. *Lancet* 1995;**345**:1455–63.
4 Dresner M, Walker JJ. Pre-eclampsia. In: Russell IF, Lyons G, eds. *Clinical problems in obstetric anaesthesia*. London: Chapman and Hall Medical,1997:11–31.
5 Editorial. The bleeding time. *Lancet* 1991;**337**(8755):1447–8.
6 Orlikowski CEP, Rocke DA, Murray WB, *et al.* Thrombelastography changes in pre-eclampsia and eclampsia. *Br J Anaesth* 1996;**77**:157–61.
7 Letsky EA. Haemotasis and epidural anaesthesia. *Int J Obstet Anesth* 1991;**1**:51–4.
8 Howell P. Spinal anaesthesia in severe pre-eclampsia: time for reappraisal, or time for caution? *Int J Obstet Anesth* 1998;**7**:217–19.
9 Ashton WA, James MFM, Janicki PK, Uys PC. Attenuation of the pressor response to intubation in hypertensive proteinuric pregnant patients undergoing caesarean section by magnesium sulphate with and without alfentanil. *Br J Anaesth* 1991;**66**:741–7.
10 Sugrue D, Blake S, MacDonald D. Pregnancy complicated by maternal heart disease at the National Maternity Hospital, Dublin, Ireland 1969–1978. *Am J Obstet Gynecol* 1981;**139**:1–6.
11 Oakley CM. Pregnancy and heart disease. *Br J Hosp Med* 1996;**55**(7):423–6.
12 Department of Health. *Report on confidential enquiries into maternal deaths in the UK 1988–1990*. London: HMSO, 1994.
13 Department of Health. *Report on confidential enquiries into maternal deaths in the UK 1991–1993*. London: HMSO, 1996.

14 Department of Health. *Report on confidential enquiries into maternal deaths in the UK 1994-1996.* London: HMSO, 1998.

15 Robson SC, Hunter S, Boys RJ, Dunlop W. Serial study of factors influencing changes in cardiac output during human pregnancy. *Am J Physiol* 1989;**256**:H1060-5.

16 Brighouse D. Anaesthesia for caesarean section in patients with aortic stenosis: the case for regional anaesthesia. *Anaesthesia* 1998;**53**:107-9.

17 Whitfield A, Holdcroft A. Anaesthesia for caesarean section in patients with aortic stenosis: the case for general anaesthesia. *Anaesthesia* 1998;**53**:109-12.

18 Yentis S, Dob D. Caesarean section in the presence of aortic stenosis. *Anaesthesia* 1998;**53**:604-13.

19 Lynch C III, Rizor RF. Anesthetic management and monitoring of a parturient with mitral and aortic valve disease. *Anesth Analg* 1982;**61**:788-92.

20 Roth A, Elkayam U. Acute myocardial infarction associated with pregnancy. *Ann Intern Med* 1996;**125**:751-62.

21 McCartney CJL, Dark A. Caesarean delivery during cardiac arrest in late pregnancy. *Anaesthesia* 1998;**53**:308-9.

22 Aglio LS, Johnson MD. Anaesthetic management of myocardial infarction in a parturient. *Br J Anaesth* 1990;**65**:258-61.

23 Slomka F, Salmeron S, Zetlaoui P, *et al.* Primary pulmonary hypertension and pregnancy: anaesthetic management for delivery. *Anesthesiology* 1988;**69**:959-61.

24 Khan MJ, Bhatt SB, Krye JJ. Anesthetic considerations for parturients with primary pulmonary hypertension. *Int J Obstet Anesth* 1996;**4**:36-42.

25 Pederson J. Weight and length at birth of infants of diabetic mothers. *Acta Endocrinol* 1954;**16**:330-42.

26 Steel JM, Johnstone FD. Guidelines for the management of insulin-dependent diabetes mellitis in pregnancy. *Drugs* 1996;**52**(1):60-70.

27 British Society for Haematology, Haemostasis and Thrombosis Task Force. Guidelines on the investigation and management of thrombophilia. *J Clin Pathol* 1990;**43**:703-10.

28 Walker ID. Management of thrombophilia in pregnancy. *Blood Rev* 1991;**5**:227-33.

29 Ginsburg JS, Hirsh J, Turner DC, Levine MN, Burrows R. Risks to the foetus of anticoagulant therapy during pregnancy. *Thromb Haemostas* 1989;**61**:197-203.

30 Grimaudo V, Gueissaz F, Hauert J, Sarraj A, Kruithoff EKO, Bachman F. Necrosis of skin induced by coumarin in a patient deficient in protein S. *BMJ* 1989;**298**:233-4.

31 Bullingham A, Strunin L. Prevention of postoperative thromboembolism. *Br J Anaesth* 1995;**75**:622-30.

32 Horlocker TT, Wedel DJ. Spinal and epidural blockade and perioperative low molecular weight heparin: smooth sailing on the *Titanic. Anesth Analg* 1998;**86**:1153-6.

33 Hynson JM, Katz JA, Bueff HU. Epidural hematoma associated with enoxaparin. *Anesth Analg* 1996;**82**:1072-5.

34 Rick ME, Williams SB, McKeown LP. Thrombocytopenia associated with pregnancy in a patient with type IIB von Willebrand's disease. *Blood* 1987;**11**:786-9.

35 Larrabee KD, Monga M. Women with sickle cell trait are at increased risk for pre-eclampsia. *Am J Obstet Gynecol* 1997;**177**(2):425-8.

36 Howard RJ. Management of sickling conditions in pregnancy. *Br J Hosp Med* 1996;**56**(1):7-10.

37 Smith JA, Espeland M, Bellevue R, Bonds D, Brown AK, Koshy M. Pregnancy in sickle cell diseaese: experience of the Cooperative Study of Sickle Cell Disease. *Obstet Gynecol* 1996;**87**(2):199-204.

38 Serjeant GR. Sickle-cell disease. *Lancet* 1997;**350**(9079):725-30.

39 Maitra AM, Palmer SK, Bachhuber SR, Abram SE. Continuous epidural analgesia for cesarean section in a patient with morbid obesity. *Anesth Analg* 1979;**58**:348-9.

40 Hodgkinson R, Husain FJ. Obesity, gravity and spread of epidural analgesia. *Anesth Analg* 1981;**60**:421-4.

41 Knight AH, Rhind EG. Epilepsy and pregnancy: a study of 153 pregnancies in 59 patients. *Epilepsia* 1975;**16**:99-110.

42 Warren TM, Datta S, Ostheimer GW. Lumbar epidural anesthesia for a patient with multiple sclerosis. *Anesth Analg* 1982;**61**:1022-3.

43 Crawford JS, James FM, Nolte H, van Steenberge A, Shah JL. Regional analgesia for

patients with chronic neurological disease and similar conditions. *Anaesthesia* 1981;**36**:821.

44 Bader AM, Hunt CO, Datta S, Naulty JS, Osthiemer GW. Anesthesia for the obstetric patient with multiple sclerosis. *J Clin Anesth* 1988;**1**:21–4.

45 Coaldrake LE, Livingstone P. Myasthenia gravis in pregnancy. *Anaesth Intens Care* 1983;**11**:254–7.

46 Tidmarsh MD, May AE. Epidural anaesthesia and neural tube defects. *Int J Obstet Anesth* 1998;**7**:111–14.

47 Russell R, Reynolds F. Backpain pregnancy and childbirth. *BMJ* 1997;**314**:1062–3.

48 Dresner M, Freeman J, Cole P. Obstetric anaesthesia for patients with chronic back problems. *Br J Anaesth* 1997;**78**:A349.

49 Jones DC. Pregnancy complcated by chronic renal disease. *Clin Perinatol* 1997;**24**(2):483–96.

50 Lindheimer MD, Katz AI. Gestation in women with kidney disease; prognosis and management. *Baillière's Clin Obstet Gynaecol* 1987;**1**(4):921–37.

51 Jakobi P, Ohel G, Szylman P, *et al*. Continuous ambulatory peritoneal dialysis as the primary approach in the management of renal insufficiency in pregnancy. *Obstet Gynecol* 1992;**79**(5):808–10.

52 First MR, Combs CA, Weiskittel P, *et al*. Lack of effect of pregnancy on renal allograft survival or function. *Transplantation* 1995;**59**(4):472–6.

53 Hughes GVR. The antiphospholipid syndrome: ten years on. *Lancet* 1993;**342**:341–4.

54 Dattel BJ. Antiretroviral therapy during pregnancy – beyond AZT (ZDV). *Obstet Gynecol Clin North Am* 1997;**24**(3):645–7.

55 Newell ML, Thorne C. Pregnancy and HIV infection in Europe. *Acta Paediatr* 1997;**421** (suppl):10–14.

56 Markovic SN, Knight PR, Murasko DM. Inhibition of interferon stimulation of natural killer cell activity in mice anesthetised with halothane or isoflurane. *Anesthesiology* 1993;**78**(4):700–6.

57 Hughes SC, Daily PA, Landers D, Dattel BJ, Crombleholme WR, Johnson JL. Parturients infected with the human immunodeficiency virus and regional anaesthesia. *Anesthesiology* 1995;**82**:32–7.

58 Halpern S, Preston R. HIV infection in the parturient. *Int Anesthesiol Clin* 1994;**32**(2):11–30.

59 Matta H, Thompson AM, Rainey JB. Does wearing two pairs of gloves protect operating theatre staff from skin contamination? *BMJ* 1988;**297**:597–8.

60 Cohen LE, di Sant'Agnese PA, Frielander J. Cystic fibrosis and pregnancy: a national survey. *Lancet* 1980;**2**:842–4.

61 Howell PR, Kent N, Douglas MJ. Anaesthesia for the parturient with cystic fibrosis. *Int J Obstet Anesth* 1993;**2**:152–7.

7: Medical emergencies in pregnancy

CAROLINE GRANGE

Pregnancy imposes differences in the recognition and treatment of medical emergencies. These include different disease entities, marked anatomical/physiological changes (with consequences on the normal physiological parameters and a reduced capacity to compensate during adverse conditions), together with considerations for fetal well-being. A poorly managed emergency may have dire consequences for both mother and baby. The principles of good management of a medical emergency in pregnancy therefore include:

- uterine displacement (>20 weeks gestation) to reduce aortocaval compression;
- aggressive correction of airway, ventilation, and circulation abnormalities;
- a multidisciplinary approach by anaesthetic, obstetric, neonatal, and midwifery teams.

This chapter aims to describe and outline the principles of treatment of the medical emergency in the obstetric patient.

Confidential Enquiries into Maternal Deaths

The Confidential Enquiries into Maternal Deaths are a series of triennial reports, currently covering a period between 1952 and 1996. The reports form the basis for monitoring both the causes and trends of maternal death in the United Kingdom. Since 1985, a combined United Kingdom report has been produced, in which anonymous cases are reviewed by a panel of assessors in obstetrics, anaesthetics, pathology, general medicine, psychiatry, and midwifery. The aim of the reports is to reduce maternal morbidity and mortality by making recommendations in order to improve clinical care. Maternal death is defined as death of women while pregnant or within 42 days of termination of pregnancy, excluding accidental or incidental causes.[1] Deaths are divided into direct (those resulting from obstetric causes) and indirect causes (those resulting from previous existing disease or disease that developed during pregnancy, which was not due to direct obstetric causes but which was aggravated by the physiological consequences of the pregnancy). The last two reports have also contained an additional category, "late deaths", in order to include those women who died as a consequence of direct or indirect causes between 42 days and one year from termination of pregnancy.

Maternal mortality has fallen exponentially since 1952, reaching a plateau at 9.9–10.1 deaths per 100 000 maternities (i.e. number of pregnancies resulting in live births or stillbirths ≥24 weeks gestation) during 1985–93. However, during the 1994–96 report,[1] improved case reporting has resulted in additional deaths becoming known to the Enquiry. Consequently, there has been an apparent increase in maternal mortality to 12.2 deaths per 100 000 maternities, resulting from an increase in both direct and indirect mortality rates. Due to the inclusion of these extra cases, meaningful comparisons of causes and trends in maternal death between the latest and the preceding reports are difficult.

The leading causes of direct maternal deaths in the 1994–96 triennium were thrombosis and thromboembolism, hypertensive disorders, amniotic fluid embolism, early pregnancy (abortions, ectopics), sepsis, and haemorrhage[1] (Table 7.1). There was a marked increase in deaths from thrombosis and thromboembolism which included 46 cases of pulmonary embolism and two cases of cerebral thrombosis. Pulmonary embolism occurred more commonly in the postpartum period (60%), the majority developing after caesarean section. Of the deaths related to pulmonary embolus in the antenatal period (40%), two-thirds occurred in the first trimester. Twenty-eight percent of deaths from pulmonary embolus had symptoms before the fatal event and were inadequately investigated and treated. Key recommendations of the report were the wider use of thromboprophylaxis, better investigation of classic signs of pulmonary embolism or deep vein thrombosis, as well as better appreciation by medical staff that pregnancy carries an increased risk of thrombosis, even in the first trimester.

Table 7.1 Causes of direct maternal death. Numbers of deaths reported to the Confidential Enquiries in the last four triennial reports

	1985–87	1988–90	1991–93	1994–96
Thrombosis/thromboembolism	32	33	35	48
Hypertensive disorders of pregnancy	27	27	20	20
Amniotic fluid embolus	9	11	10	17
Early pregnancy (abortions/ectopics)	22	24	18	15
Genital tract sepsis excluding abortion	6	7	9	14
Haemorrhage	10	22	15	12
Genital tract trauma	6	3	4	5
Anaesthesia	6	4	8	1

Trends in mortality due to hypertensive disorders remained unchanged from the 1991–3 triennium.[2] Although there was evidence of improved blood pressure control with a continued reduction in deaths from cerebral haemorrhage, inappropriate fluid management and the development of adult respiratory distress syndrome played an important role in maternal demise.

The effect of recommendations by the Royal College of Obstetricians and Gynaecologists on thromboembolism prophylaxis[3] and the evidence on the use of magnesium from the Collaborative Eclampsia Trial,[4] both published in 1995, may improve the statistics in the next triennium.

Alarmingly, deaths due to amniotic fluid embolism showed a dramatic rise in the latest triennium, which may be partly related to the increasing age of the parturient population. Although it was suggested that death from amniotic fluid embolus could be reduced by avoidance of uterine overstimulation and the prompt diagnosis of obstructed labour, this only appears to apply to a small number of the reported cases. Over 50% of the cases collapsed suddenly and died despite acceptable resuscitative attempts and of those that survived longer (6 hours–3 days), only one case had substandard care after delivery. Specific advice to improve these statistics was therefore difficult.

The mortality rate related to sepsis increased during the latest triennium, with the majority occurring after vaginal delivery. The report emphasised the need for medical staff to remain vigilant for symptoms and signs of infection, to enable appropriate investigation and treatment. Although only two women died after caesarean section, the use of prophylactic intraoperative antibiotics was stressed.

The number of deaths from haemorrhage showed an improvement from the last triennium. The main criticisms of management of the reported cases were inexperienced operators for high-risk patients (with particular reference to placenta praevia) and poor communication between the labour ward and the blood bank and between the accident and emergency department and the duty obstetrician. Key recommendations emphasised the avoidance of the above factors, in addition to the need for protocols and the regular practice of emergency drills for major haemorrhage.

Anaesthesia was the seventh and eighth commonest cause of maternal death in the 1991–93 and 1994–96 triennia respectively. The death rate associated with anaesthesia fell from 3.5 to 0.5 deaths per million maternities during this period. Of the 14 cases reported in the 1991–93 triennium, eight were directly due to anaesthesia. All of the direct deaths associated with caesarean section involved the use of general anaesthesia and most resulted from hypoxia and airway obstruction. Only one death, which was associated with anaesthesia, involved an epidural. During the 1994–96 triennium, there was only one anaesthetic death, which was related to an unconventional combined spinal-epidural technique. Hypotension,

241

dyspnoea, and subsequent cardiac arrest were associated with intrathecal bupivacaine, alfentanil, and clonidine in combination with epidural bupivacaine. Ignoring this unusual case, improved trends in anaesthetic-related mortality may be related to the increased number of regional anaesthetics now administered for instrumental and operative delivery. However, despite the apparent vindication of regional anaesthesia, it should be remembered that caesarean section requiring general anaesthesia is still on occasion necessary and is more likely to occur in more urgent and less well-prepared patients and in situations where regional anaesthesia is contraindicated.

In the latest report, indirect maternal deaths were mainly due to cardiac causes (29%) (particularly ischaemic heart disease, cardiomyopathy, and thoracic aortic aneurysms) and diseases of the central nervous system (35%), with increases in deaths associated with epilepsy and subarachnoid haemorrhage. Deaths from psychiatric causes (i.e. suicide and substance abuse) also played a significant role.

Throughout the last report underlying events leading to death included substandard care, failure of consultant involvement, lack of clear policies for the treatment of certain conditions, and delay in ITU admission. Although much valuable information can be obtained from these audits, direct correlation between the triennia is hampered by different population groups (for example, increased age at first birth, increased incidence of multiple gestation), different methodology of collection of data, uncertainty of denominators (for example, total number of anaesthetics, caesarean sections, and pregnancies) together with inadequate information about certain cases. It is hoped that standardisation of data collection and denominator information will improve this situation in the future.

Cardiopulmonary resuscitation

Cardiac arrest in pregnancy is rare, occurring in one in 30 000 pregnancies.[5] Although this incidence may be increasing due to the prevalence of high-risk parturients, obstetric teams will still have limited experience in dealing with this problem. Fundamental differences occur with cardiac arrest during pregnancy, which include aetiology of event, anatomical and physiological changes in the parturient hindering successful resuscitation, fetal influences, and modifications in basic and advanced life support.

Initial management principles of cardiopulmonary resuscitation are similar, regardless of the aetiology of the event. Cardiac arrest in the non-pregnant population is more likely to be due to a primary cardiac event, whereas those occurring during pregnancy have other causes (Box 7.1). It is important to diagnose rapidly and correct potentially reversible events (for example, haemorrhage, dysrhythmias due to local anaesthetic or magnesium toxicity) to optimise maternal and fetal outcome. Resuscitation in

---

Box 7.1 Aetiology of cardiac arrest during pregnancy

Pulmonary embolus
Severe pregnancy-induced hypertension
Hypovolaemia – for example, haemorrhage
Amniotic fluid embolus
Hypoxaemia – for example, anaesthetic related (failed intubation, aspiration)
Drug overdose/toxicity:
    local anaesthetics (high spinal, toxicity)
    hypermagnesaemia
    tocolytics
    drugs abuse (cocaine)
Pre-existing or pregnancy-related heart disease
Anaphylactic/anaphylactoid reactions
Usual reasons for cardiac arrest in non-pregnant state

---

the parturient is more difficult due to anatomical and physiological changes occurring during pregnancy (Table 7.2). Although cardiopulmonary resuscitation should follow the 1998 European Guidelines for Adult Basic and Advanced Life Support,[6,7] certain modifications should be applied[8,9] (Box 7.2).

Table 7.2 Anatomical and physiological changes in pregnancy influencing successful CPR

Change	Implication
Aortocaval compression ($\geq$20 weeks gestation)	Decreased aortic outflow Decreased venous return Decreased uteroplacental blood flow Effective CPR more difficult
Enlarged breasts Oedema Increased body mass	Intubation more difficult
Decreased functional residual capacity Increased oxygen consumption Increased carbon dioxide production	Increased susceptibility to hypoxia and acidosis
Respiratory alkalosis with partial renal compensation	Decreased bicarbonate ion concentration resulting in less buffering capacity
Decreased lung compliance	Increased difficulty with cardiac massage and artificial ventilation
Increased cardiac output Increased heart rate, stroke volume Decreased systemic vascular resistance	Less ability to adapt to adverse conditions Need for increased cardiac output during CPR
Reduced oesophageal sphincter tone Increased intragastric pressure Reduced gastrointestinal motility	Increased risk of aspiration

Box 7.2   Modifications of the standard ALS guidelines

Relieve aortocaval compression (≥20 weeks gestation)
Consider possible aetiologies
Airway protection (cricoid pressure, early intubation)
Consider perimortem caesarean section within five minutes of cardiac arrest, if resuscitation attempt is unsuccessful
Involvement of obstetric/neonatal staff

Reduction of aortocaval compression

The effectiveness of cardiac massage is reduced due to aortocaval compression by the gravid uterus, which becomes significant after 20 weeks gestation. The severity of aortocaval compression increases with advancing gestation and with the maternal supine position. As external cardiac massage is most effective in the supine position and aortocaval compression least severe in the full lateral position, the best compromise is achieved with the patient wedged at an angle of 27°. Methods of reducing aortocaval compression include the use of a left lateral wedge, a lateral tilting surface or manual displacement of the uterus.

Consideration of potential aetiology

Reversible causes of cardiac arrest should be rapidly identified and appropriately treated. There should be a high index of suspicion for haemorrhage, which may be occult. Suspected magnesium toxicity may be treated with calcium chloride and bupivacaine-induced ventricular tachyarrhythmias with bretylium.

Airway protection

Pregnancy produces an increased risk of aspiration, hypoxia, and acidosis (Table 7.2). Early intubation is important to protect the airway from gastric contents and also to produce the most effective artificial ventilation.

Perimortem caesarean section

Caesarean section should be performed within five minutes of cardiac arrest, if resuscitation is unsuccessful in any parturient after 20 weeks gestation.[10] Even if the fetus is not viable, there will be significant advantages for the mother, namely, improvements in aortocaval compression, a reduction in oxygen requirements, and a reduction in carbon dioxide production. For optimal survival of the baby, the delivery should be within five minutes of an arrest, although intact infant survival after more than 20 minutes has been reported.[11]

Other dilemmas

Although ventricular fibrillation is a less common initial rhythm during pregnancy, standard advanced life support defibrillation guidelines should apply. Defibrillation has been used in pregnancy without adverse effects; the fetal heart may be protected from ventricular fibrillation due to its inadequate critical myocardial mass. Stimulation of uterine contractions has not been reported.

During cardiopulmonary resuscitation, adrenaline is used to maintain peripheral vascular constriction and adequate cerebral and coronary filling pressures. Adrenaline should be used as per standard advanced life support protocol, despite concerns over its potential for uteroplacental vasoconstriction. Fetal survival is improved if the maternal circulation is restored within five minutes of the cardiac arrest, particularly if the fetus is not independently viable. In addition, severe uteroplacental vasoconstriction is already likely to be present in established cardiac arrest even without exogenous adrenaline use. Although acidosis may occur more rapidly in the parturient, sodium bicarbonate should only be used in severe documented acidosis (pH <7.1).

Major obstetric haemorrhage

Haemorrhage remains an important cause of maternal mortality. In the 1994–96 triennium, 12 deaths were directly due to haemorrhage (approximately 60% antenatal and 40% postnatal). Sixty-six percent of cases were judged to have received substandard care. The report emphasised the importance of experienced operators for high-risk cases, accurate estimation of blood loss, prompt recognition and treatment of clotting disorders, use of adequately sized intravenous cannulas, central venous pressure monitoring, early involvement in patient management of consultants in obstetrics, anaesthesia, and haematology and good communication between labour ward and blood bank. The need for protocols and regular practice of emergency drills for major haemorrhage were also stressed.

As the uteroplacental unit receives 12% of the cardiac output at term, it forms a potential source of major haemorrhage. Haemorrhage results in a reduction in the oxygen supply to both fetus and maternal organs, following the loss of circulating volume and red cell mass. Consequent cellular hypoxia and acidosis may lead to organ dysfunction. The uteroplacental circulation is at particular risk during haemorrhage due to:

1 compensatory selective vasoconstriction resulting in diversion of blood from less vital maternal organs (i.e. skin, gut, muscle, kidney, uteroplacental unit) to maintain perfusion of the more critical organs (i.e. heart, brain)

245

2 absent autoregulatory capacity; reduction in maternal blood pressure results in a decrease in the uterine blood flow with detrimental effects on the fetus.

Therefore during haemorrhage, rapid restoration of maternal blood volume with adequate oxygen-carrying capacity and treatment of the underlying cause improves fetal well-being.

Management strategies for the treatment of major haemorrhage include:

- assessment of severity;
- determination of aetiology;
- treatment of haemorrhage, including resuscitation of the patient and control of bleeding site;
- reassessment of the patient including the effectiveness of resuscitation and continuing blood loss.

For these strategies to be implemented, adequate staff, including anaesthetists, obstetricians, midwives, haematologists, neonatologists, laboratory staff, and auxiliary workers, as well as adequate facilities need to be available.

Assessment of blood loss

Obstetric haemorrhage is defined as an acute blood loss of greater than 500 ml. The average blood loss at vaginal delivery is 320–400 ml and that at caesarean section about 500 ml although occasionally it may be considerably more.[12] The severity of haemorrhage is dependent on both the actual blood loss and the rate of haemorrhage. The greater the blood loss, the greater the discrepancy between the actual and estimated volumes. In addition, assessment of blood loss in pregnancy may be difficult (Box 7.3). An

---

Box 7.3   Pitfalls in assessment of blood loss in obstetric patients

- Physiological anaemia: ↑ plasma volume >> ↑ red blood cell mass. Therefore larger blood volume loss before compensatory mechanisms occur
- Cardiovascular physiology altered in normal pregnancy: increased heart rate, decreased systemic vascular resistance. Therefore classic signs of acute blood loss may be affected
- Patients generally young and healthy. Therefore may compensate without cardiovascular parameter changes
- Blood loss may be concealed (contained in uterus)
- Effects of autotransfusion from contraction of uterus. Therefore decompensation may be slowed
- Amniotic fluid contamination with blood. Therefore visual assessment of blood loss may be inaccurate

---

Table 7.3   Classification of haemorrhagic shock

Acute % blood loss	Clinical findings
15–20	None
20–25	Respiratory rate 14–20/min ↑ Heart rate (100/min) Mild hypotension Peripheral vasoconstriction
25–35	Respiratory rate 20–30/min ↑ Heart rate (100–120/min) Hypotension 80–100 mmHg Restlessness Oliguria
>35	Respiratory rate >35/min ↑ Heart rate (>120/min) Hypotension (<60 mmHg) Altered consciousness Anuria

Blood volume = 100 ml/kg during 3rd trimester

estimate of blood loss may be obtained from visual assessment and the clinical features of shock[13] (Table 7.3).

Aetiology

The source of bleeding should be identified (Table 7.4) and controlled. Fetal concerns will have management implications, if haemorrhage occurs during the antenatal period. The commonest cause of antenatal haemorrhage is placental abruption,[14] whereas in the postpartum period 90% of cases are due to uterine atony. Patients at risk of haemorrhage should be identified early (Box 7.4) to ensure rapid implementation of treatment.

Table 7.4   Aetiology of obstetric haemorrhage

	Antepartum	Postpartum
Uterine causes	Placenta praevia Placental abruption	Uterine atony Retained placenta Placenta accreta Uterine inversion
Non-uterine causes	Lower genital tract lesions Coagulopathy	Lower genital tract lacerations Coagulopathy Haematoma

Treatment

During major haemorrhage initial resuscitation of the patient is similar to that of the non-pregnant patient (Box 7.5). Resuscitation and control of

---

Box 7.4   Increased risk of postpartum haemorrhage from uterine atony

Multiple gestation
Polyhydramnios
Multiparity
Macrosomia
Prolonged augmented labour
Tocolytic therapy
Chorioamnionitis

---

bleeding should occur simultaneously. The immediate concern is that of replacing blood volume before that of correction of haemoglobin or coagulation.

Intravenous fluids should be administered using two large-bore cannulas (14 or 16 gauge). The debate regarding crystalloid or colloid resuscitation remains unresolved.[15] The advantages of crystalloids (normal saline 0.9%, Ringer's lactate) include cost, availability, and absence of allergic reactions. However, pulmonary oedema may be precipitated due to fluid equilibration into the interstitial space, as 2–4 times the volumes of crystalloid compared to colloid are needed to produce equivalent haemodynamic responses. Hypotonic solutions (5% dextrose) should not be used as intravascular expansion is poor due to equilibration with interstitial and intracellular spaces. Hyperosmotic sodium chloride solutions have not been shown to be better than conventional regimes.

Colloids, such as human albumin solution, dextrans, polygelatins (Haemacel, Gelofusine), and hydroxyethyl starch, produce a greater and more sustained increase in plasma volume with an improvement in oxygen transport. However, disadvantages include expense and potential for allergic reactions. Also, if capillary permeability is increased, there is an increased risk of pulmonary oedema due to increased extravascular oncotic pressure, following the escape of the colloid particles into the interstitial compartment. Other disadvantages are associated with specific colloids: for example, hydroxyethyl starch with coagulation abnormalities and dextrans with crossmatching difficulties. Human albumin should not be used to treat hypovolaemia as it offers no advantages over synthetic colloids and recent evidence suggests there may be an increased mortality with its use.[16] Crystalloid solutions (20 ml/kg) for the initial resuscitation, followed by colloid and blood products if there is continued need for volume replacement, are recommended.

Although fully crossmatched blood is preferable, the type of blood given to the patient is dependent on the urgency of the situation. In an emergency where over 35% of the blood volume has been lost, blood group O Rh (D)

Box 7.5 Management of major obstetric haemorrhage (scheme assumes continuing bleeding; many steps should occur simultaneously)

1. **Call for help**
   Anaesthetists/obstetricians/midwives

2. **Ensure adequate oxygenation/ventilation**
   Maintain patent airway
   Supplemental oxygen (FiO_2 1.0 by non-rebreathing face mask)
   Intubate trachea if loss of consciousness, respiratory failure or cardio-vascular collapse

3. **Restore circulating volume and cardiac output**
   Lateral wedge if antepartum
   Two large intravenous cannulae (16/14 gauge)
   Expand circulating volume (1–2 l crystalloid plus additional colloid/blood – consider warmed fluid and use of pressurised infusion devices)
   Treat severe hypotension with vasoconstrictors (ephedrine 5–50 mg, phenylephrine 50–200 µg intravenously)

4. **Order 6–10 units of blood**
   Crossmatched, type specific, O Rh negative depending on urgency
   Baseline investigations – full blood count, platelet count, electrolytes, coagulation screen, ionised calcium

5. **Monitoring**
   Patient colour, respiratory rate, capillary return, consciousness, ECG, BP, oximetry, urine output, fetal heart rate (if appropriate)

6. **Rapid assessment**
   Severity of blood loss (Table 7.3), aetiology (Table 7.4)
   Brief history (including anaesthetic history) and examination

7. **Treat cause**
   Medical (oxytocics with atony)
   Surgical (exploratory operation, remember aspiration prophylaxis prior to rapid-sequence induction)

8. **Call for further help**
   Extra anaesthetic/obstetric/auxiliary personnel

9. **Reassess**
   Continuing blood loss/effectiveness of resuscitation
   Consider insertion of central venous pressure line/temperature probe
   Consider further blood and blood products (fresh frozen plasma, platelets, cryoprecipitate)

10. **Continuing care**
    Intensive care admission
    Monitoring
    Treatment of complications, e.g. coagulopathies, adult respiratory distress syndrome, acute tubular necrosis

negative can be given. If the patient's blood group is known, "type-specific" blood (i.e. that comparable with patient's ABO and Rhesus blood groups) is desirable. All patients at risk of haemorrhage should have ABO/Rh groups and other red cell isoantibodies determined. If additional isoantibodies are present, blood should be crossmatched in anticipation of transfusion needs, as crossmatching will be time consuming.

The use of intraoperative blood salvage should also be considered, as previous concerns over contamination with amniotic fluid and subsequent disseminated intravascular coagulation and cardiovascular collapse have not been substantiated.[17] During massive transfusion, a haematologist is invaluable, not only for advice on product replacement, but also to supervise the logistics of component availability. Coagulopathies can occur rapidly from dilutional effects, as well as concomitant consumptive coagulopathies associated with certain obstetric disorders. In addition, the extended shelf-life of homologous blood results in minimal platelet function and considerably reduced quantities of factors V and VIII at the time of the transfusion. Coagulation components should only be transfused in patients with continuing microvascular bleeding together with confirmatory laboratory tests.

Fresh frozen plasma (15 ml/kg) should be considered with prothrombin and partial prothrombin times in excess of 1.5 times normal values. If bleeding is largely a result of hypofibrinogenaemia (fibrinogen <1 g/l) the administration of cryoprecipitate is useful.[18] Platelet transfusion can be considered with platelet counts below 50×10^9/l. Transfusion should consist of one unit per 10 kg; for each unit transfused, the peripheral platelet count should increase by $5-10 \times 10^9$/l, assuming no consumptive coagulopathy is present.

Intravenous calcium supplementation may be required after massive blood transfusion. Ionised plasma calcium is reduced because of absorption of calcium ions by the citrate used as an anticoagulant in the transfused blood and impairment of citrate conversion to bicarbonate in conditions associated with liver dysfunction and hypothermia. Further reduction may occur in patients receiving magnesium. Calcium can be administered as a dose of 8 mg calcium chloride per kg body weight, after confirming plasma levels.

In addition to resuscitation, operative intervention may be required to establish the cause of bleeding and to control ongoing blood loss. Anaesthetic technique depends on the maternal haemodynamics, coagulation results, urgency of situation, and surgical procedure required. The risks and benefits of each technique should be evaluated. If bleeding has been controlled and the patient is haemodynamically stable, careful extension or instigation of a regional block may be possible. However, continued rapid blood loss will necessitate the use of or conversion to a general anaesthetic, enabling airway control. Ketamine and etomidate are useful as induction agents as minimal hypotension is produced. Ketamine also increases uterine tone, with the additional advantage of reducing haemorrhage caused by atony. All halogenated inhalational agents cause progressive relaxation of the uterus at increasing concentrations and may have to be discontinued to prevent worsening haemorrhage. Uterine tone is unaffected by isoflurane at concentrations up to 0.5 MAC (minimum alveolar concentration) and is therefore the drug of choice. However, in certain circumstances (for example, removal of retained placenta or uterine inversion), the reduction of uterine tone may be useful to aid initial corrective treatment.

Control of bleeding obviously depends on the underlying cause. As uterine atony is the commonest cause of postpartum haemorrhage and also often occurs with antepartum causes (for example, placental abruption, placenta praevia), it is important to be aware of possible treatment options. Normally in the postpartum period uterine contraction compresses the vessels of the placental bed and uterine wall, so achieving haemostasis. If the uterus fails to contract adequately this mechanism does not occur. Methods of achieving contraction consist of bimanual uterine compression and oxytocics (Fig 7.1). The side-effects of drugs used to control postpartum haemorrhage are shown in Table 7.5. As ergometrine and the prostaglandins may cause severe hypertension, vasoconstriction and bronchoconstriction, care should be taken in administering these drugs to patients with pre-eclampsia, ischaemic heart disease, asthma or collagen diseases. Treatment of patients suffering from collagen diseases may precipitate digital necrosis. The use of intramyometrial injections may be beneficial. In the hypovolaemic patient, intramuscular injections may result in

Table 7.5   Oxytocic drugs for use in postpartum haemorrhage

Drug	Dose	Side-effects
Oxytocin	5–10 units IV and 10–50 units/1000 ml normal saline IV at sufficient rate to produce atony	Hypotension (peripheral vasodilation) Water intoxication/hyponatraemia (mild ADH effect)
Ergometrine	0.25 mg IM or 0.25 mg diluted in 10 ml normal saline IV (slowly) or intramyometrial injection	Nausea/vomiting Severe vasoconstriction Severe hypertension Coronary artery spasm Bronchospasm
Prostaglandin 15-methyl $F_{2\alpha}$	0.25 mg IM or 0.25 mg diluted with 10 ml normal saline for intramyometrial injection (use long needle, multi-sites)	Nausea and vomiting Severe hypertension Bronchospasm Increased intrapulmonary shunt
Prostaglandin E_2	5 mg/500 ml normal saline ie 10 µg/ml IV at 5–20 µg per minute	Bronchodilation Hypotension (peripheral vasodilation) Reports of severe hypertension after IV administration

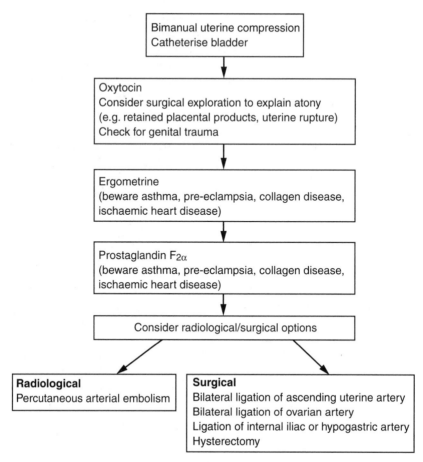

Fig 7.1   Control and treatment of postpartum haemorrhage

poor absorption, in addition to the reduced quantities of the drug reaching the target organ due to decreased uterine blood flow. Conversely, intramyometrial injections enable direct administration to the target organ, together with reduced systemic absorption due to compensatory vasoconstriction in hypovolaemic conditions. Consequently adverse side-effects are minimised. Exclusion of intravenous administration by aspiration prior to intramyometrial injection reduces the systemic effects.

Failure of the above methods to produce uterine contraction necessitates reevaluation of the situation and consideration of surgical or radiological options.[19] Reports have emphasised the usefulness of percutaneous arterial embolisation involving the insertion of gelatin sponge into the offending vessels after identification with angiography.[20] This procedure requires the patient to be haemodynamically stable and radiological facilities to be available. It offers advantages in those patients with severe intra-abdominal adhesions where surgery would be difficult. Surgical methods include ligation of uterine, ovarian, hypogastric or internal iliac arteries. Embolisation and ligation have the additional advantage of preservation of fertility. However, where these methods fail, hysterectomy should be considered as definitive treatment for postpartum haemorrhage.

Reassessment of the patient

Patients should be reassessed to evaluate both the adequacy of the resuscitation and continuing blood loss. Adequate resuscitation is indicated by heart rate <100/min, systolic blood pressure >100 mmHg, urine output >0.5 ml/kg/h, capillary refill time <2 seconds and central venous pressure 5–10 cmH$_2$O. Appropriate post haemorrhage facilities, such as a high-dependency unit, should be available to monitor the patient and treat any complications that may develop.

Amniotic fluid embolism

Amniotic fluid embolism results from the entry of amniotic fluid into the maternal circulation, producing primarily cardiovascular and haematological dysfunction. Its incidence has been estimated at between one in 8000 and one in 80 000 pregnancies;[21] the exact incidence being difficult to establish due to the diversity of the clinical presentation and the problems of obtaining a definitive diagnosis. However, despite its apparent rarity, it remains the third commonest cause of maternal death in the United Kingdom,[1] with 50% of patients dying within one hour of presentation.

Aetiology and pathophysiology

The exact aetiology and pathophysiology of amniotic fluid embolism remains unresolved. It is postulated that in order for amniotic fluid to enter the maternal circulation, the following conditions must be present: laceration of fetal membranes, laceration of uterine or cervical vessels and a pressure gradient sufficient to drive the amniotic fluid into the maternal circulation.

Early research suggested that the primary pathological change was severe pulmonary hypertension, secondary to either occlusive or vasospastic changes in the pulmonary circulation and resulting in right ventricular dysfunction. However, the mechanical obstruction theory has largely been abandoned, as postmortem studies have shown poor correlation between the quantity of particulate matter and clinical signs. Later studies, using invasive haemodynamic monitoring, revealed elevated pulmonary artery occlusion pressures and left ventricular dysfunction without elevated central venous or pulmonary artery pressures in patients with amniotic fluid embolism. Clark postulated the biphasic theory to incorporate these results.[22] He suggested an initial transient phase of pulmonary vasospasm (approximately 30 minutes) resulting from the release of vasoactive substances and producing severe hypoxia with high mortality. A secondary phase subsequently occurred in the survivors of the initial response, resulting in left ventricular failure with normalisation of right ventricular function. He suggested that, due to the delay in pulmonary artery catheter insertion in the acute resuscitation period, the initial supporting cardiovascular data for his theory were missed.

Although the cause of left ventricular dysfunction remains unclear, current work focuses on the role of cellular mediators. An anaphylactic response has been suggested whereby amniotic fluid triggers the release of maternal endogenous mediators such as histamine, prostaglandins, and leukotrienes. Others believe that metabolites of arachidonic acid present in amniotic fluid may cause the cardiovascular and haematological problems.

Similar controversy remains regarding the aetiology of the coagulopathy. It is thought that circulating trophoblast may be responsible. The amniotic fluid may also have a direct uterine relaxant effect resulting in massive haemorrhage with subsequent consumptive and dilutional effects contributing to the coagulopathy.

Clinical features

The majority of cases of amniotic fluid embolism present during labour and the immediate postpartum period. However, cases have been documented during first and second trimester abortions, up to 48 hours postpartum and even spontaneously during a pregnancy at 20 weeks gestation.

Suggested risk factors for amniotic fluid embolism include increasing maternal age, high parity, use of uterine stimulants, short duration of labour, intense contractions, and multiple pregnancy. However, only increasing maternal age (>25 years) has been consistently present in the cases documented in successive United Kingdom triennium maternal mortality reports.[1]

Clinical presentation may be variable, although over half of the cases present with severe dyspnoea, cyanosis, and hypotension. Progression to cardiopulmonary arrest may occur rapidly. Of those patients that survive the initial insult, pulmonary oedema develops in 24–70%, seizures in 10–20%, and coagulopathy in 40% of cases. Bleeding related to coagulopathy is the initial presentation in 10–15% of cases.[23] Multiple organ involvement may ensue, resulting in renal, hepatic, myocardial, and neurological dysfunction.

The differential diagnosis includes thromboembolism, air embolism, aspiration pneumonitis, shock (secondary to haemorrhage, sepsis or anaphylaxis), eclampsia, toxic reaction to local anaesthetic, and acute cardiac

Table 7.6 The diagnosis of amniotic fluid embolism

Clinical presentation	Dyspnoea, cyanosis, hypotension, coagulopathy, seizures
Arterial blood gases	Hypoxaemia, metabolic acidosis, compensatory respiratory alkalosis
Coagulopathy	Reduction in platelets, fibrinogen Elevation in prothrombin, activated partial thromboplastin times, fibrin degradation products
Chest X-ray	Enlargement of right atrium/ventricle Prominent proximal pulmonary artery Pulmonary oedema/infiltrates/ effusions
ECG	Right ventricular strain ST segment/T wave changes Rhythm abnormalities
Antemortem investigations	Antibodies to human keratin, amniotic fluid-derived mucin Zinc coproporphyrin (derived from meconium) in maternal blood Microvascular pulmonary artery samples of anucleate squamous epithelial cells, mucin, hair, fat
Postmortem investigations	Sections of lung specimens containing fetal debris in maternal arterioles and capillaries

failure (secondary to pre-existing cardiac disease or tocolytic therapy). Diagnosis, made by exclusion, is based on clinical presentation and supporting laboratory results as there is no single definitive diagnostic test. The supportive evidence for the diagnosis of amniotic fluid embolism is shown in Table 7.6. Although the presence of anucleate squamous epithelial cells (fetal squames) in the pulmonary microvascular circulation is supportive of amniotic fluid embolism, it is not pathognomonic. Squamous cells have been found in the pulmonary circulation of both pregnant and non-pregnant women without evidence of amniotic fluid embolism.[24] Obviously, a definitive diagnosis becomes increasing likely if other additional fetal debris (mucin, hair, fat) is found. New supportive tests for antenatal diagnosis include identification of antibodies to human keratin or amniotic fluid-derived mucin and zinc coproporphyrin levels (derived from meconium) in the blood, although the sensitivity and specificity of these tests have not been clearly defined.

Management

The treatment of amniotic fluid embolism is entirely supportive. The goals include ensuring adequate oxygenation, treating cardiovascular collapse, and combating the coagulopathy. Cardiopulmonary resuscitation should be instigated immediately, if indicated. Aortocaval compression should be reduced by left uterine displacement if amniotic fluid embolism occurs in the antenatal period. Due to the dramatic presentation of amniotic fluid embolism, most patients require oxygen therapy, endotracheal intubation, and positive pressure ventilation to ensure adequate oxygenation. A large-bore intravenous cannula should be sited and intravenous fluids rapidly infused to increase the preload. Blood samples should be taken for baseline full blood count, urea and electrolytes, clotting screen and also for cross-matching. Central venous pressure monitoring is useful to assess the adequacy of the patient's circulating volume and to enable titration of further intravenous fluids. Pulmonary artery catheterisation is helpful for treatment of continuing hypotension despite adequate right ventricular filling pressures or in the face of pulmonary oedema. Manipulation of intravenous fluid administration and vasopressors according to haemodynamic measurements may then be used to optimise left ventricular dysfunction. In antenatal situations, urgent delivery by caesarean section may improve resuscitation and also prevent further amniotic fluid embolism.

Aggressive management of coagulopathy, including transfusion of blood, platelets, fresh frozen plasma, and cryoprecipitate, is important. Cryoprecipitate may be particularly useful, as it contains high concentrations of fibronectin in addition to fibrinogen and other clotting factors. Fibronectin aids the clearance of cellular and particulate matter from the circulation by the reticuloendothelial system, with potential improvement in outcome. Uterine atony may accompany coagulopathy and should be treated as described above. In the event of severe hypoxaemia, ergometrine and prostaglandin 15-methyl $F_{2\alpha}$ should be used cautiously due to additional bronchoconstrictive properties of these drugs. Indwelling epidural catheters should only be removed when coagulopathy has been corrected. The use of heparin and ε-aminocaproic acid may be helpful in the treatment of disseminated intravascular coagulopathy unresponsive to product replacement. Intravenous corticosteroids have been reported to be of benefit in some cases, but efficacy has not been proved. Continuous arteriovenous haemofiltration has also been used successfully in amniotic fluid embolism.[25] It is speculated that substances playing an important role in respiratory and left ventricular dysfunction may be removed during filtration.

Coagulopathy

Haemostasis initially requires local vasoconstriction with simultaneous dilation of the adjacent arterioles in order to divert blood away from the site of haemorrhage. Sequential platelet plug formation and initiation of the coagulation cascade with deposition and stabilisation of fibrin are necessary. Finally due to fibrinolysis, fibrin is removed and blood flow reestablished.

During normal pregnancy there is an associated blood hypercoagulability, which helps to reduce blood loss at delivery. Hypercoagulability results from increased concentrations of coagulation factors (fibrinogen, VII, VIII, IX, X, XII), decreased levels of coagulation inhibitors (protein S), and a reduction in fibrinolytic activity. This is reflected in a mild reduction in pro-thrombin time, activated partial prothrombin time, thrombin time, and bleeding time as compared to the non-pregnant state.

Bleeding diatheses can result from abnormalities of the blood vessels, platelets or the coagulation system. The commoner coagulopathies occurring in pregnancy are shown in Box 7.6.

Box 7.6   Aetiology of obstetric coagulopathies

Disseminated intravascular coagulation secondary to:
    placental abruption
    amniotic fluid embolus
    massive blood transfusion
    pre-eclampsia/eclampsia
    chorioamnionitis
    prolonged intrauterine death
    sepsis
Dilutional secondary to:
    massive blood transfusion
HELLP syndrome
Iatrogenic secondary to:
    warfarin
    heparin and LMWH
Pre-existing coagulopathy secondary to:
    von Willebrand's disease
    haemophilia (A – factor VIII, B – factor IX)
    autoimmune thrombocytopenic purpura

Assessment

Haemostatic assessment should include a detailed history of previous excessive bruising or bleeding with minor trauma, surgery or dental work. Family history of similar events should also be noted. Drug history, including recent ingestion of heparin, warfarin, aspirin or NSAIDs, should be recorded. Patients should be examined for signs of bleeding or bruising with particular reference to the mucous membranes, intravenous sites, recent surgical incisions, and beneath blood pressure cuffs. Evidence of chronic bleeding disorders such as arthritic deformities and hepato-splenomegaly may be apparent. Coagulopathies due to platelet dysfunction tend to produce more superficial bruising than those due to coagulation factor deficit.

Laboratory haemostatic evaluation may include platelet count, activated

257

partial thromboplastin time, prothrombin time, thrombin time, and fibrin degradation products.

The platelet count is useful as spontaneous bleeding can occur at levels below 20×10^9/l and severe intraoperative bleeding with counts below 70×10^9/l. The activated partial thromboplastin time indicates changes in the intrinsic and common pathways of the coagulation cascade (i.e. all factors except VII and XIII). However, prolongation will only occur when factors have fallen to 30% of the normal levels[26] or rarely by the inhibition of the intrinsic pathway such as by the lupus anticoagulant. The prothrombin time assesses the extrinsic and common pathways of the coagulation cascade (i.e. factors II, V, VII, X, and fibrinogen). Prolongation occurs when factors V, VII or X are reduced by 50%, factor II (prothrombin) is reduced by 70% or fibrinogen is reduced to less than 1 g/l.[26] Thrombin time evaluates the last step in the common pathway, the conversion of fibrinogen to fibrin by the action of thrombin. Either fibrinogen deficiency or the presence of inhibitory substances such as heparin or fibrin degradation products can cause a prolongation of the result. Prolongation of thrombin time unrelated to heparin administration is suggestive of disseminated intravascular coagulation. Fibrin degradation products are formed from the cleavage of both fibrin and fibrinogen by plasmin. Although elevated levels are found in pregnancy, liver disease, renal disease, and thromboembolism, increased levels are also found with disseminated intravascular coagulation. A more accurate test for the products of plasmin cleavage, with fewer false-positive results, is the D dimer test.

The use of bleeding time for individual patients has largely been abandoned as it is not a specific *in vitro* indicator of the platelet function or a predictor of the risk of haemorrhage.[27]

The involvement of a haematologist may be necessary to provide advice on the usefulness of additional investigations such as those for platelet function or coagulation factor assay.

Thrombelastography provides a global assessment of haemostatic function including information on subsequent clot stability and fibrinolysis, rather than results from isolated areas of the coagulation profile. Its use, both in the assessment of coagulopathy in the pregnant patient and also for guidance of blood component replacement, is gaining acceptance.[28]

Management

Management and treatment priorities for the bleeding obstetric patient with a coagulopathy are the same as those described in relation to massive haemorrhage (see above).

The use of blood and coagulation component replacement is determined by continued blood loss together with laboratory assessment of coagulation dysfunction. Acquired coagulopathies also require treatment of the precipitating cause, such as sepsis or intrauterine fetal death in the case of disseminated intravascular coagulation. It should also be remembered that the cause of the coagulopathy may be multiple. For example, massive blood transfusion may be accompanied by coagulopathies produced by both dilutional effects as well as disseminated intravascular coagulation.

Disseminated intravascular coagulopathy (DIC)

DIC is triggered by a procoagulant stimulus in a wide variety of obstetric and non-obstetric conditions. The result is uncontrolled intravascular fibrin deposition and haemorrhage associated with depletion of clotting factors and platelets. Subsequent activation of the fibrinolytic system produces fibrin degradation products with additional anticoagulant properties. The clinical presentation of DIC ranges from asymptomatic to life-threatening haemorrhage or thrombosis.

Obstetric triggers for DIC include tissue thromboplastin (placental abruption, amniotic fluid embolus), endothelial damage (HELLP syndrome) or hypotensive conditions (Gram-negative septicaemia, massive haemorrhage). Fulminant DIC carries a high mortality which may be related to the underlying cause (sepsis), haemorrhage or end-organ failure. Diagnosis of DIC includes clinical presentation with confirmatory laboratory tests. Although there is no single pathognomonic test for DIC, the following *in vitro* findings may occur.

1 Prolongation of coagulation tests (thrombin, activated partial thromboplastin and prothrombin times).
2 Decreased fibrinogen and antithrombin III concentrations.
3 Reduced platelets.
4 Increased fibrin degradation products, D dimers.

Fibrin degradation products may be normal in up to 15% of patients with DIC and because of their long half-life, clinical improvement may not be reflected in a reduction in their concentration for some time. Antithrombin III is probably the most sensitive index of DIC but as the assay is complex, its measurement may not be a practical option.

Treatment

Treatment of the condition is directed towards removing the underlying cause.[29] If the DIC is attributable to a gravid uterus, as in the case of pre-eclampsia, placental abruption or intrauterine death, delivery of the baby may be necessary. Regional anaesthesia is clearly contraindicated in a patient with a significant coagulopathy because of the risk of haematoma and spinal cord compression.

Supportive treatment is necessary to correct concurrent hypotension, anaemia, hypoxia, acidosis, and electrolyte imbalance. This may include the use of intravenous fluids, inotropes, blood transfusion, ventilation, and haemofiltration. Correction of coagulation abnormalities should be attempted with fresh frozen plasma, cryoprecipitate, factor concentrates, and platelets.[30] Due to the consumptive nature of the disease process, it is difficult to predict the quantities of coagulation component replacement needed. Laboratory test results help to select the most effective blood products and to monitor doses required. However, in cases of dramatic haemorrhage with DIC, empiric coagulation component replacement may be needed in the initial treatment period.

Fresh frozen plasma should be given in situations of microvascular bleeding and activated partial thromboplastin time, prothrombin time, and thrombin time in excess of 1.5 times normal values. Each unit of fresh frozen plasma consists of 150–300 ml of plasma containing all clotting factors and a fibrinogen level of 2–5 mg/ml. The usual initial dose of fresh frozen plasma is 15 ml/kg. However, if the fibrinogen level is less than 1 g/l, the level can only be effectively increased by giving cryporecipitate. Each unit of cryoprecipitate consists of 10–20 ml of plasma and contains factors I, V, VIII, and XIII with a fibrinogen content of 150–300 mg/unit. The initial adult dose is 15 units which contains 3–4 g of fibrinogen. As outlined earlier, platelets should be considered with platelet counts below 50×10^9/l. Each unit of 40–60 ml contains at least 55×10^9 platelets and should be given at an initial dose of one unit per 10 kg body mass.

The use of heparin is controversial, although it may be advocated where intravascular thrombosis rather than haemorrhage is the major problem. Heparin stimulates the production and activity of antithrombin III which forms a complex with activated thrombin, so preventing the conversion of fibrinogen to fibrin. Factor X is also prevented from inducing the conversion of prothrombin to thrombin.

Pre-eclampsia and eclampsia

Hypertensive disorders of pregnancy are the second most common cause of maternal mortality in the United Kingdom.[1] Although there has been a reduction in mortality attributable to cerebral haemorrhage, there has been an increased number of deaths due to adult respiratory distress syndrome. Poor control of fluid balance and circulatory overload were evident in over 25% of the cases reviewed.

Pre-eclampsia or gestational proteinuric hypertension is a multisystem disorder of unknown aetiology occurring after 20 weeks gestation unless associated with a hydatidiform mole. Both mother and baby face potential dangers as a consequence of pre-eclampsia. Maternal problems include seizures, cerebral haemorrhage, pulmonary oedema, coagulopathy, hepatic dysfunction, renal dysfunction, and increased maternal mortality. In addition, the fetus is at risk of intrauterine growth retardation, placental abruption, prematurity, and increased perinatal mortality.

Life-threatening complications may occur in pre-eclampsia without prior warning symptoms or signs. Despite this, it is important to determine those with severe pre-eclampsia who can be identified and who are at increased risk of maternal/perinatal morbidity and mortality.

Severe pre-eclampsia is diagnosed in the presence of one or more of the following.

- Hypertension (systolic pressure ≥160 mmHg or diastolic ≥110 mmHg)
- Proteinuria (≥5 g/24 hours or ≥3+ on dipstick)
- Oliguria
- Cerebral problems (seizures, headache, visual symptoms, altered consciousness)
- Respiratory dysfunction (pulmonary oedema)
- Hepatic dysfunction (impaired liver function tests, right upper quadrant/epigastric pain, hepatic rupture)
- Thrombocytopenia
- HELLP syndrome (Haemolysis, Elevated Liver enzymes, Low Platelets)

Pre-eclampsia occurs in 6–7% of all pregnancies, with approximately 1% having severe disease. Eclampsia, the occurrence of seizures in the pre-eclamptic patient, occurs in approximately 0.05% of pregnancies in the United Kingdom.[31]

The goals in the management of the patient with severe pre-eclampsia include maintenance of maternal well-being together with the delivery of a live infant in optimal condition. The decision, as well as the urgency of delivery, depends on both maternal and fetal condition.[32] The anaesthetist may be involved in certain emergency situations with these patients including maternal hypertensive crises, seizures, oliguria, coagulopathy (including DIC and HELLP syndrome), and emergency delivery.

Management of severe pre-eclampsia

These patients should be admitted to a high-dependency area in order to adequately monitor maternal parameters and fetal well-being.

Acute hypertensive episodes

Severe hypertensive episodes should be treated in order to attenuate the risk of intracranial haemorrhage, hypertensive encephalopathy, acute renal failure, and placental abruption.[33] It is recommended that blood pressure in excess of 170/110 should be treated urgently, although the rate of increase in the blood pressure may be more important than the absolute level. Over-enthusiastic reductions in blood pressure may result in coma, stroke, acute renal failure, myocardial infarction or decreased uteroplacental perfusion.

The cause of hypertension in pre-eclampsia was originally thought only to be due to a high systemic vascular resistance. However, studies have shown variable haemodynamics in these patients. Untreated patients have been shown to have normal or increased systemic vascular resistance, reduced or normal central venous pressure, reduced or normal pulmonary artery occlusion pressure, and reduced or normal cardiac output. Poor correlation exists between central venous pressure and pulmonary artery occlusion pressure in patients with severe disease. Findings in treated patients (i.e. mild vasodilation/intravascular volume expansion) have included normal or high cardiac output, systemic vascular resistance, and pulmonary artery occlusion pressure. This means that although hypertension is usually the result of increased systemic vascular resistance, it may also be due to a hyperdynamic left ventricle.

Treatment of acute hypertension usually involves the use of vasodilators to combat the elevated systemic vascular resistance and potential organ ischaemia. Careful prior intravascular volume expansion with fluids is necessary to prevent precipitous falls in blood pressure. Although a variety of drugs have been used, all have advantages and disadvantages and no single drug has proved to be superior (Table 7.7). Labetalol, with its combined α- and β-blocking effects, has the potential advantage of combating the elevated systemic vascular resistance as well as the hyperdynamic left ventricle. However, its β-blocking action may impair the capacity of the fetus to respond to intrauterine stress. Ideal drug properties include rapid onset, short offset (in the event of overtitration), ability to titrate to the desired blood pressure and to produce an improvement in uteroplacental perfusion. During the treatment of an acute hypertensive episode, continuous fetal heart rate monitoring should be applied in order to determine any detrimental fetal effects.

Eclampsia

Treatment of convulsions is important in order to reduce maternal and fetal hypoxia resulting from loss of consciousness, airway obstruction, and aspiration. Most eclamptic seizures occur postnatally (44%), although 38% occur antenatally and 18% during labour.[31] Seizures are the result of severe cerebrovasospasm resulting in ischaemia and oedema. Management goals are:

1 maintenance of an unobstructed protected airway;
2 cessation of the convulsion (either with magnesium or benzodiazepines);
3 reduction in aortocaval compression by left lateral tilt;
4 maintenance of adequate maternal and fetal oxygenation (with respiratory support if necessary);
5 prevention of subsequent convulsions (by the use of magnesium);
6 maintenance of fluid balance;
7 control of blood pressure if necessary;
8 consideration of delivery once the maternal situation has been stabilised.

Table 7.7 Acute antihypertensive treatment in pre-eclamptic patients

Agent	Dose	Action	Advantage	Disadvantage
Hydralazine	5–10 mg IV	Direct arteriolar vasodilation	Extensive use in parturients, good safety record	Slow onset (10–20 min) Long duration (4–6 h) Tachycardia
Nifedipine	10 mg SL	Calcium channel antagonist	Rapid onset (<5min) Uterine relaxation	Tachycardia Interaction with magnesium ($\downarrow\downarrow$ BP)
Labetalol	5–10 mg IV	α/β antagonist	Rapid onset $\downarrow$SVR/CO Rare to overshoot target BP	Variable efficacy Contraindications (asthma, pulmonary oedema) Reduced fetal heart rate variability
Sodium nitroprusside	Initial IV infusion 0.25 µg/kg/min	Direct vasodilator	Rapid onset (<1 min) Short duration (<10 min)	Cyanide/thiocyanate toxicity Direct arterial BP monitoring required
Nitroglycerin	Initial IV infusion 10 µg/min	Direct vasodilator	Rapid onset (<1 min) Short duration (<10 min)	Methaemoglobinaemia Direct arterial BP monitoring required

Magnesium sulphate has been shown to be superior to phenytoin or diazepam in the prevention of recurrent seizures in eclamptic patients.[4] It has also been shown to reduce the incidence of convulsions in hypertensive parturients as compared to phenytoin[34] or placebo.[35] Although definitely indicated in eclampsia, its prophylactic use in pre-eclampsia is controversial. Widespread use in pre-eclamptic patients would necessitate many patients receiving the drug, with the inherent risk of side-effects, in order to combat the relatively low incidence of eclampsia found in the United Kingdom. Also, approximately 40% of eclamptic patients are not identified before their first convulsion[36] and therefore will not receive the benefit of prophylaxis.

Although magnesium may be used in the acute control of seizures, it has not been shown to be superior to diazepam. Therefore either drug may be used, although controversy exists regarding the optimum dose of magnesium. The Royal College of Obstetricians and Gynaecologists suggest a loading dose of 4 g over 5–10 minutes, followed by a maintenance dose of 1 g/h continued for at least 24 hours after the last convulsion. Recurrent seizures should be treated with further 2 g boluses of magnesium.[37]

The postulated mechanisms of action of magnesium are NMDA blockade, calcium antagonism, and cerebral vasodilation. Magnesium is only effective in the treatment of eclamptic seizures, having no effect on other convulsions. Additional beneficial effects are improvement in uterine and renal blood flow, reduction in platelet adhesiveness, and tocolysis. However, side-effects include negative inotropic properties, nausea, flushing, neuromuscular blockade, and fetal effects (decreased fetal heart rate variability and neonatal neuromuscular depression).[38,39] Its use in myasthenia gravis is contraindicated. Magnesium sulphate has a narrow therapeutic window (2–4 mmol/l) and awareness of signs of increasing toxicity is important. These include nausea, flushing, diplopia, slurred speech, weakness, loss of tendon reflexes, muscular paralysis and ultimately respiratory and cardiac arrest. Toxicity should be monitored by hourly deep tendon reflexes, respiratory rate, and oxygen saturation. If deep tendon reflexes become absent, the magnesium infusion should be terminated until serum levels are known. As magnesium is excreted by the kidneys, serum levels should be monitored regularly during oliguria to enable an appropriate reduction in dosage. The acute effects of toxicity can be managed by supportive means in addition to 10 mmol of intravenous calcium chloride.

The use of magnesium has further implications for the anaesthetist. Magnesium inhibits the release of neurotransmitters at all nerve terminals, including that of acetylcholine at the motor endplate. Consequently, as well as inherent neuromuscular blocking properties, it has been shown to potentiate both depolarising and non-depolarising muscle relaxants. However, its effect on depolarising muscle relaxants has been refuted. As fasciculations after suxamethonium may be absent, they should not be relied on to indicate acceptable intubation conditions. Normal doses of suxamethonium for intubation may be used. However, if repeated doses are administered, there is an increased risk of phase II block and subsequent potentiation by magnesium. Approximately one-fifth of the normal dose of non-depolarising muscle relaxants should be used and to enable the safe use of additional doses, neuromuscular function must be monitored.

Due to the vasodilator properties of magnesium, its use in conjunction with regional anaesthesia may increase the risk of hypotensive episodes. Clinically this does not seem to be problematic with judicious use of intravenous fluids and ephedrine. If patellar reflexes are used to determine neuromuscular weakness, it should be remembered that their disappearance may be related to increasing epidural blockade and not magnesium toxicity.

Once seizures are controlled, hypotension corrected, and severe hypertension treated, delivery can be expedited. Vaginal or caesarean delivery can be considered depending on the clinical condition. If the patient is stable and without contraindications to regional anaesthesia, an epidural can be established. However, if the patient is obtunded or has evidence of increased intracranial pressure, an opioid/relaxant general anaesthetic technique is necessary.

Oliguria

Oliguria in the pre-eclamptic patient can result from inadequate intravascular volume, reduced renal perfusion or renal failure (acute tubular necrosis or cortical necrosis). Fluid management in these patients is complicated by altered haemodynamics and the risk of pulmonary oedema, due to both cardiogenic and non-cardiogenic causes. Pre-eclamptic patients are at particular risk of pulmonary oedema because of a reduction in intravascular colloid osmotic pressure (due to increased protein loss in urine/interstitial tissue and reduced hepatic synthesis), increased permeability of the pulmonary capillary endothelium (due to damage), increased intravascular volume without corresponding vasodilation (due to iatrogenic fluid overload, postpartum mobilisation of extravascular fluid or renal dysfunction) as well as ventricular dysfunction.

Initial maintenance intravascular fluid should be initiated at 1 ml/kg/h. However, this should be reviewed after assessment of the patient's condition, urine output and other additional fluid losses. If oliguria (≤ 0.5 ml/kg/h) occurs, a fluid challenge of 2 ml/kg of crystalloid may be considered. Although there are few randomised controlled studies on the use of fluid regimens in these patients, there is no evidence that colloid is superior to crystalloid replacement. On face value, colloid replacement would seem more appropriate due to the low intravascular colloid osmotic pressure found in these patients. However, in situations of increased capillary permeability, the colloid may be lost into the extravascular space, thereby exerting a reversed osmotic gradient and worsening the situation. It

265

is important that repeated unmonitored fluid challenges are not attempted and central venous pressure monitoring considered if oliguria persists. Due to associated coagulopathy in pre-eclampsia, the insertion of a central venous line is best achieved using a peripheral route (such as the antecubital fossa) or using the internal jugular rather than the subclavian route, so that local pressure can be applied in order for haemostasis to occur.

Absolute values of central venous pressures are not as important as their change in response to fluid challenges. Aggressive fluid preloading to central venous pressures of 6 cmH$_2$O (zeroed to right atrium) or more should be avoided in these patients due to the increased risk of pulmonary oedema.[36] Instead, cautious preloading should be used to convert central venous pressures from a negative to a positive value (such as 2–4 cmH$_2$O). Pulmonary artery catheter insertion should be considered in those patients with pulmonary oedema or renal failure. Fluid administration can then be given, based on the clinical signs of poor perfusion such as oliguria, decreased central venous or pulmonary artery occlusion pressures, increased systemic vascular resistance or decreased cardiac output. Intravenous fluid should be restricted in the presence of hypervolaemia as indicated by increased central venous or pulmonary artery occlusion pressures and normal systemic vascular resistance or in the presence of pulmonary oedema. If pulmonary oedema occurs treatment includes supplemental oxygen, diuretics, reduction in preload and afterload, fluid restriction, and ventilation. Persistent oliguria with deteriorating renal function should be managed with fluid restriction (volume infused per hour = urine output during previous hour + 30 ml). Low-dose dopamine and haemodialysis or filtration may be required.

Coagulopathy

Coagulopathy associated with pre-eclampsia may be the result of isolated thrombocytopenia, DIC (see above) or HELLP syndrome. Thrombocytopenia occurs in 15–30% of pre-eclamptic patients due to increased consumption and shortened platelet lifespan. In addition, platelet dysfunction may occur, although recent evidence has cast doubt over this.

HELLP syndrome, a subgroup of pre-eclampsia, occurs in up to 20% of those with severe disease.[36] It is characterised by microangiopathic haemolytic anaemia (due to the destruction of red blood cells after passage through damaged vessels), elevated liver enzymes (due to periportal or focal parenchymal hepatic necrosis), and low platelets (due to consumption and reduced lifespan). The syndrome represents a continuum from mild to life-threatening forms with patients at risk being white, multiparous, and of increased age. Hypertension and proteinuria may not be immediately apparent. Two-thirds of cases occur antenatally and common symptoms include general malaise or flu-like symptoms (90%), right upper quadrant or epigastric pain (90%), and nausea and vomiting (50%). The anaesthetist should have a high index of suspicion in patients complaining of these symptoms and ensure adequate evaluation, especially of haemostatic status, is performed.

Maternal mortality occurs in up to 24% of patients and perinatal mortality in up to 60%.[40] This is related to associated complications such as haemorrhage, DIC, severe hypoglycaemia, placental abruption, acute renal failure, hepatic failure, and rupture.

The decision for delivery depends on the maternal condition and severity of disease as well as fetal gestational age and well-being. Conservative management has been used in those with mild disease or with a premature fetus if the maternal condition allows.

Blood components, including red blood cells, platelets, and fresh frozen plasma, should be readily available. The nadir of thrombocytopenia can occur within 1–3 days of delivery and may not recover for up to 11 days postpartum. Platelet transfusion has been recommended if the platelet count is $<50 \times 10^9/l$ for caesarean section and $<20 \times 10^9/l$ for vaginal delivery.

Although regional anaesthesia would not be considered with severe coagulopathy, controversy exists as to the safe lower limit of thrombocytopenia. Haljamäe recommends that regional anaesthesia may be considered safe in pre-eclamptic parturients if prothrombin time is $\geq 50\%$, activated partial thromboplastin time is at the upper normal limit, platelet count is $\geq 80 \times 10^9/l$ and with no symptoms of bleeding tendency.[41] If, however, there has been a rapid decline in platelets (e.g. from 120 to $80 \times 10^9/l$) during the preceding four hours, regional anaesthesia is probably unsafe. It is important to evaluate the risks and benefits of regional anaesthesia in the individual patient.

Emergency delivery

There is a choice of regional (spinal, extension of epidural block or combined spinal epidural) or general anaesthesia for urgent caesarean section. However, emergency situations such as severe fetal distress or maternal haemorrhage may necessitate the use of a general anaesthetic. Additional hazards associated with general anaesthesia in pre-eclamptic patients include difficult intubation, pressor responses related to laryngoscopy, intubation and extubation, and problems with neuromuscular relaxants after magnesium administration.

Difficult intubation may be related to generalised or largyngeal oedema. Assessment of facial oedema and history of hoarseness or stridor is important before induction. Difficult intubation equipment and a wide range of smaller, differently sized endotracheal tubes should be available. Blood pressure should be controlled before induction, as discussed earlier in the chapter. Despite this, exaggerated pressor responses may occur in pre-eclamptic patients due to intubation with risk of cerebrovascular accident, increased myocardial oxygen requirements, pulmonary oedema, and reduced uterine blood supply. These responses may be attenuated with alfentanil 10 μg/kg, magnesium sulphate 40 mg/kg or labetalol 5–10 mg. At extubation the pressor responses also need to be obtunded but without depression of conscious level or airway reflexes. Antihypertensive agents such as labetolol 5–10 mg or esmolol 1.5 mg/kg may be useful.

The concurrent use of magnesium sulphate potentiates the action of non-depolarising muscle relaxants and may also prolong the action of suxamethonium. Atracurium is the non-depolarising muscle relaxant of choice as renal or hepatic clearance is not required. Isoflurane is the optimal volatile due to minimal hepatic metabolism. In the presence of laryngeal oedema, continued intubation should be considered until a leak occurs around the endotracheal tube once the cuff is deflated.

Where caesarean section is urgent but not immediate, spinal or extension of a pre-existing epidural block can be considered. Use of regional anaesthesia in the presence of coagulopathy has already been discussed. Spinal anaesthesia is often precluded because of the perceived risks of severe hypotension in pre-eclamptic patients. However, recent evidence indicates that spinals may not produce significantly more hypotension than epidurals.[42] Before regional anaesthesia, careful preloading with 500–1000 ml of intravenous fluid reduces the risk of hypotension and fetal distress. Ephedrine can be used to treat hypotension; however, as pre-eclamptic patients are more sensitive to vasopressors, reduced doses should be titrated to required response.

Fetal distress

Fetal distress results from inadequate oxygen delivery to the baby and represents one of the major indications for emergency caesarean section. It is therefore vital that the anaesthetist should understand the diagnosis, aetiology, and management of fetal distress in order to implement a safe anaesthetic plan and avoid unnecessarily urgent deliveries being performed without adequate evaluation and preparation.

During inadequate oxygen delivery, the fetus adapts by releasing catecholamines inducing a tachycardia and redistribution of blood flow from peripheral to more central vital organs (including the brain, heart, and placenta). Anaerobic metabolism occurs resulting in hypoxaemia, hypercarbia, and acidosis. Progressive reduction in fetal heart rate variability occurs and the initial tachycardia is replaced by bradycardia.

Diagnosis

The most widely used methods for detecting intrapartum fetal distress include fetal heart rate and scalp pH monitoring. Although these methods rarely fail to identify a compromised baby, the large false-positive rate may result in obstetric intervention being undertaken unnecessarily. Other assessment techniques, including intrapartum oximetry, umbilical artery blood velocity waveform, and computerised fetal heart rate analysis, may be found to be more accurate predictors of neonatal outcome.

Fetal heart rate monitoring consists of assessment of baseline rate, variability and the relationship of accelerations and decelerations to uterine contractions. The normal fetal heart rate pattern includes a rate of 120–160/min and variability of 10–15/min and shows accelerations in response to uterine contractions. During labour, early decelerations in heart rate may occur. Assuming the decelerations fall by less than 20 beats/minute and are synchronous with the uterine contraction, the pattern is reassuring of adequate oxygenation and no further action need be taken. However, in the presence of a non-reassuring heart rate pattern, a fetal scalp pH blood sample should be taken to confirm or exclude acidosis. Non-reassuring heart rate patterns include profound bradycardia (<80/min for ≥3 min), late decelerations where onset and offset occur 10–30 seconds after uterine contractions or unexplained poor or absent baseline variability.

To interpret fetal pH results correctly, the maternal acid-base status should be known. Otherwise maternal hyperventilation can normalise the results obtained from an acidotic fetus or a healthy fetus may appear compromised due to maternal acidosis. Assuming maternal acid-base status is known, a fetal scalp blood pH >7.25 is considered normal, pH 7.2–7.25 necessitates repeat sampling, and pH <7.2 indicates the need for immediate delivery.[43] However, pH assessment is irrelevant in the presence of an agonal fetal heart rate pattern such as prolonged bradycardia or late deceleration without variability and recovery, as immediate operative delivery is necessary.

Aetiology

Fetal distress can be caused by reduced maternal oxygenation as well as poor oxygen transport via the uterine vessels. Reductions in uterine blood flow can result from:

1 decreased uterine arterial pressure caused by maternal hypovolaemia, hypotension or cord entrapment;
2 increased uterine venous pressure caused by uterine contractions, vena caval compression or the Valsalva manoeuvre;
3 increased uterine vascular resistance resulting from the release of endogenous catecholamines during stress, from exogenous vasoconstrictors such as phenylephrine and ephedrine or due to disease states such as pre-eclampsia.

269

Table 7.8   Categories of emergency caesarean section

Urgency of delivery	Preferred anaesthetic technique	Example
Stable: delivery within 2 hours	Epidural/spinal/CSE	Chronic uteroplacental insufficiency Previous caesarean section in active labour
Urgent: delivery within 1 hour	Extension of existing epidural/spinal/CSE	Failure to progress Severe pre-eclampsia
Emergency: delivery within 30 minutes	Extension of existing epidural/single-shot spinal/general anaesthesia	Severe fetal heart rate abnormality Fetal blood sample pH <7.20
Immediate: delivery as soon as possible	General anaesthesia ?Extention of pre-existing epidural	Cord prolapse with fetal distress Ruptured uterus Massive maternal haemorrhage

Management

Anaesthetic management during fetal distress includes identification and treatment of reversible causes and formation and implementation of an anaesthetic plan to ensure the safety of both mother and infant. Good communication between obstetrician and anaesthetist is necessary to ensure the urgency of the delivery is clearly defined.

The degree of urgency determines the choice of anaesthetic, as time is the critical factor (Table 7.8). Before caesarean section, treatment should be directed towards correcting reversible causes of fetal distress (Table 7.9). This may also reduce the urgency of delivery, allowing more time for patient preparation and evaluation before anaesthesia.

All parturients with acute fetal distress should be treated with supplemental oxygen, alteration of maternal position in order to alleviate cord compression and reduce aortocaval compression, and the discontinuation of any oxytocics. Fetal distress associated with uterine hyperactivity can also be improved by active tocolysis as uteroplacental perfusion only occurs between contractions. Tocolysis is usually achieved with β-agonists including ritodrine or terbutaline. However, prolonged side-effects may be produced such as tachycardia, palpitations, tremor and tocolysis (with potential effects on the subsequent course of labour and postpartum blood loss). Recent evidence suggests 60–90 µg of intravenous nitroglycerine may relieve severe intrapartum fetal distress related to uterine hyperactivity.[44] Side-effects including mild hypotension can be rapidly corrected with the use of ephedrine. Nitroglycerine may be the drug of choice due to its rapid onset and offset.

All parturients undergoing emergency caesarean section should receive aspiration prophylaxis such as metoclopramide and ranitidine and, when general anaesthesia is required, sodium citrate. Fetal heart rate monitoring should be continued until delivery as any changes in fetal condition may

Table 7.9   Treatment of fetal distress

Aetiology	Management
Decreased maternal oxygenation, for example pneumonia	Administer supplemental oxygen
Hypotension	Administer supplemental oxygen Lateral tilt to reduce aortocaval compression Intravenous fluid bolus Vasoconstrictors (for example, ephedrine)
Prolonged uterine contraction	Discontinue oxytocin Administer tocolytics (for example, ritodrine 6 mg IV, terbutaline 0.25 mg IV, nitroglycerin 50–100 µg IV)
Umbilical cord compression	Change position to relieve compression Consider amnioinfusion if indicated (for example, with thick meconium-stained amniotic fluid or oligohydramnios)
Umbilical cord prolapse	Push fetal head off pelvic floor and deliver
Chronic antepartum fetal distress	Epidural in labour may improve uteroplacental blood flow and can be used for anaesthesia if surgical delivery becomes necessary

require re-evaluation of the anaesthetic plan.

General anaesthesia usually provides the most rapid means of anaesthesia for a immediate caesarean section. Other beneficial effects include abdominal and uterine relaxation, which may be important in prematurity. Disadvantages of general anaesthesia include depressant effects of anaesthetic drugs in an already compromised baby, in addition to the risks of failed intubation, aspiration, and awareness.

Extension of an epidural (providing pre-existing block already exists) using 2% lignocaine with adrenaline has been used in emergency caesarean section to provide adequate operating conditions within 12.5 minutes.[45] If anaesthesia is initially inadequate for surgery, additional anaesthesia can be achieved using local infiltration or analgesics such as increments of ketamine 10 mg intravenously. Advantages of epidural blockade include the relatively slow onset of action with its consequent lower incidence of severe hypotension. The sympathetic blockade may also be useful in reducing uterine vasoconstriction providing hypotension does not exist. All patients considered at high risk for fetal distress should be encouraged to have epidural analgesia in labour.

The advantages of spinal anaesthesia in the presence of fetal distress are the speed of onset and the minimal drug effects on the baby. However, the risk of hypotension may be higher than for epidural blockade, although fluid preloading and the availability of vasoconstrictors may reduce this problem.

271

Neonatal resuscitation

Although most babies are born in good health, 6% require life support in the delivery suite and 0.12% need chest compressions or pharmacological resuscitation.[46,47] Resuscitation is more likely in those pregnancies considered to be high-risk deliveries (Table 7.10). The anaesthetist's prime role is to provide care to the mother; however, in an emergency situation he or she may be required to briefly assist in the resuscitation of the newborn.

Certain anatomical/physiological changes occur in the newborn during the transition to extrauterine life that are paramount to the understanding of neonatal resuscitation. As many of these changes are initially reversible, they can revert during conditions associated with hypoxia, acidosis, and hypothermia, with detrimental effects on the newborn.

Table 7.10   Babies at increased risk of requiring resuscitation

Maternal	Obstetric related disease, e.g. pre-eclampsia
	Pre-existing chronic disease, e.g. diabetes mellitus, cardiac disease, renal disease
Fetal	Preterm <35 weeks gestation
	Postterm >42 weeks gestation
	Oligohydramnios/polyhydramnios
	Congenital abnormalities
	Intrauterine complications (growth restriction, infection)
	Multiple pregnancy
Labour/delivery	Fetal distress
	Complications of labour/delivery (e.g. antepartum haemorrhage, prolapsed umbilical cord)
	Abnormal presentations
	Assisted delivery (caesarean section, forceps)

Cardiovascular system

The placenta is the site of gas exchange in the fetus, with minimal blood flow going to the lungs where pulmonary vascular resistance is high. As a consequence of this, various shunts are required to deliver oxygenated blood from the placenta to the rest of the body. These include:

1 the ductus venosus (between the placenta and the inferior vena cava);
2 the foramen ovale (between right and left atrium);
3 the ductus arteriosus (between the pulmonary outflow tract and descending aorta).

At birth, as the umbilical cord is clamped (or exposed to cold), there is an increase in the systemic vascular resistance as placental blood flow ceases and the ductus venosus closes. The right atrial pressure decreases due to the reduction in the venous return from the inferior vena cava. As the lungs expand there is a reduction in pulmonary vascular resistance, with an elevation in left atrial pressure, as increased quantities of blood return from the pulmonary circulation. As a result of left atrial pressure becoming greater than right atrial pressure, the foramen ovale closes. The ductus arteriosus also closes because of the increase in partial pressure of oxygen due to the increase in pulmonary oxygenation.

Respiratory system

Asphyxia from cessation of oxygenated blood is the major stimulant of respiration. The type II pneumocytes in the alveoli are then stimulated by lung distension to produce surfactant, which decreases surface tension and prevents alveolar collapse during expiration. During the first breath, an intrapleural pressure in excess of −70 mmHg has to be generated, in order to expand the lungs and overcome the viscosity of the fluid-filled airways and surface tension in the alveoli, in addition to the elastic recoil and compliance of the chest wall, airways, and lungs. Surfactant production is reduced in conditions of hypothermia, hypoxia, and acidosis, resulting in an increase in the work of breathing with further increases in intrapulmonary shunt.

Thermal regulation

Hypothermic neonates can only produce heat by non-shivering thermogenesis from brown fat metabolism. This process involves the release of noradrenaline with a subsequent increase in systemic vascular resistance, oxygen consumption, carbon dioxide production, and acidosis. A vicious circle is produced as these conditions favour fetal circulation reversion with pulmonary vascular constriction and further hypoxaemia. Maintaining a warm environment and adequate drying of the newborn should be emphasised to prevent these detrimental effects occurring.

Vital signs of a neonate at term are shown in Table 7.11. Apgar scores have been used widely to evaluate neonatal well-being by assessment of heart rate, respiratory activity, reflex irritability, muscle tone, and colour. However, the European Resuscitation Council[48] now suggests that the need for resuscitation can be more rapidly and accurately predicted by the assessment of heart rate, respiratory activity, and colour without the other

Table 7.11   Term neonatal vital signs

Heart rate (awake)	100–180/min
Respiratory rate	30–60/min
Systolic blood pressure	39–59 mmHg
Diastolic blood pressure	16–36 mmHg

Table 7.12   Initial assessment and resuscitation of newborn

Group	Clinical findings	Actions
1	Good respiratory efforts Centrally pink HR >100/min	Dry Keep warm
2	Respirations inadequate or absent Centrally cyanosed HR >100/min	Tactile stimulation (drying, flicking soles of feet) ± facial oxygen ± basic life support
3	Respirations inadequate or absent Pale/white (poor cardiac output, peripheral vasoconstriction) HR <100/min	Basic life support Intubation Positive pressure ventilation
4	Respirations inadequate or absent Pale/white (poor cardiac output, peripheral vasoconstriction) No detectable HR, although documented up to 20 minutes before delivery	Basic life support Advanced life support (positive pressure ventilation, chest compressions, resuscitation drugs)

parameters. Neonates can then be divided into four groups based on the clinical signs and the need for resuscitation (Table 7.12).

Hypothermia can be reduced by maintaining a warm (25°C), draught-free delivery room and placing the baby under a preheated radiant warmer. Rapid drying of the neonate and wrapping in a warm towel is also important.

Life support in the neonate follows the usual routine of assessment and correction of problems with the airway, breathing, and circulation. Basic life support should be initiated if the neonate has a heart rate <100/min, has failed to cry by 30 seconds or has failed to establish regular respiration by one minute. Advanced life support should be started if basic life support fails to produce a prompt improvement and there is either inadequate neonatal respiration or the heart rate remains less than 100/min despite adequate ventilation.

Figures 7.2 and 7.3 document the essentials of basic and advanced life support in the neonate. It is critical to initially expand the lungs adequately. It is recommended that inspiration should be maintained for 2–3 seconds and for 1–2 seconds for the subsequent 2nd–6th breaths. After these initial breaths the lungs should be ventilated at a rate of 30–40 breaths per minute.

The management of meconium aspiration is controversial, although general consensus is for an active approach. The oropharynx should be sucked out at birth and direct laryngoscopy performed. If there is meconium staining in the trachea, the newborn should be intubated and suction applied directly to the endotracheal tube. Providing the heart rate remains above

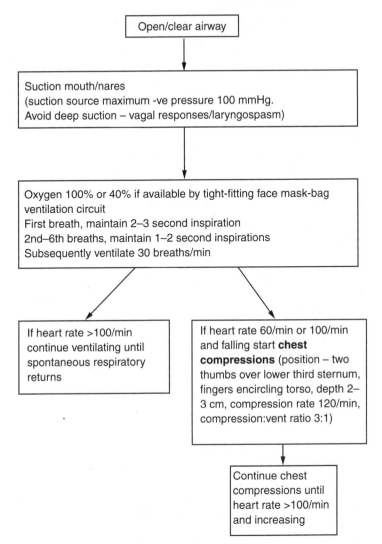

Fig 7.2 Neonatal basic life support

100/min, this procedure should be repeated before giving further respiratory support.

Oxygen in neonatal resuscitation

The use of 100% oxygen in resuscitation has been questioned, as this may increase organ damage due to increased oxygen free radicals. Studies comparing neonatal resuscitation using either 100% oxygen or room air have

275

If no response to basic life support

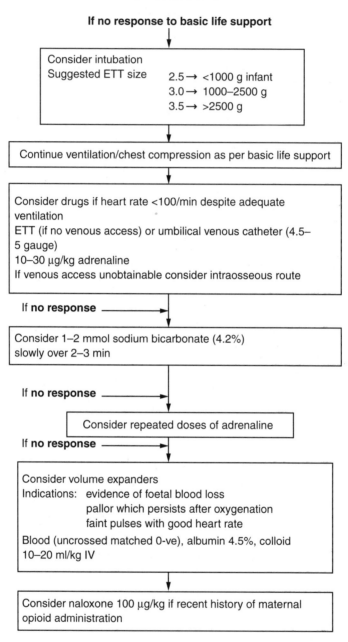

Consider intubation
Suggested ETT size   2.5 → <1000 g infant
                      3.0 → 1000–2500 g
                      3.5 → >2500 g

Continue ventilation/chest compression as per basic life support

Consider drugs if heart rate <100/min despite adequate ventilation
ETT (if no venous access) or umbilical venous catheter (4.5–5 gauge)
10–30 µg/kg adrenaline
If venous access unobtainable consider intraosseous route

If **no response**

Consider 1–2 mmol sodium bicarbonate (4.2%)
slowly over 2–3 min

If **no response**

Consider repeated doses of adrenaline

If **no response**

Consider volume expanders
Indications: evidence of foetal blood loss
               pallor which persists after oxygenation
               faint pulses with good heart rate
Blood (uncrossed matched 0-ve), albumin 4.5%, colloid
10–20 ml/kg IV

Consider naloxone 100 µg/kg if recent history of maternal opioid administration

ETT = endotracheal tube

Fig 7.3   Neonatal advanced life support

shown no differences in outcome.[49] Therefore, unnecessarily high concentrations or prolonged exposure of oxygen should be avoided.

Laryngeal mask airway

The size 1 laryngeal mask airway has been used to ventilate successfully neonates requiring resuscitation at birth.[50] Peak inflation pressure averaged 37 mmHg without problems related to gastric distension. The laryngeal mask may be useful during resuscitation as a means of avoiding intubation and its associated complications.

Route of drug administration

Resuscitation guidelines suggest endotracheal administration of certain drugs if intravenous access cannot be established rapidly. Suggested doses of adrenaline for intravenous or endotracheal routes are similar. However, effective doses via the endotracheal route may be much higher, as absorption may be reduced due to fluid-filled lungs, right-to-left intracardiac shunts, and a smaller pulmonary surface area to body mass ratio compared to the adult. Dose recommendations for resuscitation in the newborn have been extrapolated from the adult values with little scientific evidence.[51]

High-dose adrenaline

High-dose adrenaline (0.2 mg/kg) is not recommended for use in resuscitation of the newborn. Acute hypertensive responses to high-dose adrenaline may be of concern due to the susceptibility of the neonatal brain to intraventricular haemorrhage.

Sodium bicarbonate

Guidelines recommend that bicarbonate should only be given with presumed or documented metabolic acidosis, after adequate ventilation has been instigated. However, volume expanders may correct acidosis as effectively as bicarbonate, without the risks of hypernatraemia and hyperosmolality producing intraventricular haemorrhage.

Naloxone hydrochloride

Guidelines recommend that naloxone should be given to the newborn in order to reverse respiratory depression after maternal opioid administration. However, severe neonatal seizures have been reported when naxolone was given to the newborn of an opioid-dependent mother. Controversy exists as to whether in this situation, the neonate should be mechanically ventilated rather than have the respiratory depression pharmacologically reversed.

Viability

Many clinicians now consider that resuscitation of a neonate less than 23 weeks gestation age should not be attempted. One study[52] showed only 15% of those born at 23 weeks gestation survived and of those that survived, 98% had severe neurological damage.

References

1 Department of Health. *Report on confidential enquiries into maternal deaths in the UK, 1994–1996.* London: HMSO, 1998.

2 Department of Health. *Report on confidential enquiries into maternal deaths in the UK, 1991–1993.* London: HMSO, 1996.

3 Royal College of Obstetricians and Gynaecologists. *Thromboembolic disease in gynaecology and pregnancy. Recommendations for prophylaxis.* London: RCOG, 1995.

4 The Eclampsia Trial Collaborative Group. Which anticonvulsant for women with eclampsia? Evidence from the Collaborative Eclampsia Trial. *Lancet* 1995;**345**:1455–63.

5 Rees GAD, Willis BA. Resuscitation in late pregnancy. *Anaesthesia* 1988;**43**:347–9.

6 Basic Life Support Working Group of the European Resuscitation Council. The 1998 European Resuscitation Council guidelines for single rescue basic life support. *BMJ* 1998;**316**:1870–6.

7 Advanced Life Support Working Group of the European Resuscitation Council. The 1998 European Resuscitation Council guidelines for adult advanced life support. *BMJ* 1998;**316**:1863–9.

8 International Liaison Committee on Resuscitation. Special resuscitation situations. *Resuscitation* 1997;**34**:129–49.

9 Special situations. In: Driscoll P, Gwinnutt C, Mackway Jones K, Wardle T, eds. *Advanced cardiac life support: the practical approach,* 2nd edn. London: Chapman and Hall Medical, 1997:181–204.

10 Dildy GA, Clarke SL. Cardiac arrest during pregnancy. *Obstet Gynecol Clin North Am* 1995;**22**:303–14.

11 Selden BS, Burke TJ. Complete maternal and fetal recovery after prolonged cardiac arrest. *Ann Emerg Med* 1988;**17**:346–9.

12 Duthie SJ, Ghosh A, Ng A, Ho PC. Intraoperative blood loss during elective lower segment Caesarean section. *Br J Obstet Gynaecol* 1992;**99**:364–7.

13 Gonik B. Intensive care monitoring of the critically ill pregnant patient. In: Creasky RK, Resnik P, eds. *Maternal fetal medicine.* 2nd edn. London: WB Saunders, 1989.

14 Suresh M, Belfort M. Antepartum hemorrhage. In: Datta S, ed. *Anesthetic and obstetric management of the high risk pregnancy.* St Louis: Mosby, 1996:76–109.

15 Velanovich V. Crystalloid versus colloid fluid resuscitation. A meta-analysis of mortality. *Surgery* 1989;**105**:65–71.

16 Cochrane Injuries Group Albumin Reviewers. Human albumin administration in critically ill patients: systematic review of randomised controlled trials. *BMJ* 1998;**317**:235–40.

17 Jackson SH, Lonser RE. Safety and effectiveness of intracesarean blood salvage. *Transfusion* 1993;**33**:181.

18 Roberts WE. Emergent obstetric management of postpartum hemorrhage. *Obstet Gynecol Clin North Am* 1995;**22(2)**:283–302.

19 Moise KJ, Belfort MA. Damage control for the obstetric patient. *Surg Clin North Am* 1997;**77(4)**:835–52.

20 Mitty HA, Sterling KM, Alvarez M, Gendler R. Obstetric hemorrhage: prophylactic and emergency arterial catheterisation and embolotherapy. *Radiology* 1993;**188**:183–7.

21 McDougall RJ, Duke GJ. Amniotic fluid embolism syndrome: case report end review. *Anaesth Intens Care* 1995;**23**:735–40.

22 Clark SL, Montz FJ, Phelan JP. Hemodynamic alterations associated with amniotic fluid embolism: a reappraisal. *Am J Obstet Gynecol* 1985;**151**:617–21.

23 Martin RW. Amniotic fluid embolism. *Clin Obstet Gynecol* 1996;**39**:101–6.
24 Clark SL, Pavlova Z, Greenspoon J, Horenstein J, Phelan JP. Squamous cells in the maternal pulmonary circulation. *Am J Obstet Gynecol* 1986;**154**:104–6.
25 Weksler N, Ovadia L, Stav A, Luchtman M, Ribac L. Continuous arteriovenous haemofiltration in the treatment of amniotic fluid embolism. *Int J Obstet Anesth* 1994;**3**:92–6.
26 Orlikowski CEP, Rocke DA. Coagulation monitoring in the obstetric patient. *Int Anesthesiol Clin* 1994;**32**:173–91.
27 Rodgers RPC, Levin J. A critical reappraisal of the bleeding time. *Semin Thromb Hemostas* 1990;**16**:1–20.
28 Sharma SK, Vera RL, Stegall WC, Whitten CW. Management of a post partum coagulopathy using thrombelastography. *J Clin Anesth* 1997;**9**:243–7.
29 Richey ME, Gilstrap LC, Ramin SM. Management of disseminated intravascular coagulopathy. *Clin Obstet Gynecol* 1995;**38**:514–20.
30 McLelland B, ed. *Handbook of transfusion medicine*. London: HMSO, 1996.
31 Douglas KA, Redman CWG. Eclampsia in the United Kingdom. *BMJ* 1994;**309**:1395–400.
32 Sibai BM, Frangieh AY. Management of severe pre-eclampsia. *Curr Opin Obstet Gynecol* 1996;**8**:110–13.
33 Barton JR, Sibai BM. Acute life threatening emergencies in pre eclampsia – eclampsia. *Clin Obstet Gynecol* 1992;**35**:402–13.
34 Lucas MJ, Leveno KJ, Cunningham FG. A comparison of magnesium sulfate with phenytoin for the prevention of eclampsia. *N Engl J Med* 1995;**333**:201–5.
35 Coetzee EJ, Dommisse J, Anthony J. A randomised controlled trial of intravenous magnesium sulphate versus placebo in the management of women with severe pre-eclampsia. *Br J Obst Gynaecol* 1998;**105**:300–3.
36 Mushambi MC, Halligan AW, Williamson K. Recent developments in the pathophysiology and management of pre-eclampsia. *Br J Anaesth* 1996;**76**:133–48.
37 Royal College of Obstetricians and Gynaecologists. *Management of eclampsia*. RCOG guidelines No. 10. London: RCOG, 1996.
38 James MFM. Magnesium in obstetric practice. *Int J Obstet Anesth* 1998;**7**:115–23.
39 Idama TO, Lindow SW. Magnesium sulphate: a review of clinical pharmacology applied to obstetrics. *Br J Obstet Gynaecol* 1998;**105**:260–8.
40 Donner A, Ullrich R, Kneifel W, et al. The HELLP syndrome. *Acta Anaesthesiol Scand* 1997;**111**(suppl):165–7.
41 Haljamäe H. Thromboprophylaxis, coagulation disorders and regional anaesthesia. *Acta Anaesthesiol Scand* 1996;**40**:1024–40.
42 Hood DD, Boese PA. Epidural and spinal anesthesia for Cesarean section in severely pre-eclamptic patients. *Reg Anesth* 1992;**17**:35.
43 Suresh MS, Belfort MA. Anesthetic management of obstetric emergencies. In: Barash PG, ed. *ASA refresher course in anesthesiology*. Philadelphia: Lippincott-Raven Publishers, 1996.
44 Mercier FJ, Dounas M, Bouaziz H, Lhuissier C, Benhamou D. Intravenous nitroglycerin to relieve intrapartum fetal distress related to uterine hyperactivity: a prospective observational study. *Anesth Analg* 1997;**84**:1117–20.
45 Price ML, Reynolds F, Morgan BM. Extending epidural blockade for emergency caesarean section: evaluation of 2% lignocaine with adrenaline. *Int J Obstet Anesth* 1991;**1**:13–18.
46 American Heart Association: Standards and guidelines for cardiopulmonary resuscitation and emergency care. *JAMA* 1992;**268**:2276–81.
47 Perlman JM, Risser R. Cardiopulmonary resuscitation in the delivery room: associated clinical events. *Arch Pediatr Adolesc Med* 1995;**149**:20–5.
48 European Resuscitation Council. Recommendations on resuscitation of babies at birth. *Resuscitation* 1998;**37**:103–10.
49 Ramji S, Ahuja S, Thirupuram S, Rootwell T, Rooth G. Saugstad OD. Resuscitation of asphyxic newborn infants with room air or 100% oxygen. *Pediatr Res* 1993;**34**(suppl 6):809–12.
50 Paterson SJ, Byrne PJ, Molesky MG, Seal RF, Finucane BT. Neonatal resuscitation using the laryngeal mask. *Anesthesiology* 1994;**80**:1248–53.

51 Ginsberg HG, Goldsmith JP. Controversies in neonatal resuscitation. *Clin Perinatol* 1998;**25**:1–15.
52 Allen MC, Donohue PK, Dusman AE. The limit of viability – neonatal outcome of infants born at 22 to 25 weeks gestation. *N Engl J Med* 1993;**329**:1597–601.

8: Postnatal assessment

ROBIN RUSSELL

Postnatal symptoms

The obstetric anaesthetist's duties do not end with delivery of the baby and placenta. Adequate recovery facilities with suitably trained staff must be available for those who have received both regional and general anaesthesia for operative delivery. High dependency or intensive care may be required for the particularly sick parturient. Whatever the input from anaesthetic staff, any mother who has been attended by an anaesthetist during delivery should be visited during the postnatal period. This provides a useful opportunity to assess the quality of care that has been provided. It gives the mother the opportunity to ask questions about the effects of analgesia and finally it allows investigation of any postpartum problems that are frequently attributed to, although seldom the result of, the use of regional blocks in labour.

At the postnatal visit, the anaesthetist should first enquire into the quality of labour analgesia. The mother should be asked about pain relief during both the first and second stages and at delivery, whether this was spontaneous, instrumental or operative. This provides information on both the success of the block and its management by the attending staff. The anaesthetist should enquire as to the health of the baby and congratulate the mother on her new arrival. Perhaps the most important aspect of the postnatal visit is assessment of postnatal symptoms.

Headache

It is possibly the greatest fear of the obstetric anaesthetist that the dura will be accidentally punctured during attempts to site an epidural catheter. Dural puncture not only carries the risks of postnatal headache (PDPH) but also, if unrecognised, total spinal anaesthesia in labour (see Chapter 4). With careful teaching of an appropriate epidural technique, the incidence of accidental dural puncture should be less than 1%, especially if saline is used to detect loss of resistance.[1] However, not every postnatal headache is the result of anaesthetic intervention.

Differential diagnosis

Up to 40% of women suffer from headache in the first week after delivery[2] and for the majority this is unrelated to labour analgesia. Migraine usually improves during pregnancy but may return once the baby is delivered. Headache is a common symptom of pre-eclampsia, which sometimes only develops in the postnatal period. Other less common causes of postnatal headache are listed in Box 8.1.[3]

Box 8.1   Differential diagnosis of postpartum headache

Non-specific headache
Postdural puncture headache
Migraine
Pre-eclampsia
Systemic infection
Meningitis
Benign intracranial hypertension
Cortical vein thrombosis
Tumour
Intracranial haemorrhage
Lactation
Caffeine withdrawal
Pneumocephalus

Postdural puncture headache (PDPH)

If the loss of cerebrospinal fluid (CSF) through a dural tear is greater than that produced by the arachnoid villi, headache results. The CSF acts as a cushion for intracranial contents and if its volume is reduced, traction on pain-sensitive structures produces headache, especially in the upright position. Pain may also result from cerebrovasodilation, a reflex response in an attempt to maintain intracerebral volume.

Symptoms

The most important feature of PDPH is its postural nature. Mothers may report no symptoms on waking but a thumping headache develops with mobilisation. The site of the headache is variable. Typically pain is felt in the fronto-occipital region, but in 25% pain may be diffuse and radiate to the neck. PDPH may be associated with auditory or visual symptoms and occasionally cranial nerve palsies (most commonly the sixth nerve). Symptoms may present in labour but more usually develop within 24–48 hours of delivery although occasionally a mother may not exhibit headache until five days after delivery.[4] Dural puncture headache may develop after a normal epidural if the dura is torn by the tip of the Tuohy needle but CSF is not seen to flow via either needle or catheter.

Epidemiology

Dural puncture, whether deliberate or accidental, produces CSF leak and, where this is significant, low-pressure headache. The incidence and severity of PDPH are related to the quantity of CSF leak which in turn is determined by size, design, and bevel direction of the needle. Postnatal mothers are at particular risk of developing PDPH as this complication is more common in younger females and maternal dehydration in labour is quite possible. Furthermore, prolonged active pushing may increase the leak of CSF and if this were not enough, changes in oestrogen, progesterone, and serotonin levels may worsen symptoms.[5]

Over 75% of mothers develop headache when the dura is breached with a 16 or 18 gauge epidural needle. Smaller gauge spinal needles produce fewer and less severe headaches. The design of the needle point also influences the incidence of headache. Cutting (Quincke) points of 25 gauge produce headaches in up to 20% of women. This figure may be reduced by using a 29 gauge cutting needle but these are technically difficult to use. An atraumatic point (Whitacre, Sprotte) of similar gauge to a cutting point is associated with significantly fewer headaches.[6] It has been suggested that the needle point stretches and separates rather than cuts the dural fibres, resulting in less CSF leak. Needles with an atraumatic point have therefore become the choice for spinal anaesthesia in obstetrics.

Headache is less likely after dural puncture when the bevel of a cutting point needle is introduced parallel to the long axis of the spine. This was originally thought to be due to the fact that dural fibres ran longitudinally, although electron microscopy has revealed that fibres are multidirectional. It is now thought that a dural tear resulting from a needle introduced with the bevel parallel to the long axis of the spine produces a hole that is under less tension. Inserting an epidural needle in such a position necessitates rotation of needle through 90° once the epidural space is located, which itself may increase the risk of dural puncture and is therefore not recommended.[7] Reports that the paramedian approach may produce fewer headaches due to the acute angle at which the dura is torn have not been confirmed.

Prophylactic measures

Once accidental dural puncture has been recognised various measures have been suggested to prevent or minimise symptoms.

Management of labour

The use of elective forceps does not reduce the incidence of headache although it may delay its onset.[4] Provided descent of the fetal head is observed during active pushing, spontaneous delivery should be permitted. However, it is wise not to permit excessive bearing down and assisted delivery after a limited period of pushing would seem a reasonable compromise.

Bed Rest

It is well recognised that enforced bed rest does not prevent the development of PDPH. Early ambulation is encouraged after delivery as hypercoagulability predisposes to venous thrombosis.

Hydration

There is no evidence that excessive hydration increases CSF production and thus prevents PDPH. However, it is wise not to allow the mother to become dehydrated as this may exacerbate symptoms should they develop.

Abdominal binders

Increasing intra-abdominal pressure and thus CSF pressure has been reported in one study to reduce the incidence and severity of PDPH.[8] Others have, however, failed to find abdominal binders successful. As they are often uncomfortable and not popular with mothers, they are rarely used.

Epidural fluids

A continuous infusion of crystalloid into the epidural space for 24 hours after delivery has been demonstrated to slightly reduce the incidence of headache.[4] Side-effects including pain in the legs, back, and neck have been reported with epidural fluid infusion. Large boluses of epidural saline have also been suggested but are best avoided as intraocular haemorrhage has been reported as a complication.

Spinal opioids

It has been suggested that addition of opioids to intrathecal local anaesthetic solutions decreases the incidence of PDPH.[9] This finding has failed to be reproduced by other workers. Epidural morphine has also been reported to reduce headache after dural puncture with a Tuohy needle. Furthermore, the low incidence of PDPH following combined spinal-epidural anaesthesia for caesarean section has been attributed to the use of postoperative epidural opioids. The mechanism by which epidural and spinal opioids reduce the incidence of PDPH, if indeed they do, has yet to be established.

Prophylactic epidural blood patch

Prophylactic epidural blood patching (see below) has been recommended by some authors,[10] although others have not found it to be as effective as delayed patching. Opinion is thus divided as to the place of prophylactic patching. Some would argue that severe headache develops in around 70–80% of mothers in whom accidental dural puncture occurs with a 16 gauge needle. Conversely, 20–30% will not develop headache. If a prophylactic blood patch is to be performed, all signs of local anaesthetic block should have worn off. This is important first because the mother must be able to report symptoms during the injection and also because total spinal anaesthesia has been reported after an epidural injection of 15 ml blood before a block had completely receded. In this case it was suggested that increased CSF pressure lead to rostral spread of the residual local anaesthetic.[11]

Treatment

It is incorrect to assume that symptoms of PDPH will resolve after several days as this is frequently not the case. MacArthur and colleagues reported that 23% of women who suffered accidental dural puncture had either long-term headache or neckache.[12] Of greater concern, however, are the reports of death due to medullary and tentorial coning and intracranial bleeding following untreated CSF leaks.

Should headache develop, its treatment depends on the severity of symptoms. Severe headache usually follows dural puncture with a 16 or 18 gauge needle and active management with blood patching is usually advised. Conservative measures may be preferable, at least in the short term when headache develops after deliberate puncture with a smaller spinal needle. However, if symptoms continue for several days or if they interfere with the mother's ability to care for her new baby, blood patching is again recommended.

Bed rest

The upright position exacerbates PDPH. Bed rest is therefore advised to obtain partial relief of symptoms. The prone position may be more effective, presumably as CSF pressure is increased.

Analgesics

Simple oral analgesics may be helpful after dural puncture with a spinal needle but are often inadequate where a larger dural tear exists. In this latter situation analgesics are purely symptomatic and do not treat the underlying cause. With the small risk of serious adverse effects of CSF leak, more active management with a blood patch is preferred.

Pharmacological agents

Cerebral vasoconstrictors have been reported to be effective in the management of PDPH. Caffeine sodium benzoate has been used although large doses may cause seizures. Theophylline and sumatriptan have also been used with some success. However, as with simple analgesics, these drugs may mask the signs of CSF leak without treating the problem.

Hydration

There is little evidence that hydration is therapeutic, although no mother with PDPH should be allowed to become dehydrated.

Abdominal binder

Although rarely used in the treatment of PDPH, the abdominal decompression test can be valuable in establishing the diagnosis.[13] Here the mother sits up and when she complains of headache, the anaesthetist grips her as tightly as possible around the waist. This produces relief of symptoms in those with PDPH.

Epidural fluids

Injection of 10–20 ml of epidural saline may temporarily relieve headache by increasing CSF pressure, although headache usually returns. Continuous infusion of saline may be tried (see above) but may require replacement of the epidural catheter. It may also be limited by pain in the legs, back, and neck. Epidural injection of dextran 40 has been reported to relieve PDPH but carries a small risk of anaphylaxis.

Epidural blood patch

Gormley, in 1960, was the first to describe the use of epidural injection of autologous blood to cure PDPH.[14] He used only 2–3 ml of blood. Further reports of high success rates with first 10 ml and then 20 ml of blood led to the widespread acceptance and practice of the technique. The mechanism of action is twofold. First, CSF and thus intracranial pressure are increased, producing almost instant relief of symptoms, whilst blood clot seals the hole in the dura and prevents further leak of CSF.

Before embarking on a blood patch, consent must be obtained. The procedure is explained and the risks of repeat dural puncture and low back pain outlined. Contraindications are similar to those for epidural analgesia in labour, but blood patching should be avoided where there is evidence of systemic infection.

Blood patching requires two operators, one to locate the epidural space and another to draw a specimen of the mother's blood. It is important that a senior anaesthetist performs the epidural as the mother may already have limited confidence in her carers and a further accidental dural puncture should, if possible, be avoided. Before starting, the mother should empty her bladder and lie in bed for about two hours to reduce the volume of CSF in the epidural space, which would dilute the injected blood.

The procedure is then best performed with the mother in the left lateral position. Both operators must observe strict asepsis. The skin over the lumbar spine and that of the antecubital fossa is prepared with a suitable antiseptic. As blood mostly tracks in a cephalad direction,[15] it is preferable to use either the same intervertebral space or the one just below. The epidural space is then located and if saline is used, the bare minimum should be injected. The second operator takes a sample of 20–30 ml of maternal blood. This is slowly injected into the epidural space until the mother reports discomfort in either her back or legs. Injection is discontinued and the pain allowed to settle and then further blood injected until symptoms return. A maximum injection of 20 ml of blood has been recommended although recently larger volumes have been reported to be more efficacious.[16] When injection is complete, 1–2 ml of saline should be used to clear the needle, minimising backtracking of blood into the soft tissues of the back producing backache. Any blood remaining may be sent for culture. The mother should rest in bed for at least two hours after the procedure to maximise the success of the blood patch,[17] following which she may mobilise slowly. She must be told to keep her back straight and avoid lifting, twisting, and straining for at least two weeks. Laxatives may be given.

Regrettably, headache may return if the blood clot sealing the hole in the dura becomes dislodged. It is all too easy to see how this may occur in a mother who has been incapacitated by severe headache since delivery. When her symptoms are cured, she may suddenly become more active in caring for her baby. Should headache recur, blood patching may be repeated and the postpatch management emphasised to the mother.

Mothers who have experienced PDPH may wish never to have an epidural in a future pregnancy. Although there have been data suggesting a blood patch may diminish the success of future epidural analgesia, more recent evidence has found this not to be so.[18]

Neurological problems

Obstetric neurological problems

Although regional blocks are often blamed for postnatal neurological symptoms, these problems may arise when neither an epidural nor a spinal needle has been remotely near a mother's back. Indeed, maternal obstetric palsy was first reported as long ago as 1838, long before the first use of regional block for labour analgesia. Neurological problems are usually caused by compression of maternal pelvic nerves by the fetal head and damage is more likely to occur when there has been a degree of cephalopelvic disproportion.

Lumbosacral trunk (L4,5)

Compression of the lumbosacral trunk as it crosses the sacral ala may produce postpartum foot drop, which is almost always unilateral.[19]

287

Examination usually reveals weakness of ankle dorsiflexion and eversion. Sensory deficit is often detected on the lateral aspect of the leg and across the dorsum of the foot. Compression of the common perineal nerve as it passes over the fibula head may produce similar symptoms, although sensory deficit is usually confined to the foot. This problem may arise if care is not taken when placing women in lithotomy poles.

Femoral nerve (L2,3,4)

Injury to the femoral nerve is most commonly the result of compression by the fetal head during its passage through the pelvis. Damage may also follow the use of self-retaining retractors during surgery or compression under the inguinal ligament in the lithotomy position.[20] Approximately 25% of cases are bilateral. It is stated that the woman may recall stabbing pain in her knee, thigh or ankle during labour. As she mobilises after delivery, she may have difficulty climbing stairs. Examination reveals reduced power in the quadriceps muscles, a sensory loss in the distribution of the femoral nerve, and an absent patella reflex.

Obturator nerve (L2,3,4)

An obturator neuropathy is usually unilateral and often combined with damage to the femoral nerve. Symptoms are limited to decreased power in the hip adductors and decreased sensation on the upper inner thigh.

Lateral Cutaneous Nerve of the Thigh (L2,3)

Entrapment of the lateral cutaneous nerve of the thigh produces an area of painful paraesthesia on the upper outer aspect of the thigh – meralgia paraesthetica. This condition may be seen in pregnancy but it may also follow hyperextension of the hips during delivery.[20]

Nerve root lesions

Nerve root lesions from disc prolapse may be observed during pregnancy or the postnatal period. Back pain radiating down one or both legs may be associated with sensory loss and absent reflexes. Diagnosis is confirmed with MRI.

Spinal cord lesions

Ishaemic damage to the spinal cord may result from inadequate blood flow. In 15% of the population the major blood supply to the conus medullaris and cauda equina arises from the internal iliac arteries. These vessels lie close to the lumbosacral trunk and are therefore at risk of compression during prolonged and obstructed labour. Should blood flow be interrupted, permanent paralysis may result.[21] Epidural vein rupture can occur spontaneously, especially during active pushing. If there is a coagulation disorder an expanding haematoma may develop, leading to cord or nerve root compression. A rare cause of postnatal neurological deficit is a spinal vascular malformation. It is possible that vasodilation from increased oestrogen secretion and increased spinal venous pressure can reduce capillary flow, leading to ischaemic neurological damage.[22]

Neurological disease may develop at any time of life and it is therefore quite conceivable that symptoms may develop in the postnatal period. Of particular interest is the progress of multiple sclerosis after childbirth. Fear of provoking relapse has made many anaesthetists wary of the use of regional blocks for delivery. However, about 40% of women suffer a relapse during the first six months after childbirth, a rate which does not appear to be related to anaesthesia or analgesia.

Neurological complications of regional blocks

Neurological sequelae of regional blocks in labour are fortunately rare but potentially catastrophic. Symptoms may be short-lived or prolonged and range in severity from small areas of paraesthesiae to permanent paraplegia. A not uncommon problem seen after the use of regional block for labour and delivery is prolonged residual anaesthesia lasting 24 hours after delivery. Such cases are usually unilateral and are associated with large doses of local anaesthetic during labour often extended for operative delivery. Although recovery is complete, prolonged block may be difficult to distinguish from more sinister and potential permanent causes of postnatal problems.

Transient sensory and motor deficits are not uncommon after delivery. They are seen more frequently after complicated labour and delivery, the very situation in which regional block is likely to be employed. Ong and colleagues looked at the incidence of neurological problems by interviewing over 23 000 women soon after delivery.[23] They discovered that, compared with those using either inhalational or no analgesia, symptoms were more common in women receiving blocks (Table 8.1). However, women requiring general anaesthesia who had not received a regional block were as likely as the epidural group to report symptoms. In this study all symptoms were transient and resolved within 72 hours.

Several other studies have been published reporting the incidence of prolonged neurological problems after regional block. The results of such

Table 8.1   Occurrence of transient neurological problems after delivery[23]

Analgesia/anaesthesia	Incidence of neurological problems
Nil	1 in 4099
Inhalation	1 in 1589
Epidural	1 in 277
General anaesthesia	1 in 288
Other	1 in 199
Total	1 in 530

investigations are often difficult to interpret as many do not relate solely to obstetric practice and include large numbers of vascular and urological patients. Moreover, with the incidence of neurological problems being extremely low, large numbers of patients need to be recruited and followed up. With such large numbers, the potential for failing to pick up all post-natal problems is increased which may then produce inaccuracies when calculating the extent of the problem. Furthermore, when cases are high-lighted the exact aetiology of the disorder is not always defined.

Most of these issues were admirably addressed by Holdcroft and col-leagues.[24] They investigated neurological complications persisting for more than six weeks after delivery. In their study population of over 48 000, there were 35 notifications of neurological problems. Further investigation revealed that only 19 in fact had neurological complications associated with pregnancy and delivery, an incidence of one in 2530. Of these 19 women, only one was considered the result of a regional block. When the number of women receiving regional block was established it was calculated that the incidence of prolonged neurological problems resulting from the use of epidurals was one in 13 007.

Despite the renewed interest in spinal block and the introduction of com-bined spinal-epidural techniques, there are as yet no accurate data to reli-ably estimate the neurological sequelae of these procedures in obstetrics. Most studies of spinal anaesthesia have combined obstetric with general surgical patients in whom one would expect a greater number of postblock problems. However, in a prospective study which included 14 856 women who received spinal anaesthesia for delivery, of whom eight reported neuro-logical complications, Scott and Tunstall reported no cases of permanent disability.[25] However, at least one woman in this report still complained of pain and numbness of the foot 10 months after delivery.

Mechanisms of injury

The mechanisms by which epidural and spinal blocks cause neurological problems are outlined in Boxes 8.2 and 8.3.

Box 8.2   Mechanisms of neurological complications after epidural block

- Paraplegia
  Space-occupying lesions   Haematoma
                                  Abscess

  Neurotoxicity   Inappropriate solutions
  Ischaemia   Hypotension
- Nerve root lesions   Trauma
- Peripheral lesions   Compression

Box 8.3   Mechanisms of neurological complications after spinal block

- Paraplegia and cauda equina syndrome
  - Space-occupying lesions   Haematoma
                                           Abscess
  - Neurotoxicity/arachnoiditis   Inappropriate solutions
                                           Detergents/antiseptics
- Infection   Meningitis
- Cranial nerve palsy   CSF leak
- Cranial subdural haematoma   CSF leak
- Coning   CSF leak
- Nerve root lesions   Trauma
- Peripheral lesions   Compressive

Paraplegia and cauda equina syndromes

Space-occupying lesions within the vertebral canal may be caused by spinal haematoma or abscess. Compression of the spinal cord, cauda equina or isolated nerves or their blood supply may lead to paraplegia, cauda equina syndrome or nerve root damage. Neurotoxicity is difficult to achieve in the epidural space where a variety of drugs have been injected either accidentally or deliberately, producing little other than a systemic effect and reversible neural blockade. There are, however, reports of neurotoxicity following epidural injection of hypertonic potassium chloride and preservative containing multidose vials. Unfortunately, the subarachnoid space is not as forgiving where nerve roots are far more vulnerable to neurolysis, while irritant solutions may produce arachnoiditis. The result may be a transient radicular irritation or more permanent damage of the cauda equina. There are many reports of neurological damage resulting from misguided subarachnoid injection.[26]

Cauda equina syndrome associated with the use of microspinal catheters led to their withdrawal by the FDA in North America.[27] In these cases the use of hyperbaric 5% lignocaine pooling around sacral nerves was implicated. The use of spinal lignocaine continues to cause concern as a number of reports have linked its use to postoperative transient radicular irritation. This presents as a dull ache or cramp in the buttocks or lower back radiating to the dorsolateral aspect of the thighs, beginning up to 24 hours after recovery from anaesthesia. It usually resolves within one week. Symptoms are thought to result from a direct neurotoxic effect of the local anaesthetic[28] although excessive stretching of the cauda equina in the lithotomy position has also been implicated. Transient radicular irritation does not appear to be associated with the use of spinal bupivacaine.

Detergents have also been linked with arachnoiditis and more recently, chemical meningitis following combined spinal-epidural analgesia has been attributed to iodine-containing skin preparation solutions.[29] It is therefore imperative not to contaminate epidural and spinal needles with antiseptic solutions used to prepare the patient's back before siting a regional block.

Ischaemic damage of the spinal cord damage is unlikely in the childbearing population but may occur if hypotension is associated with arterial constriction, compression or disease.[30] Anterior spinal artery syndrome has been described in association with a labour epidural.[31] This risk would be increased with a large-volume top-up in the presence of a vascular malformation, disc protrusion or spinal stenosis.

Nerve root lesions

During epidural insertion, either needle or catheter may cause nerve root damage if they stray from the midline. Transient paraesthesia is not uncommon during catheter insertion and usually signals that a sensory nerve root has been touched. Trauma is much less common and produces pain in the associated dermatome and occasionally paraesthesia lasting several weeks or months. The use of stiletted catheters has been reported to cause more prolonged dysfunction. Nerve roots may also be damaged by spinal needles producing more protracted and severe damage.

Peripheral lesions

Obstetric pelvic entrapment neuropathies as described above may all follow labours in which regional blocks have been used. These problems are often wrongly attributed to anaesthetic intervention. Compressive neuropathy may be associated with regional blocks if a mother lies in the same position for a prolonged period. Symptoms may pass unrecognised due to effective sensory block and immobility attributed to motor block from the epidural.[30] Pressure sores on the heels and over ischial tuberosities have also been reported after prolonged immobility with epidural blockade.[32]

Meningitis

There have been recent concerns regarding a number of cases of meningitis following spinal and combined spinal-epidural blocks in labour. Whether dural puncture represents an increased risk to the mother remains to be established. These reports emphasise the need for meticulous care and strict aseptic technique when performing regional blocks.

CSF leak

The dangers of CSF leak, such as cranial nerve palsy, subdural haematoma, and coning, have been discussed under dural puncture.

Assessment

When assessing a mother with a postnatal neurological problem there are a few key things to remember. There is a tendency for staff and patients to attribute all neurological symptoms to regional blocks. As the anaesthetist may potentially be viewed with some hostility, it may be prudent for a senior member of staff to be present and conduct the assessment. This saves further referrals and repeated visits by anaesthetists, reinforcing the mother's beliefs that the epidural caused all her problems. A thorough history must be elicited following which a detailed examination is made, documenting any neurological deficit. Prompt referral to a neurologist or neurosurgeon is advised for an impartial opinion of site of the lesion and its further management.

Backache

Postnatal backache is a very common symptom and may result from a variety of causes. It may simply be a continuation of antenatal backache. Up to 50% of women suffer with backache during pregnancy with 10% prevented from working due to the severity of pain.[33] In over a third of pregnant women, backache interferes with their daily life. Pain is usually non-specific and produced by an increasing lumbar lordosis with joint laxity from elevated levels of the hormone relaxin. Sacroiliac joint dysfunction is also often present and occasionally disc prolapse and spondylolisthesis may be observed. The more severe the backache during pregnancy, the longer it continues into the postnatal period. Fortunately, for many mothers, backache resolves during the first few days and weeks after delivery. Treatment should include education on how best to nurse the new baby with attention to posture. Mothers should be reassured that symptoms usually improve and where necessary, oral analgesics may be prescribed. Referral to a physiotherapist may be helpful if symptoms persist.

New backache that develops after delivery is usually either a local tenderness or a more generalised ache. Following regional block, localised tenderness at the site of needle insertion is relatively common, occurring in up to 50% after an epidural and 30% of those who receive a spinal. The incidence is related to needle size and ease of insertion. Mothers can be reassured that in almost all cases symptoms resolve in a few days. Very occasionally localised tenderness may persist for several weeks or even months. This is most likely to represent a slowly resolving soft tissue haematoma.[32] More generalised short-term backache is also often observed after delivery. Most likely of musculoskeletal origin, it is reported by 20% of women who receive epidural analgesia and 40% of those using other forms of pain relief. Other more esoteric causes of short-term backache have been reported, including thoracic aneurysms, spinal cord tumours, and osteitis condensans ilii.

The possibility that epidural analgesia in labour may be linked to new long-term backache after childbirth has been suggested in two retrospective studies.[34,35] It was suggested that stressed positions in labour exacerbated by muscular relaxation and the abolition of pain resulted in postural backache.

Furthermore, such stressed positions may be maintained for prolonged periods because of difficulty moving during epidural analgesia with excessive motor block and because changing position requires assistance, thus compounding the problem. Unfortunately, these retrospective studies required that women were asked about their symptoms months or years after delivery. As a result of this delay many women probably forgot that their symptoms actually started before or during pregnancy rather than after delivery. Indeed, the incidence of antenatal backache was reported to be only 9% in one retrospective study and 25% in the other. When followed prospectively through pregnancy, as many as 50% of women have reported gestational backache with the more severe backache persisting longer after delivery.[33]

Several published prospective studies have failed to demonstrate a link between new long-term backache and the use of epidural analgesia in labour.[36,37,38] More accurate documentation of antenatal backache has revealed that new long-term backache is no more common after epidural analgesia than other forms of pain relief. When searching for predictive factors for long-term backache, only pre-existing backache has been found to be significant.[36] Excessive motor block associated with more concentrated local anaesthetics was not shown to affect the incidence of backache. The aetiology of long-term backache is probably multifactorial, but in many it is a non-specific musculoskeletal problem, although cases of sacroiliac joint dysfunction and disc prolapse may be seen.

Investigation of a group of pregnant women with pre-existing backache of varying cause has failed to demonstrate any deterioration of symptoms after delivery where regional block was used.[39] Indeed, the reverse was true with mothers who avoided epidurals in labour reporting more problems at postnatal assessment.

Bladder dysfunction

It is not uncommon for labouring women to have difficulty passing urine, especially when receiving regional analgesia. Local anaesthetics may produce bladder atonia by blocking sacral nerve roots whilst opioids inhibit sacral parasympathetic outflow, resulting in detrusor muscle relaxation. If the bladder is allowed to become overdistended, not only can labour be prolonged but there is also a possibility of postnatal atonia leading to urinary retention.

Long-term urinary dysfunction has not been linked to the use of epidural analgesia in labour. MacArthur and colleagues demonstrated that stress incontinence developed in 15% of women following childbirth.[40] Although there was a weak association with epidural analgesia, this disappeared with multivariate analysis. New long-term urinary frequency was not found to be associated with regional blocks.

Risk management

Risk management is a systematic process for the identification, analysis, and control of actual and potential risks and their resource implications.[41] Such risks are both clinical and non-clinical, but it is the former that is becoming increasingly important in the field of obstetric anaesthesia and analgesia. Most anaesthetists have in fact been practising risk management for years guided by standards produced by the Association of Anaesthetists of Great Britain and Ireland. More recently, however, a greater emphasis has been put on risk management with the introduction in 1995 of the Clinical Negligence Scheme for Trusts (CNST). This scheme underwrites claims for clinical negligence against hospital trusts and has superseded Crown indemnity. As part of the CNST, risk management policies and standards are now required.

Much of the service commitment in obstetric anaesthesia is still carried out by trainees. It is therefore important that they are supported in their work by senior staff. On arrival at a new obstetric unit, there should be a formal induction programme. House rules and clinical responsibilities must be made clear and written protocols and guidelines issued. Trainees must at all times work under supervision, either directly or indirectly, and so there must be a system whereby senior assistance can be contacted immediately for serious clinical problems. It is also the responsibility of the trainee to report any clinical incident to the duty consultant.

Many aspects of clinical risk management represent nothing more than good clinical practice. For the obstetric anaesthetist, this starts in the antenatal period when high-risk cases are referred from the obstetrician. A list of potential anaesthetic problems should be widely circulated to all those providing antenatal care and there should be a recognised process for referral for anaesthetic assessment. Such consultation may take place in an antenatal anaesthetic clinic or on a less formal *ad hoc* basis. After establishing the problem, labour analgesia and anaesthesia may be discussed and a suitable plan of action drawn up. Informed consent for regional block may be obtained after discussion of risks and benefits at a time when labour pain does not make full explanation of certain procedures difficult or impossible. When anaesthetic assessment is made, clear and precise notes with a plan of action for further anaesthetic management should be documented so that those attending the woman in labour are aware of the proposed management. Where necessary, further discussion between anaesthetist, obstetrician, and other relevant specialists may be arranged to plan the optimum time and method of delivery.

For those women booked for elective caesarean section, it is helpful to arrange a preoperative visit to the delivery suite the week before surgery, avoiding the last-minute rush of admission shortly before surgery. Preoperative visiting allows anaesthetic choice to be discussed and procedures, with their complications, explained. The obstetrician also has the opportunity to explain surgical aspects of caesarean section and check that the relevant blood tests and ultrasound scans have been performed.

When anaesthetic services are required in labour, as always there must be meticulous attention to detail and a careful clinical technique. Record keeping is most important and for regional analgesia in labour, this is best done after the block has been sited. Many units have forms for recording details although not all necessary information may be included. For the purposes of risk management it is advisable to document the following.

- The date and time of the procedure.
- Potential complications discussed with the mother.
- Precise details of the procedure.
- Immediate complications.
- Further management of the block.
- Who and when to call in the event of a problem.

Should the anaesthetist be called, further interventions must also be carefully documented.

If operative delivery is necessary, adequate recovery facilities must be available. The recovery facilities for many obstetric units are distant to main operating theatres and they are often staffed by midwives, some of whom may be unfamiliar with care of the postoperative patient. This is particularly relevant after general anaesthesia, as many members of staff may not be confident or competent to deal with an unconscious patient. In such circumstances the anaesthetist must stay with the patient until she is fully awake. After regional anaesthesia it is also important that mothers are kept under close observation and physiological parameters should be measured and documented regularly.

Postnatal visiting also forms an important part of risk management (see above). Issues from labour and delivery may be discussed although where significant problems have occurred, women may be reluctant to discuss them with medical staff (see below). Should the woman consider that her care has been unsatisfactory, complaints may be made. Common causes of complaints are lack of informed consent, delay in finding the anaesthetist, pain during siting of the block and failure of the block to provide analgesia.[13] Anaesthetists must be able to respond quickly to such complaints and should take time to listen sympathetically to patients' concerns and offer explanation for labour management. This may be insufficient for some mothers and legal proceedings may sometimes follow (see below).

Medicolegal issues

Many women now have unrealistically high expectations of childbirth and thus disappointment may result when their experiences fall short of these preconceived ideals. Should this occur, complaints may be made and occasionally litigation may follow.

It is difficult to be certain of the number and nature of medicolegal claims against obstetric anaesthetists in the UK. Data from the American Society of Anesthesiologists Closed Claims Project Database provide interesting information.[42] There are, however, limitations to these data. It is not possible to know how often claims are filed or the incidence of adverse events. There may also be a substantial time period between opening and closing a file and so these data are always somewhat out of date and relate to practice up to 10 years ago. They do, however, provide a reasonable representation of medicolegal claims in the USA. The most common injuries in the obstetric anaesthetic files are listed in Table 8.2. It is interesting to note that there are more claims associated with the use of regional anaesthesia when compared with general anaesthesia, although the total numbers of each are not known.

Table 8.2   Most common injuries in obstetric anaesthetic files[42]

	Obstetric files (%) (n=434)	Regional anaesthesia (%) (n=290*)	General anaesthesia (%) (n=133*)
Maternal death	19	11	39
Newborn brain damage	19	18	21
Headache	15	21	2
Nerve damage	10	13	4
Pain during anaesthesia	9	12	0
Back pain	8	12	0
Maternal brain damage	7	6	11
Emotional distress	7	8	6
Newborn death	6	6	6
Aspiration pneumonitis	5	1	14

*In some cases anaesthetic type was not specified.

When compared to non-obstetric files, the pattern of claims against obstetric anaesthetists is somewhat different (Table 8.3). There are a greater percentage of claims for postnatal symptoms including headache, backache, and emotional distress as well as pain during surgery. Postnatal headache is more common after dural puncture in the childbearing population, but the association between backache and regional blocks may now be refuted. Emotional distress may be the result of unrealistic expectations. Pain during surgery is usually associated with regional block for caesarean section and probably reflects inadequate anaesthesia with a reluctance to convert to general anaesthesia for fear of difficult intubation and pulmonary aspiration.[42]

Awareness during both general and regional anaesthesia accounts for a substantial number of claims.[43] Severe psychiatric sequelae may result from

Table 8.3   Maternal injuries compared to similar injuries in non-obstetric files[42]

	Obstetric files (%)	Non-obstetric files (%)
Death	23	36
Headache	18	2
Nerve damage	12	17
Pain during anaesthesia	10	1
Back pain	10	1
Brain damage	9	13
Emotional distress	9	4
Aspiration pneumonitis	6	2

awareness, especially if accompanied by pain.[44] Fortunately, the frequency of awareness during general anaesthesia has fallen.[45] Fears of uterine relaxation and depression of the newborn have been overstated. Indeed, administering minimal doses of induction agents and low concentrations of volatile anaesthetics in the hope of improving the condition of the baby is nonsensical. Light planes of anaesthesia lead to increased levels of endogenous catecholamines and vasoconstriction of the uterine arteries. This may produce asphyxia in the newborn, an undesirable outcome. Alternatively, adequate amounts of induction and volatile agent may produce a degree of anaesthesia in the newborn but this is an entirely reversible process. To ensure lack of maternal awareness under general anaesthesia, many anaesthetists now use the technique of overpressure. This method was described by McCrirrick and colleagues for isoflurane anaesthesia during caesarean section.[46] Following intravenous induction, anaesthesia was maintained for the first five minutes with 2% isoflurane in 33% oxygen with nitrous oxide. This concentration of isoflurane was reduced to 1.5% for the next five minutes, after which it was decreased to 0.8%.

Of greater concern are cases of pain during caesarean section performed under regional block. In most cases this is due to failure to check that the upper level of the block is adequate. Various block heights have been suggested although the method by which this should be assessed is rarely described. The three methods commonly used are cold, pinprick, and light touch. Although an absence of cold sensation to T4 has often been quoted, it does not ensure pain-free surgery. Likewise, pinprick cannot be relied upon to confirm the adequacy of the block. Complete absence of sensation, assessed by light touch, is the best method for testing a block before surgery. Russell found that no women with an anaesthetic block that was maintained above T5, assessed by light touch, experienced intraoperative pain.[47] Unfortunately, this method of testing is not always employed, leading to reported rates of intraoperative pain of up to 10%.

To minimise problems women should be warned preoperatively that pain or discomfort during surgery is a possibility when caesarean section is performed under regional anaesthesia. This is especially important in the emergency situation where surgery may commence before the block has spread to its furthest limits. An appropriate dose of local anaesthetic must be used and upper and lower levels of the block should be tested. The extent of the block and the means by which it was assessed must be documented. Should the mother then experience pain, surgery should be temporarily stopped and inhalational, intravenous or epidural analgesia given. Where this is inadequate, general anaesthesia should be offered. If intraoperative pain is reported, it is essential that a full account of the procedure be recorded in the notes for future reference. A postnatal visit is vital to explain the problem and apologise for any distress caused.

Neurological problems after delivery are frequently attributed to the use of regional blocks and occasionally result in claims against the anaesthetist. However, nerve damage is more often due to childbirth itself rather than labour analgesia (see above). Headache is another common cause of complaint and litigation. These problems may be minimised by a sympathetic postnatal visit with prompt and effective treatment of symptoms.

Audit

Medical audit is a systematic analysis of the quality of medical care, the resources used, and the resulting outcome for the patient. The aim of medical audit is thus to improve patient care and it has now become an important part of clinical practice. Audit is necessary to identify strengths and weaknesses of an obstetric anaesthetic service, to ensure adequate training of junior anaesthetists, and to guarantee effective use of resources. Information collected by audit, such as accidental dural puncture rates, may be compared with other units. If the performance of a department does not meet accepted standards, the reasons for this may be identified and changes implemented. Finally, audit can be useful for teaching and research purposes. Indeed, all anaesthetic trainees should keep a logbook so that the adequacy of training may be assessed.

Collection and analysis of data form part of all medical audits. This must, however, be performed in a systematic way to answer specific questions relating to various aspects of anaesthetic practice. Different forms of audit may be used to assess certain areas.[48] The accurate knowledge of service provided by obstetric anaesthetists is important to ensure an appropriate level of staffing. As well as providing labour analgesia and anaesthesia for operative procedures, obstetric anaesthetists are becoming increasingly involved in providing antenatal education of pregnant women and antenatal assessment clinics for high-risk patients. Time is needed for teaching and training of junior anaesthetists and midwives, research and administration, and to perform audit itself.

Data collection can be a laborious task and has been performed somewhat haphazardly in the past.[49] Many units now use computerised audit packages to collect and analyse their service commitment. This facilitates production of annual statistics providing information on the use of regional blocks in labour and the type of anaesthesia used for both elective and emergency caesarean section. Without the aid of computerised audit packages, even the most basic information may be difficult to obtain. This was highlighted by Brown and Russell who attempted to gather information from all UK units on the method of anaesthesia used for both elective and emergency caesarean section.[50] Nearly two-thirds of obstetric anaesthetic units were unable to provide such data. Where computerised audit facilities exist, it is useful to gather further details on the choice of equipment and techniques used and anaesthetic agents administered. The success or otherwise of the procedure and the incidence of complications should be recorded so that accurate information can be given to mothers about obstetric anaesthetic services in their hospital.

More serious complications should be examined as part of morbidity and mortality audits. It is essential that each department holds regular meetings during which management of difficult cases may be discussed. It is vital that this should not take the form of a witch-hunt but should be seen as a means of education, thus improving patient care. A Critical Incident Register should be kept and any event that may possibly result in an adverse outcome for patients should be recorded. Such events should also be discussed at departmental meetings.

Maternal mortality data have been assessed nationally in England and Wales since 1952 and throughout the UK since 1985 (see Chapter 7). The most recent report examined the years 1994–96,[51] during which time 376 deaths were submitted to the Enquiry. Although completion of case reports is not compulsory the final report was considered to have covered approximately 95% of maternal deaths during this period. The major causes of direct deaths were thromboembolic disease, hypertensive disorders of pregnancy, and haemorrhage. Only one death was directly related to anaesthesia involving a somewhat unorthodox CSE technique. In previous reports anaesthetic deaths were predominantly associated with the use of general anaesthesia for emergency caesarean section.

Medical audit may also examine specific aspects of clinical practice for the purpose of improving standards. Such standards may be agreed within a department, such as an acceptable incidence of postoperative nausea and vomiting. Data are then collected and analysed and where appropriate, causes of non-achievement of standards identified. This may result in change in clinical practice following which the process is repeated. Thus audit is not a static process but an ongoing assessment.

The Obstetric Anaesthetists' Association and Association of Anaesthetists have produced guidelines on the provision of obstetric anaesthesia services.[52] These guidelines include standards of staffing, service, response times, monitoring, consent and anaesthetic assistance. The OAA is now setting up a National Obstetric Anaesthesia Database that aims to collect figures on various obstetric anaesthetic outcomes from all units in the UK. This will permit individual units to audit their own service and compare their figures with the national average.

References

1 Reynolds FR. Dural puncture and headache. Avoid the first but treat the second. *BMJ* 1993;**306**:874–6.
2 Stein G, Morton J, Marsh A, *et al.* Headache after childbirth. *Acta Neurol Scand* 1984;**69**:74–9.
3 Weeks S. Postpartum headache. In: Chestnut DH, ed. *Obstetric anesthesia.* St Louis: Mosby, 1994:606–20.
4 Stride PC, Cooper GM. Dural taps revisited. *Anaesthesia* 1993;**48**:247–55.
5 Capogna G, Celleno D. Post-dural puncture headache. In: Russell IF, Lyons G, eds. *Clinical problems in obstetric anaesthesia.* London: Chapman & Hall Medical, 1997:187–200.
6 Halpern S, Preston R. Postdural puncture headache and spinal needle design. *Anesthesiology* 1994;**81**:1376–83.
7 Miekeljohn BH. The effect of rotating the epidural needle. *Anaesthesia* 1987;**42**:1180–2.
8 Mosavy SH, Shaft M. Prevention of headache consequent upon dural puncture in obstetric patient. *Anaesthesia* 1975;**30**:807–9.
9 Johnson MD, Hertwig L, Vehring PH, Datta S. Intrathecal fentanyl may reduce the incidence of spinal headache. *Anesthesiology* 1989;**71**:A911.
10 Cheek TG, Banner R, Sauter J, Gutsche BB. Prophylactic extradural blood patch is effective. *Br J Anaesth* 1988;**61**:340–2.
11 Leivers D. Total spinal anesthesia following early prophylactic epidural blood patch. *Anesthesiology* 1990;**73**:1287–9.
12 MacArthur C, Lewis M, Knox EG. Accidental dural puncture in obstetric patients and long term symptoms. *BMJ* 1993;**306**:883–5.
13 Reynolds F. They think it's all over. In: Reynolds F, ed. *Pain relief in labour.* London: BMJ Publishing Group, 1997:220–41.
14 Gormley JB. Treatment of postspinal headache. *Anesthesiology* 1960;**21**:565–6.
15 Beards SC, Jackson A, Griffiths AG, Horsman EL. Magnetic resonance imaging of extradural blood patches: appearances from 30 min to 18 h. *Br J Anaesth* 1993;**71**:182–8.
16 Pratt SD, Sarna MC, Soni AK, Oriol NE. Efficacy of greater than 20 cc volume for epidural blood patch. *Anesthesiology* 1996;**85**:A875.
17 Martin R, Jourdain S, Clairoux M, Tetrault JP, Duration of decubitus position after epidural blood patch. *Can J Anaesth* 1994;**41**:23–5.
18 Blanche R, Eisenach JC, Tuttle R, Dewan DM. Previous wet tap does not reduce success rate of labor epidural analgesia. *Anesth Analg* 1994;**79**:291–4.
19 Donaldson JO. *Neurology of pregnancy*, 2nd edn. Philadelphia: WB Saunders, 1989.
20 Russell IF. Postpartum neurological disorders. In: Russell IF, Lyons G, eds. *Clinical problems in obstetric anaesthesia.* London: Chapman & Hall Medical, 1997:140–60.
21 Bademosi O, Osuntokun BO, van der Werd JH, Bademosi AK, Ojo OA. Obstetric neuropraxia in the Nigerian African. *Int J Gynaecol Obstet* 1980;**17**:611–14.
22 Bromage PR. Neurologic complications of labor, delivery and regional anesthesia. In: Chestnut DH, ed. *Obstetric anesthesia.* St Louis: Mosby, 1994:621–39.
23 Ong BY, Cohen MM, Esmail A, Cumming M, Kozody R, Palahniuk RJ. Paresthesias and motor dysfunction after labor and delivery. *Anesth Analg* 1987;**66**:18–22.
24 Holdcroft A, Gibberd FB, Hargrove RL, Dawkins DF, Dellaports CI. Neurological complications associated with pregnancy. *Br J Anaesth* 1995;**75**:522–6.
25 Scott DB, Tunstall ME. Serious complications associated with epidural/spinal blockade in obstetrics. *Int J Obstet Anesth* 1995;**4**:133–9.
26 Russell R, Reynolds F. Long term effects of epidural analgesia. *Baillière's Clin Anaesthesiol* 1995;**9**:607–22.
27 Rigler ML, Drasner K, Krejcie TC, *et al.* Cauda equina syndrome after continuous spinal anesthesia. *Anesth Analg* 1991;**72**:275–81.

301

28 Fenerty J, Sonner J, Sakura S, Drasner K. Transient radicular pain following spinal anesthesia: review of literature and report of a case involving 2% lignocaine. *Int J Obstet Anesth* 1996;5:32–5.
29 Harding SA, Collis RE, Morgan BM. Meningitis after combined spinal-extradural anaesthesia in obstetrics. *Br J Anaesth* 1994;73:545–7.
30 Silva M, Mallinson C, Reynolds F. Sciatic nerve palsy following childbirth. *Anaesthesia* 1996;51:1144–8.
31 Ackerman WE, Juneja MM, Knapp RK. Maternal paraparesis after epidural anesthesia and cesarean section. *South Med J* 1990;83:695–7.
32 Crawford JS. Some maternal complications of epidural analgesia for labour. *Anaesthesia* 1985;40:1219–25.
33 Russell R, Reynolds F. Backpain, pregnancy and childbirth. *BMJ* 1997;314:1062–3.
34 MacArthur C, Lewis M, Knox EG, Crawford JS. Epidural anaesthesia and long term backache after childbirth. *BMJ* 1990;301:9–12.
35 Russell R, Groves P, Taub N, O'Dowd J, Reynolds F. Assessing long-term backache after childbirth. *BMJ* 1993;306:1299–302.
36 Russell R, Dundas R, Reynolds F. Long-term backache after childbirth: prospective search for causative factors. *BMJ* 1996;312:1384–8.
37 Breen TW, Ransil BJ, Groves PA, Oriol NE. Factors associated with back pain after childbirth. *Anesthesiology* 1994;81:29–34.
38 MacArthur A, MacArthur C, Weeks S. Epidural anesthesia and long-term back pain after delivery: a prospective cohort study. *BMJ* 1995;311:1336–9.
39 Dresner M, Freeman J, Cole P. Obstetric anaesthesia for patients with chronic back problems. *Br J Anaesth* 1997;78:A349.
40 MacArthur C, Lewis M, Knox EG. *Health after childbirth.* London: HMSO, 1991.
41 Association of Anaesthetists of Great Britain and Ireland. *Risk management.* London: AAGBI, 1998.
42 Chadwick HS. An analysis of obstetric anesthesia cases from the American Society of Anesthesiologists closed claims project database. *Int J Obstet Anesth* 1996;5:258–63.
43 Aitkenhead A. The pattern of litigation against anaesthetists. *Br J Anaesth* 1994;73:10–21.
44 MacLeod AD, Maycock E. Awareness during anaesthesia and post traumatic stress disorder. *Anaesth Intens Care* 1992;20:378–82.
45 Lyons G, Macdonald R. Awareness during caesarean section. *Anaesthesia* 1991;46:62–4.
46 McCrirrick A, Evans GH, Thomas TA. Overpressure isoflurane at Caesarean section: a study of arterial isoflurane concentrations. *Br J Anaesth* 1994;72:122–4.
47 Russell IF. Levels of anaesthesia and intraoperative pain at caesarean section under regional block. *Int J Obstet Anesth* 1995;4:71–7.
48 Crowhurst JA, Simmons SW. Standard setting and practice audit in obstetric anaesthesia. *Baillière's Clin Anaesthesiol* 1995;9:713–33.
49 Reynolds F. Auditing complications of regional analgesia in obstetrics. *Int J Obstet Anesth* 1998;7:1–4.
50 Brown GW, Russell IF. A survey of anaesthesia for caesarean section. *Int J Obstet Anesth* 1995;4:214–18.
51 Department of Health. *Report on confidential enquiries into maternal deaths in the UK 1994–1996.* London: HMSO, 1998.
52 Association of Anaesthetists of Great Britain and Ireland and the Obstetric Anaesthetists Association. *Guidelines for obstetric anaesthesia services.* London: AAGBI/OAA, 1998.

9: Anaesthesia for gynaecological surgery

KYM OSBORN, SCOTT SIMMONS

The problems for the anaesthetist presented by gynaecological surgery may be as challenging as those encountered in any area of modern practice. At one extreme, the patient may be a fit and healthy young woman who does not perceive herself as being "sick" and having the most minor of procedures. In this situation, the expectation is for as little disruption to the normal pattern of life as possible and often anaesthesia is perceived as of much greater concern than surgery. At the other end of the spectrum is the elderly patient, with possibly a host of complicating medical problems. She may be having surgery for carcinoma with the prospect of a protracted hospital stay and of significant perioperative complications, including death. To deal appropriately with this sort of variation over the full range of gynaecological surgery, the perioperative care team must not only be able to provide an efficient service for same-day surgery but must have the full back-up of inpatient facilities. This includes having sufficient numbers of appropriately trained nursing staff, an acute pain service, blood transfusion and laboratory services, and adult intensive care capabilities.

Preoperative assessment

Preoperative anaesthetic assessment has two broad purposes. First, it allows the anaesthetist the opportunity to take an appropriate history, perform an examination, and evaluate any potential complicating factors which may adversely affect outcome. Such factors may be medical or social and require further investigation and work-up before the day of surgery. Of equal importance, it gives the patient the opportunity to receive information regarding treatment options, to ask questions and ultimately meaningfully engage in the process of informed consent. Furthermore, there should be provision of basic information defining the admission process and any postoperative management issues, including common side-effects and implications for return to work.

The processes involved in the above may vary in complexity and use a variety of tools. As a part of this, in our institution we use a form which incorporates a patient questionnaire with a section for the anaesthetist to record relevant information (Fig 9.1).

	WOMEN'S & CHILDREN'S HOSPITAL GYNAECOLOGY ANAESTHETIC CHECK LIST	
	Please complete and bring this questionaire with you on the day of your pre-anaesthetic visit.	PATIENT LABEL

YES	NO	
		Have you ever had any anaesthetics before?
		Have you ever had any problems with your local or general anaesthetics?
		Have any of your blood relatives had anaesthetic problems?
		Are you suffering from, or have you ever had:
		Heart trouble or palpitations?
		Chest pain after exercise or climbing stairs?
		Asthma, a collapsed lung or other breathing problems?
		Convulsions, fits, blackouts or a stroke?
		Diabetes?
		Jaundice, hepatitis or liver disease?
		Peptic ulcers, heart-burn or indigestion?
		Kidney trouble?
		Psychiatric treatment?
		Or been in contact with infectious disases?
		Any other serious illness?
		A cold or flu in the last 2 weeks?
		Any neck or jaw stiffness?
		Any cortisone–related drugs in the last 6 months?
		Any aspirin in the last 2 weeks?
		Are you taking any medication?
		If yes, specify
		Do you have any allergies?
		Do you have any caps, crowns or dentures?
		Do you have any loose or chipped teeth?
		Do you have any contact lens, hearing aids or prostheses?
		Do you smoke? How much per day?
		Do you drink alcohol? How much per day?
		Are you left-handed?

PREANAESTHETIC ASSESSMENT

	YES	NO			
			PROCEDURE PLANNED:		AGE:
PROBLEMS WITH ANAES.			ALLERGIES:		WEIGHT:
FAMILY HISTORY					
ALLERGIES					
CARDIOVASCULAR DIS.					
RESPIRATORY DIS.					
OTHER MEDICAL DIS.					
GASTRIC REFLUX					
CONSENT SIGNED					

PREMED.		SEEN PREOP	AIRWAY ASSESSMENT	ISSUES COVERED	YES	NO	INVESTIGATIONS
NONE	0		MALLAMPATI 1 2 3 4	FASTING			
TEMAZEPAM	1	YES	THYROMENT. DIST.	MEDICATION			
MIDAZOLAM	2	TIME:	JAW	ANAES. RISKS			
RANITIDINE	3	DATE:	CERVICAL SP.	N.S.A.I.D.S			
ANTACID	4	BY:	TEETH	P.C.A.			
VENTOLIN	5			REGIONAL			
OTHER	6	NO:	ASA E 1 2 3 4 5	D/C ARRANGS.			
				D/C DRUGS			

Fig 9.1   Preanaesthetic gynaecology questionnaire and form

At the end of this phase the anaesthetist should have formulated a management plan appropriate for each patient, taking into account the nature of surgery, relevant past history, any concurrent medical problems, and patient preferences. In addition, the patient should be happy with this plan, having been informed of any alternatives and their relative risks and benefits. Also, clear instructions should be given regarding such issues as fasting requirements, taking of medications and, for day surgery patients, admission and discharge times and locations (Fig 9.2).

Anaesthetic techniques

The choice of anaesthetic method will be determined by an evaluation of risks and benefits based around the following considerations.

1 The nature and duration of surgery.
2 Patient preference.
3 Medical complications.
4 The knowledge and experience of the anaesthetist.
5 Availability of postoperative care.
6 Mode of postoperative analgesia.

There has been very little evaluation of whole techniques with respect to appropriate outcomes, although it is possible to draw some conclusions about discrete areas; for example, drug selection to reduce postoperative nausea and vomiting (PONV) (see below). Some general principles for the more common types of surgery are set out below.

Day-case procedures

Included within this group are hysteroscopy, termination of pregnancy (TOP), large loop excision of transformation zone (LLETZ) procedure, and endometrial ablation.

These are generally minor procedures where the duration of surgery is usually less than 30 minutes and postoperative pain, nausea, and vomiting are significantly less than with more invasive cases. They may be carried out in an operating theatre but an increasing proportion is being performed in outpatient clinics or consulting rooms under various permutations of local anaesthesia, with or without sedation. Local techniques may include paracervical block or topical anaesthesia with transcervical endocavitary instillation of local anaesthetic. For short, minimally invasive procedures such as vaginal termination of pregnancy, it may be tempting to consider general anaesthesia as unnecessary. However, there is no evidence that local blockade with sedation provides a better outcome than a well-conducted general anaesthetic with currently available drugs. For example, in a study of TOP when paracervical block was compared with general anaesthesia under a

305

Date of Surgery	**WOMEN'S AND CHILDREN'S HOSPITAL**
Time of Admission	*INSTRUCTIONS FOR GYNAECOLOGY PATIENTS*

FASTING INSTRUCTIONS

If your operation is in the morning, do not eat anything after midnight on the night before your operation.
If your operation is in the afternoon, you may have a light breakfast (tea and/or juice and toast) before 7.00 a.m.
Up to 3 hours prior to your operation you may drink a cup (200ml) of clear fluid per hour (e.g. water, apple juice, black tea or coffee – no milk).
Nothing further should be taken by mouth in the 3 hours prior to the scheduled time of your operation, apart from regular medications as indicated below.

MEDICATION INSTRUCTIONS

Please bring with you all your medication that you take regularly.
You should take your usual morning medication (tablets, capsules, etc.) with a sip of water before leaving home on the day of your operation, unless indicated otherwise by your anaesthetist.

SMOKING

It is recommended you stop smoking 2–3 days before your operation. DO NOT smoke on the day of surgery.

ADMISSION

Patients are admitted in a staggered fashion to minimise waiting.
Please present to the Admissions Department, Ground Floor, Queen Victoria Building, at your appointed time.

PERSONAL BELONGINGS

Do not wear jewellery or bring valuables.
Bring a case for your glasses, contact lenses or dentures.

DRESSING

Dress sensibly and be comfortable. Do not wear high heels, make-up or nail polish.
You will not need sleeping attire or a dressing gown, but please bring a pair of socks and toilet items.

DISCHARGE ARRANGEMENTS FOR GYNAECOLOGY DAY SURGERY PATIENTS

YOU MUST NOT DRIVE HOME AFTER YOUR OPERATION. You should make

arrangements for a responsible person to accompany you home after your operation. He/she should telephone the Gynaecology Surgery Unit (8204 7540) approximately 2 hours after your scheduled surgery time to determine when you are able to be discharged. Most patients can go home between 2.00 and 6.00 p.m.
Journeys longer than 1–1¹/₂ hours drive are not recommended. If this is the case, it is recommended that you make arrangements to stay overnight in Adelaide. If this is not possible, admission can be arranged.

POSTOPERATIVE CARE

You should also arrange for a responsible person to stay with you overnight, following your operation, to assist you should a complication arise.

IMPORTANT POSTOPERATIVE INSTRUCTIONS

Although after 3 or 4 hours you may feel that you have fully recovered from your general anaesthetic or intravenous sedation, your ability to think normally or to carry out simple tasks may in fact be impaired for a much longer period.
For your own safety, therefore, it is recommended that you:

1. **DO NOT** drive a motor car or use machinery
2. **DO NOT** have exposure to hazards (e.g. heights, hot stoves, chemicals)
3. **DO NOT** sign legal documents or make important decisions
4. **AVOID** alcohol and sedative drugs which will greatly prolong your recovery
   until the morning after your operation.

QUESTIONS

If you have any questions telephone 8204 7550 between 7.00 a.m. & 6.00 p.m. Monday to Friday.
If you develop a cold or any other illness during the 48 hours prior to the day of surgery, please telephone the Duty Gynaecology Anaesthetist on 8204 7000 as it may be advisable to alter your arrangements.

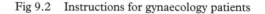

Fig 9.2   Instructions for gynaecology patients

combination of propofol, alfentanil, and nitrous oxide, there was no difference in recovery between groups.[1] In addition, 8% of the regional patients remembered pain during the procedure in spite of supplemental sedation with alfentanil (0.01 mg/kg) and midazolam (0.1 mg/kg IV). Deep paracervical blockade with carbonated lignocaine can also be used but pain scores are unacceptably high.

Central neural blockade in the form of spinal, lumbar epidural or caudal blocks in principle is appropriate for these types of procedures. In general, however, there is no benefit in terms of recovery and there are potential problems with patient preference and postdural puncture headache.

Overall, regional techniques are viable alternatives in motivated individuals who decline general anaesthesia but there seems little advantage for routine use where general anaesthesia is available. Heavy sedation mandates the presence of an anaesthetist with appropriate monitoring and airway management equipment. In addition, alternatives to general anaesthesia are not without problems such as local anaesthetic toxicity and vasoconstrictor effects, as well as longer turnover times.

For conduct of general anaesthesia in these and other day procedures as below, propofol is used extensively because of presumed benefits in recovery and PONV. Jakobsson et al. compared propofol, thiopentone, and methohexitone in various combinations with ketamine or fentanyl.[2] The propofol/fentanyl combination resulted in shorter discharge times compared with thiopentone (approximately 20 minutes less) but no difference from those with methohexitone. The latter group, however, reported a higher incidence of pain. Also, satisfaction as reported directly by patients was highest in the propofol/fentanyl group. The method of propofol administration as either repeat bolus or continuous infusion has no influence on outcome when combined with alfentanil and nitrous oxide. However, the use of propofol as part of a technique of total intravenous anaesthesia (TIVA) may have benefits at limiting PONV (see below).

Propofol has become popular for these cases and now has an extensive track record of safe use in a vast number of patients. Nonetheless, no drug is entirely without problems. Propofol has been associated with pain on injection, convulsions, transient desaturation, asystole, and sexually inappropriate, disinhibited behaviour. Furthermore, it should not be used in the context of an ongoing pregnancy on the basis of teratogenic findings in animals.

Recent attention has focused on sevoflurane as an alternative to propofol because of its capacity for rapid emergence. Initial experience suggests no clear advantage in this regard and it may be inferior with respect to PONV (see below). There is also the potential for volatile agents to increase blood loss due to reduction of uterine tone. This has been demonstrated for TOP with isoflurane and consideration should be given to avoiding or limiting volatiles in these patients.

Although a common practice, the merit of adding an opioid such as fentanyl for these procedures has been questioned. In a study by Cade and Ross, fentanyl in a dose of approximately 1 µg/kg in combination with either propofol or methohexitone and nitrous oxide had no effect on analgesic requirements in recovery or on nausea and vomiting.[3] Nonetheless, moderate postoperative pain is common (35–40% of women) and simple analgesics alone such as prophylactic oral paracetamol may be inadequate.

Laparoscopy

This includes day surgery procedures such as sterilisation, division of adhesions, cystectomy, and investigation of infertility or pelvic pain. More complex procedures such as assisted vaginal hysterectomy (LAVH) or myomectomy may also be perfomed with the aid of the laparoscope.

Although gaseous distension of the abdomen in the Trendelenburg position to examine the pelvis dates from the early 1900s, the technique was only popularised in the 1960s. Several early papers from that era describe the fundamental physiological changes associated with head down position and the presence of a pneumoperitoneum with pressures of the order of 2.7 KPa.[4] In essence, in the spontaneously breathing individual there is decreased diaphragmatic movement, increased dead space, and associated hypoventilation. This led to recommendations for the use of endotracheal intubation and positive pressure ventilation. Further concerns regarding raised intra-abdominal pressure and risk of aspiration while head down reinforced this view.

With the advent of the laryngeal mask airway (LMA) and increasing desire for early mobilisation and discharge, there has been a trend away from these principles.[5] This has led some workers to recommend guidelines for the use of the LMA for laparoscopy by appropriate patient selection and management. These include selecting only non-obese patients, short procedures (<15 minutes), avoidance of high intra-abdominal pressures or steep head down tilt and correct LMA insertion with adequate depth of anaesthesia.[6] However, aspiration pneumonia has been reported in a 60 kg supine woman undergoing cholecystectomy using positive pressure ventilation with the LMA.[7] In addition, the likelihood of reflux was increased in a group of patients having cataract surgery under positive pressure ventilation with the LMA compared with those where the trachea was intubated.[8]

Technological advances have made some of these issues less relevant. Several workers have reported laparoscopic procedures without the need for pneumoperitoneum using a variety of retraction systems for procedures ranging from simple diagnostic work to LAVH, adhesiolysis, and myomectomy. In addition, there are now several series, using 2 mm laparoscopes, where intravenous sedation plus local infiltration have been used successfully for diagnostic and procedural work including sterilisation and lysis of adhesions. However, it would appear that patient selection is crucial for these techniques to be successful, as there needs to be a high level of motivation and a significant requirement to convert to more conventional techniques after the procedure has commenced. Overall, the incidence of low or equivocal patient satisfaction may be of the order of 15%.[9]

Management of postoperative pain and limitation of PONV are essential considerations when dealing with this group. More detailed discussions of PONV and the use of non-steroidal anti-inflammatory drugs (NSAIDs) are given elsewhere but some other pertinent issues are worth raising at this point. In particular, the pain of laparoscopic tubal ligation is more severe than that of diagnostic laparoscopy.[10] Pain in both cases is due to a number of factors including surgical incision and injury related to peritoneal stretching which ultimately includes shoulder tip pain experienced for several days postoperatively. Surgical technique remains the prime factor for these contributors. Attempts at alleviating these sources have included provision of small transumbilical peritoneal drains and the use of topically applied lignocaine, but benefits appear to be short-lived and these have not been widely accepted.

The main difference between these two procedures is presumably largely as a result of tubal damage and spasm, but even most of this difference has disappeared 24 hours after surgery. On this basis, however, techniques have been described for directly attenuating tubal pain. These include the application of topical bupivacaine to the fallopian tubes, application of lignocaine gel, bupivacaine infiltration of the mesosalpinx, and intravenous glycopyrrolate. However, in almost all these instances, whilst some differences can be demonstrated in the immediate postoperative period, it is questionable whether these changes are clinically relevant. For example, Tool et al. showed a significant reduction in pain scores 30 minutes after tubal sterilisation using topical bupivacaine compared with placebo.[11] Unfortunately, there was no difference in requirements for supplemental analgesia, postoperative vomiting or length of time in recovery.

Inpatient procedures

This group includes abdominal hysterectomy, vaginal surgery, and surgery for malignancy. The approach to anaesthesia should apply the same basic principles as for other major abdominal cases. The main considerations lie with attention to temperature loss, fluid balance, blood loss, and adequate analgesia. Specific issues of PONV, postoperative analgesia and dealing with the problems of malignancy are covered elsewhere in this chapter.

Postoperative nausea and vomiting

Postoperative nausea and vomiting is a significant cause of morbidity with a multifactorial basis.[12,13] In the day surgery setting, it is a factor contributing to prolonged stay in recovery and increased overnight admission rates. The incidence and severity of PONV in the group of young women, predominantly ASA 1 or 2, having same-day gynaecological surgery is so high that this group is often the subject of clinical trials for new antiemetic therapies. Indeed, research in this area could possibly be deemed unethical when the study protocol includes a placebo arm where the baseline incidence is known to be of the order of 50–100%.[14]

Patient factors

- *Gender*: the incidence in females is two to three times that in males.[15]
- *Age*: rates are generally low at the extremes of life but higher within the range applicable to this group.[16]
- *History of PONV*: a positive history is associated with a threefold increased risk.[17]
- *History of motion sickness*: this has been questioned by some but the main body of opinion would support a significant role for a positive history being contributory.[13] It is also possible that the emetic effects of some drugs, particularly morphine, initially satisfactory in the immediate postoperative recovery phase, may become most pronounced only in association with the motion of travelling home after surgery.
- *Anxiety*: anxious patients are probably at increased risk secondary to such factors as greater drug dosage requirements and air swallowing.
- *Phase of menstrual cycle*: some work has suggested incidence increases during menstruation,[18] but this has not been a consistent finding and may in any event be difficult to put into clinical practice.

Surgical factors

- *Peritoneal injury or stimulation*: this is more likely to be associated with PONV and includes stretching related to pneumoperitoneum performed under high pressure, failing to remove distending gas, and irritation from blood.
- *Surgical trauma*: excessive handling of the gut and possibly the use of Fallope rings as opposed to clips for sterilisation may increase the incidence of PONV.
- *Duration of surgery*: procedures longer than one hour have been seen to be associated with higher incidences of PONV although the basis of this is probably multifactorial.

Anaesthetic factors

Homeostatic regulation

Maintenance of normal body temperature, hydration, and blood glucose will contribute to more rapid recovery, at least in part due to reduced PONV.

Drugs used for induction and maintenance of general anaesthesia

Propofol has become the principal intravenous induction agent for day surgery – this is both as a result of decreased recovery time as well as decreased incidence of PONV. In particular it has been promoted as the drug of choice, as part of the technique of total intravenous anaesthesia for patients at high risk, over alternatives employing volatile agents plus or minus nitrous oxide.[14]

With respect to any differences between various volatile agents, there has been recent interest in sevoflurane both as compared to established volatiles such as isoflurane and also by comparison with propofol.[19] Experience in the gynaecological population is still very small and it is too early to draw conclusions.

In a study involving non-gynaecological day-care surgery, Raeder et al. showed a more rapid emergence with sevoflurane after propofol induction compared with propofol alone but there was significantly more nausea and vomiting in the first 24 hours postoperatively in the sevoflurane group.[20]

Nitrous oxide has the potential to be emetogenic through such mechanisms as bowel distension and middle ear effects. Many small studies over a number of years have not demonstrated any consistent action but in a meta-analysis by Divatia et al. a clear risk reduction was demonstrated.[21] In a pooled evaluation of 24 studies over almost 30 years up until 1994, the omission of nitrous oxide resulted in an overall reduction of risk of PONV of 28%. Moreover, in the subgroup of female patients this effect was most marked, being of the order of 50%.

Muscle relaxants per se seem to have little effect on the incidence and severity of PONV but reversal agents are potentially more important. Neostigmine has been associated with an increased incidence of PONV.[22] However, small doses of atropine may be beneficial, particularly in the context of the relative bradycardia that may follow vagal stimulation.

Drugs used for prophylaxis and treatment of PONV

Given the extent of the problem and complexity of the underlying mechanisms producing nausea and vomiting, it is not surprising that there is a plethora of drugs and drug combinations that have been evaluated and are now in common use. A detailed review of the basic pharmacology of these drugs is beyond the scope of this chapter and the reader is referred to a more general text.

The agents subjected to recent evaluation include:

- 5HT$_3$ receptor antagonists: ondansetron, tropisetron and granisetron;
- droperidol;
- metoclopramide: has been widely used in a dose of 10 mg despite little evidence to support its efficacy;[23]

- ephedrine: may be of benefit in doses of 0.5 mg/kg IM or 3–6 mg IV, particularly with increased risk of postural hypotension;[24]
- cyclizine;
- dexamethasone;
- other – ginger root, scopolamine patches, and acupuncture.

Of the above, ondansetron has probably received greatest recent attention and has been shown to be of benefit for both outpatient and major inpatient gynaecology surgery.[25] A meta-analysis by Tramer *et al.* evaluated seven trials from the period 1991 to 1996 for established nausea and vomiting; more than 80% of patients in these trials were women.[26] They concluded that ondansetron is more efficacious than placebo in about one in four patients. However, there was no difference with regard to low-dose droperidol (15–20 µg/kg) and metoclopramide (although in the latter case, from one trial only). In addition, there appeared to be no clear dose-response relationship over the range of 1–8 mg.

Some studies have specifically evaluated prophylactic therapy. In a placebo-based trial, Malins *et al.* compared ondansetron (4 mg) with metoclopramide (10 mg) in day case laparoscopy, including follow-up for the first 48 hours after surgery.[27] They showed a virtual halving of the incidence of nausea and vomiting with ondansetron compared with placebo rate of 50%. However, the number who experienced symptoms for the first time only after leaving hospital was the same in all groups, implying that any actual differences were in the immediate postoperative period. With regard to the endpoint of unplanned admission, there was only one patient who was admitted.

In a more recent study Sniadach and Alberts compared the prophylactic use of ondansetron (4 mg) with droperidol (20 µg/kg), looking at nausea, vomiting, and sedation.[28] There were no differences between groups except for a higher incidence of vomiting in the ondansetron group on the first postoperative day. These authors further evaluated cost-effectiveness which was clearly in favour of droperidol as it was less than one-tenth of the cost of ondansetron.

Taking this concept further, Tang *et al.* described an elaborate model for evaluating cost-effectiveness when comparing ondansetron and droperidol for outpatient gynaecology.[29] They looked at a number of outcome parameters and took into consideration such factors as acquisition cost, additional time spent in recovery, rate of unplanned admission, and return to work. They concluded that prophylactic droperidol at a dose of 0.625 mg was as effective as ondansetron at limiting PONV. In addition, they estimated that droperidol would be more cost-effective as long as the relative acquisition costs for the two drugs remained in the ratio of 1:2.5 or greater in favour of droperidol. Prophylaxis with droperidol was also more cost-effective than waiting to treat established PONV provided the baseline incidence was at least 13%. This contrasted with ondansetron where the incidence would have to be 30%. Finally they were unable to show any difference between the two drugs with respect to discharge readiness or return to work.

More recent additions to the list such as tropisetron and granisetron have only been evaluated in a few studies. Capouet et al. have reported on a multicentre trial from Belgium evaluating the relative effectiveness of 0.5, 2, and 5 mg of tropisetron for prophylaxis for a diverse group of patients;[30] 2 mg appeared to be the optimal dose with regard to both efficacy and side-effects. In addition, when compared with droperidol (1.25 mg) for prophylaxis of PONV for inpatient gynaecological surgery, tropisetron (5 mg) has been shown to be more effective with fewer side-effects.[31] However, it is probable that when used in higher dose and in an older population, such as in this study, predictable adverse effects of droperidol such as anxiety and sedation become more prominent. Droperidol has been used effectively for minor outpatient gynaecology in doses as low as 0.25 mg and it would appear reasonable to limit dosages to less than 1 mg.

Presumed benefits of tropisetron and also granisetron are somewhat longer durations of effectiveness than with ondansetron or the cheaper alternatives. This is particularly relevant for dealing with persistent residual effects and any effects related to travel home. In this regard, efforts have been made to extend the duration of antiemesis by addition of steroids. Dexamethasone has been used successfully for both chemotherapy and in children after tonsillectomy. In a study involving major gynaecology surgery, Fujii et al. showed that the combination of granisetron 40 μg/kg and dexamethasone 8 mg was more effective than droperidol (1.25 mg) and metoclopramide, with or without dexamethasone in a group with a history of motion sickness.[32]

In summary, this patient group has a well-documented problem with respect to both high incidence and severity of PONV. A number of drugs, including droperidol and the 5HT₃ antagonists, have been shown to be significantly better than placebo at both prevention and treatment. Individual drugs vary considerably in cost in different parts of the world, although in general, newer agents will be more expensive. Cost-benefit decisions should be made in the context of local conditions and consider all ramifications of any changes.

Postoperative analgesia

Day-case procedures

Management of pain in the day surgery setting is geared toward limitation of PONV and early mobilisation and discharge. Many of the relevant issues are discussed elsewhere. Opioids should be limited where possible and in particular, morphine appears to increase motion-induced vomiting.

Fentanyl and alfentanil in moderate doses are satisfactory and are indicated for more invasive procedures such as minor operative laparoscopic work, including tubal sterilisation. The addition of NSAIDs is common but evidence for routine use is tenuous. Supplemental techniques involving local anaesthetic infiltration or application are generally of short-term benefit but should be considered where appropriate; for example, topical bupivacaine to fallopian tubes at sterilisation.

Since techniques are generally aimed at early emergence and a desire to limit opioid side-effects there is a potential for patients to initially experience significant pain immediately after general anaesthesia. Consideration should therefore be given to the implementation of a simple procedure for administration of small, incremental doses of an analgesic in the immediate recovery period, for example 20–40 µg boluses of IV fentanyl, every five minutes against a verbal pain score.

Inpatient procedures

The nature of the surgical stimulus and the priorities for discharge are quite different in this group compared with those for day surgery procedures. It is appropriate to consider more extensive and invasive analgesic techniques for more prolonged periods. This includes the use of intravenous and epidural infusions and patient-controlled analgesia (PCA). As with day surgery, however, non-opioid analgesics such as NSAIDs and paracetamol have been tried in an attempt to limit opiate side-effects.

Intravenous PCA with any of the potent opioids is an entirely suitable technique. However, there is little evidence that any agent is significantly better than another. For example, in a direct comparison of morphine and pethidine after elective total abdominal hysterectomy (TAH), Stanley et al. found no difference in pain scores, patient satisfaction, vomiting, antiemetic requirements, and postoperative sedation.[33] The mean drug consumption in the first 24 hours was 70 mg of morphine and 660 mg of pethidine. The dosing schedule for PCA should reflect these rates of consumption but in addition should be sufficiently flexible to allow for the very wide range of dosing requirements that have now been recognised. Overall, the best predictor of IV PCA morphine in the first 24 hours is given by the equation: mean 24 hour morphine requirement (mg) = 100 − age, and the interpatient variability in each age group is approximately 10-fold.[34]

In an attempt to tailor morphine dosing to limit PCA requirements, different dosing schedules have been evaluated. Mansfield et al. showed that an induction dose of 0.3 mg/kg significantly reduced PCA usage compared with 0.15 mg/kg at both induction and at the end of surgery, although the total 24-hour morphine dose was only reduced from 77 mg to 63 mg and pain scores were the same in all groups.[35] A similar insignificant result has been found for dosing with morphine up to two days before surgery.

With a view to reducing opioid side-effects, NSAIDs such as ketorolac and diclofenac have been used as part of the analgesic technique. Whilst several studies have been able to show analgesic effect, the results have been inconsistent and positive benefits for various clinically significant outcome parameters are not great. For example, in one study after TAH, rectal diclofenac was associated with a substantial reduction in morphine consumption compared with placebo but there was no evidence of any reduction in the incidence of nausea and vomiting.[36] Similarly, Balestrieri *et al.* have evaluated the effectiveness of intravenous ketorolac with IV PCA morphine after TAH and myomectomy.[37] Despite using rather large doses of ketorolac, there were no significant reductions in adverse events or median times to recovery, in spite of decreased morphine use. Furthermore, there appears to be no clinical value in a preemptive approach.

In principle, some benefit may be gained by adding other simple analgesics to NSAIDs when used with opioids. Montgomery *et al.* showed that a combination of rectal paracetamol (1.5 g) and diclofenac (100 mg) after abdominal hysterectomy was better than either alone for reduction of total morphine use.[38] Morphine consumption was approximately 40 mg in the first 24 hours in this group, although again there was no difference between groups with respect to nausea and vomiting which ranged from 26% to 40%.

Both epidural and subarachnoid techniques have also been employed in order to reduce side-effects. In an intriguing study from Northwick Park Hospital, the possibility of pre-emptive benefits using spinal blockade was evaluated by comparing PCA morphine requirements after spinal bupivacaine given either before or at the completion of surgery.[39] There was very little difference between the groups other than an increased requirement in the preoperative spinal patients at 12 hours. Furthermore, there appears to be no clinical value in a preemptive approach using low thoracic epidural bupivacaine combined with diclofenac.[40] The whole issue of preemptive analgesia is contentious. Other work suggests that for any benefits to be derived, blockade must be continued well into the postoperative period and this may not be a practical option. There is, however, some evidence that epidural anaesthesia and postoperative analgesia offer an improvement in both analgesia and more rapid recovery than general anaesthesia and intravenous morphine.[41] This benefit may translate to earlier hospital discharge as a result of decreased duration of postoperative ileus. However, the safe conduct of epidural techniques on general wards is not without hazards and should not be undertaken without appropriate consideration of levels of nursing supervision and protocols of management.

NSAIDs in gynaecological surgery

Many different drugs fall within this group of agents and they have gained increasing popularity and are now used extensively for postoperative pain relief. However, whilst numerous studies have demonstrated analgesic efficacy, relative potency and the capacity for side-effect reduction through opioid sparing have not been so clearly established. Indeed, these drugs are not without their own side-effects, including gastrointestinal upset and ulceration, renal dysfunction, precipitation of asthma in susceptible individuals, and coagulation problems.

In a study comparing fentanyl and ketorolac for analgesia after minor gynaecological procedures such as dilation and curettage (D&C) and cone biopsy, ketorolac alone was shown to be inadequate and inferior to fentanyl.[42] In addition, the combination of ketorolac and fentanyl was not associated with any reduction in recovery time or postoperative side-effects compared to fentanyl alone. Similar results have been found for laparoscopic sterilisation with either ketorolac or ibuprofen in combination with fentanyl, including "pre-emptive" administration. Similarly, in a multi-centre trial in which oral ketorolac was compared with a hydrocodone-paracetamol mixture for treatment of postoperative pain after laparoscopic sterilisation, there was no difference in analgesic efficacy between the groups, with neither being effective.[43] There are several other studies showing a similar lack of effectiveness for ketorolac, diclofenac, ketoprofen, tenoxicam, and indomethacin.

However, by contrast with the above, there are some reports of a significant benefit from intraoperative use of NSAIDs through reduction of side-effects and shorter recovery time after laparoscopy, this having been reported for both ketorolac,[10] and diclofenac.[44]

In summary, it is difficult to make a clear recommendation for routine use of these drugs, there being inconsistent clinical results and potential for significant side-effects. The most sensible use would appear to be for those patients with documented sensitivity to opioids. In any event, use should be after an appraisal of the potential for side-effects, including renal injury, gastrointestinal bleeding, coagulopathy and asthma, as stated in the manufacturer's recommendations and by such bodies as the Royal College of Anaesthetists. Ideally, each hospital should have documented guidelines defining contraindications and dosing schedules.

The laryngeal mask airway

The LMA is widely used in gynaecological anaesthesia. Pollard and Cooper surveyed 386 anaesthetists in 15 centres in the United Kingdom and found that 23% used the LMA for laparoscopy with positive ventilation and 18% with spontaneous ventilation.[45]

The lithotomy position, head down tilt, gas insufflation of the peritoneal cavity and stimulation of the peritoneum all have the potential to increase the risk of regurgitation of gastric contents and pulmonary aspiration. The work of breathing during laparoscopic surgery is also increased in the spontaneously breathing patient. A working party convened in 1978 by the Royal College of Obstetricians and Gynaecologists recommended that patients for gynaecological laparoscopy should be intubated and ventilated.[46] As noted in the study by Jansen et al., surgical complications occurred at a rate of 5.7 per 1000 and almost 50% of these occurred with insertion of the trocar.[47] Intubation and ventilation with endtidal CO_2 monitoring allows for early detection of gas embolism. Furthermore, delay in diagnosis and management by use of a face mask technique has been the subject of medicolegal action.

Joshi et al., in a study comparing LMA with tracheal intubation in 381 patients undergoing peripheral surgery, found that there was no difference in the times to "home readiness" although the duration of the time in the postanaesthesia care unit and time to mobilise were significantly shorter in the LMA group.[48] They also demonstrated a significant reduction in sore throats in the LMA group. In patients undergoing laparoscopy, Swann et al. found that patients with an LMA, either breathing spontaneously or with assisted ventilation, reported significantly more nausea and vomiting when compared with intubated and ventilated patients, possibly due to gastric insufflation.[5] The incidence of regurgitation as detected by methylene blue dye is of the order of 25% during general anaesthesia with a LMA, although with this technique aspiration has not been observed. However, other methods such as hypopharyngeal pH measurements have shown no evidence of pharyngeal regurgitation.

In the first 5000 Australian Incident Monitoring Study (AIMS) reports there were 133 documented aspiration incidents, of which 27 involved the use of the LMA (M Kluger, personal communication). Brimacombe and Berry performed a meta-analysis of the published data on the incidence of aspiration with the LMA and gave a final incidence of two per 10 000 cases (three cases in the 12 901 patients).[49] Malins et al. reported that they had used the technique on about 3000 cases without serious morbidity. As well as careful patient selection, they limited the intra-abdominal pressure to between 1.6 and 2 KPa and the amount of tilt to no more than 15°(see Anaesthetic techniques above).[27]

In summary, anaesthesia with a LMA for laparoscopy is a technique in use in carefully selected patients. It does not, however, protect the airway which may need to be secured should there be a surgical or anaesthetic incident requiring resuscitation.

Positioning for surgery

Lithotomy

When positioning a patient in the lithotomy position, each lower limb is flexed at the hip and knee and both legs are elevated simultaneously and separated. For most vaginal surgery, the patient's thighs are flexed about 90° to the trunk and the knees are bent sufficiently to maintain the lower legs parallel to the floor. Major vessels may be compressed by more acute flexion at either the hip or knee joint. When access to the abdomen is required, as in laparoscopic surgery, the degree of thigh elevation is only 30–45°. This reduces perfusion gradients to and from the lower extremities. The legs are supported in leg supports or stirrups. To avoid torsion stress on the lumbar spine, when lowering the legs at the end of the procedure, the legs should be first brought together in the sagittal plane at the knees and ankles. The arms are either extended laterally to less than 90° on arm boards or flexed across the chest.

Trendelenburg

To improve the exposure of pelvic organs, the head down position is commonly used. In the past, a steep 30–45° tilt was used. This is referred to as the Trendelenburg position as it was popularised by Friedrich Trendelenburg of Leipzig. Shoulder braces were required to prevent the patient sliding off the table. These braces were implicated in brachial plexus injury. The tilt is now usually limited to 10–15°, obviating the need for patient restraints. This, in fact, more closely corresponds to the scultetus position, after the German surgeon, Johann Schultes (1595–1645).

In the head down position, preload to the heart is increased which may stress a compromised right ventricle. Cerebral perfusion pressure may decrease, as will the arterial pressure to the legs.[50] The cephalad movement of the abdominal viscera causes a cephalad displacement of the diaphragm and obstruction of its caudal movement in inspiration. As the head down tilt increases, the normal upright pressure gradient is reversed and the pleural pressure gradient is greater at the apex than at the base. The apex of the lung then has the alveoli with smaller volumes, which makes them more compliant. The abdominal contents also push into the bases, making them less compliant. Consequently, ventilation of the apices is favoured over the bases, functional residual capacity decreases, pulmonary compliance decreases, and the work of breathing increases. This may aggravate atelectasis and cause hypoxaemia, particularly in the obese and the elderly. As the mediastinum moves cephalad, the lungs and carina can also shift, causing the tip of the endotracheal tube to migrate distally into the right mainstem bronchus. Ventilation of both lungs should be confirmed whenever a patient is placed head down.

Nerve injury

The lithotomy position is associated with an increased risk of lower limb neuropathy. Warner et al. examined the perioperative courses of 198 461 consecutive patients who underwent 56 surgical procedures in the lithotomy position at the Mayo Clinic, Minnesota, from 1957 to 1991.[51] Persistent neuropathies of the lower limbs associated with motor deficit and lasting at least three months occurred at a rate of one per 3608. Of the 55 affected patients, 43 had a common peroneal nerve lesion, eight sciatic nerve problems, and in four the femoral nerve was damaged. The obturator and saphenous nerves may also be affected. Direct pressure on the calf muscle has the potential to cause the rare complication of compartment syndrome. Particular care should be taken that ankles, knees and elbows are padded to prevent pressure injury to the peroneal nerve as it crosses the head of the fibula and the ulnar nerve at the elbow and that the arms are not abducted greater than 90°.[50] This is especially so when the theatre lights are dimmed. The surgeon may inadvertently lean against the arm board and abduct it when operating.

Day-case anaesthesia

With the advance of clinical methods and the economic pressures of the modern health system, there has been a return to the practices of almost a century ago whereby time in hospital is limited to the bare minimum. This has meant that the recent relatively conservative practice of limiting day surgery to only fit patients having minor procedures has been progressively expanded. Indeed, one of the basic principles of achieving "street fitness" before discharge is perhaps becoming less relevant in this context as individuals are discharged home or to "hotel" facilities for a level of ongoing postoperative care only just short of that available in the acute hospital setting. In passing, it should be noted that this has increasingly shifted the burden of care to the community and providers of day surgery services must be conscious of what is available, as not all health planners or administrators have necessarily addressed this issue appropriately.

When considering the issues pertinent to delivery of a same-day service for gynaecology, the following issues should be addressed.

1 Patient selection and preparation
2 Fasting requirements
3 PONV (see above)
4 Pain relief (see above)
5 Perioperative fluids
6 Organisational issues
7 Management of discharge

Patient selection and preparation

This should follow the principles defined above (Preoperative evaluation). In general, patients of ASA grades 1, 2, and possibly 3 are suitable. The surgery should be less than one hour in duration and with a level of postoperative pain able to be controlled by oral medication. Patients should be identified as being able to be discharged to a place no more than approximately 90 minutes away from the facility and into the care of a responsible adult.

Management of the preoperative evaluation can be addressed in several different ways and is probably a function as much of available resources as fundamental principle. All patients should be evaluated sufficiently in advance of surgery for investigation or management of medical problems and to appropriately determine a plan of management. In doing this before the day of surgery, the admission process and running of lists on the day can be greatly facilitated. However, this will require specifically allocated outpatient time and ideally the anaesthetic consultation should be conducted by the individual who will actually administer the anaesthetic. Realistically, for a busy service these ideals may not be achievable due to insufficient resources and the direct matching of each anaesthetist with their prospective patients may be logistically difficult. By way of compromise, it has been common to adopt a "screening" process to identify higher risk patients who in the broadest sense would benefit from seeing the anaesthetist before the day of surgery. The elements of this process may include:

1 using a preoperative questionnaire to identify, at low threshold, any issues which need to be addressed;
2 using appropriately trained nursing staff to conduct preoperative interviews or review questionnaires and refer only those of concern to be seen by an anaesthetist;
3 providing patients with written information in the form of a simple booklet through the gynaecology clinic or rooms which includes advice on seeking further information in the light of particular problems;
4 educating surgeons about the need for appropriate preanaesthetic evaluation;
5 developing practice guidelines within the anaesthetic department or group which enable consistency in approach with respect to evaluation and advice regarding the method of anaesthesia. This should not (and need not) be overly prescriptive nor limit diversity.

Fasting requirements

Advice regarding fasting requirements must be provided and understood. Recommendations as to the appropriate duration of fasting have been revised in recent years with a general acceptance of a reduction, particularly in relation to clear fluids.[52] Several studies have shown no difference in gastric emptying amongst elective patients with no gastrointestinal disease or other drug effects where free fluids have been allowed up to two or three hours before anaesthesia compared with those with longer fasting times.[53,54] Indeed, there is some evidence that the volume of clear fluids ingested does not correlate with the residual gastric volume and that other factors are more significant. On this basis, it is appropriate to allow patients to drink clear fluids up to three hours before anaesthesia. Traditional recommendations regarding fasting from food for six hours are still generally applied and there is no evidence to change this.

Pregnancy may be a confounding factor, particularly for first and second trimester termination and for procedures in the immediate postpartum period. Whitehead et al. observed no difference in gastric emptying, as demonstrated by paracetamol absorption, for any of the three trimesters.[55] In addition, Lam et al. concluded that oral water could be given safely 2–3 hours preoperatively to women more than one day postpartum, there being no difference in intragastric volume and acidity compared with their non-pregnant counterparts.[56] Nonetheless, simple gastric emptying is not the only determinant of aspiration risk. It would be appropriate to employ longer fasting times and other measures such as preoperative H_2-receptor blockers and even rapid-sequence induction with intubation when there is a history of reflux, obesity or opioid use and for women more than 20 weeks pregnant.

Perioperative fluids

Numerous studies have been conducted to determine possible benefits of perioperative fluid administration with respect to less nausea and vomiting, less dizziness, and earlier discharge. In general, some marginal improvements can be demonstrated with volumes of the order of 15–20 ml/kg.[57] In principle, any such benefits are more likely in circumstances such as after more prolonged fasting, in hotter weather or with longer surgical procedures. There is little evidence in this group that one form of crystalloid confers substantial benefits over another. Overall, it is appropriate in this group for whom PONV is a significant risk to provide fluids as part of a total technique to limit morbidity. Additionally, where TIVA is employed, it would seem sensible to establish a free-flowing intravenous line to ensure reliable drug delivery, particularly when low drug infusion rates are used.

Organisational issues

Various aspects of the management of day surgery have been defined as influencing total outcome.[58] In particular, the admixture of day surgery patients and inpatients significantly increases recovery times for day-case procedures and has been associated with higher unplanned admission rates. Such mixed facilities also have longer preoperative waiting times and this contributes to reduced patient satisfaction. Even if day surgery is performed within a general facility, consideration should be given to providing for separation of day cases and inpatients both on operating lists and in recovery.

Management of discharge

Discharge criteria for day surgery patients have also been steadily revised in the light of experience. For example, the requirement to be able to drink before going home has been accepted as not only unnecessary but actually counterproductive due to increasing the likelihood of postoperative vomiting. Patients should only be allowed to leave once there is physiological stability, side-effects have been controlled and appropriate information has been provided for immediate care and further follow-up. A discharge checklist used in our unit is presented as Fig 9.3.

Consistent with the fundamental principles of auditing of service delivery, there should also be some process for communication with patients in the first 1–2 days after surgery.

	Yes	No	N/A	Comments
Anti-D/Rhogam				
Rubella vaccine				
Appts/follow up/other investigations				
Discharge medication/contraception				
Discharge letter				
Sick certificate				
Risk form				
Check dressing/PV loss				
Drains removed				
IV access removed/site checked				
ECG dots removed				
When to remove sutures				
General discharge information given				
Specific information given				
Valuables returned				
Discharge criteria met				

Date/Time Discharged: _____ **RN/EN Signature:**

Fig 9.3   Discharge checklist and record

Gynaecological procedures

Hysteroscopy and endometrial ablation

The hysteroscope is used for diagnosis and surgical treatment. As a diagnostic tool it is used in the investigation of abnormal bleeding, evaluation of infertility and recurrent miscarriages and the location and removal of embedded intrauterine contraceptive devices.[59]

Hysteroscopic surgical techniques

Hysteroscopic techniques can be used for resection of submucous fibroids, intrauterine adhesions, and septa as well as endometrial ablation. In the management of selected women with menorrhagia, endometrial ablation has several advantages over hysterectomy.

1 Shorter surgical time.
2 Fewer complications..
3 Reduced analgesia requirement.
4 Shorter convalescence and time to return to work.
5 Hysteroscopic endometrial ablation appears to avoid the need for hysterectomy in about 80% of the women treated.[60]

There are several methods of endometrial ablation available. The use of Nd-YAG laser photovaporisation to ablate the endometrium was first described in 1981. The laser beam passes down fine flexible quartz fibres and is directed via an operating hysteroscope onto the endometrial surface. The Nd-YAG laser causes necrosis to a depth of 5–6 mm. If lasers are used for any procedure it is essential that protocols and procedures for safe use are in place.

Later in the 1980s, electrodiathermy using wire-loop resection and "rollerball" coagulation techniques were described. These later methods use simple and cheaper electrosurgical equipment.[60]

All three of the above methods use a hysteroscope in conjunction with fluid infused into the uterine cavity under pressure to provide the operator with a clear view. Endometrial ablation by laser and rollerball is significantly better than wire-loop resection with less risk of immediate haemorrhage and uterine perforation.[60]

Radiofrequency endometrial ablation was reported in 1990. This is a non-hysteroscopic treatment. A radiofrequency source is connected to an intrauterine probe. The radiofrequency energy, delivered at a frequency of 27 Hz, induces a rapid oscillation of charged particles in the tissues directly around the probe, heating the endometrial surface to approximately 60°C. A belt electrode around the patient's waist ensures a closed circuit by way of a return cable to the radiofrequency source. Each treatment takes about 20 minutes but does not require distending fluids, thereby avoiding the complications associated with their use (see below).[61]

Radiofrequency equipment is expensive and special training is required. A strict safety protocol must be followed. Particular care must be taken to prevent radiofrequency burns by careful placement of electrocardiography electrodes and avoiding patient–metal contact. Radiofrequency-induced heating of the pulse oximeter probe is avoided by a common mode choke. This consists of a ferrite ring core through which the pulse oximeter cable is wound several times.[61] Similarly, metal-containing airway equipment should not be used because of the risk of burns. Other complications include superficial skin burns, finger burns from non-approved pulse oximeters, vesicovaginal fistulae, thermal injury of the bowel, and thermal damage to the cervix and anterior fornix. General anaesthesia, epidural, and spinal anaesthesia have all been used with this technique. Same-day surgery is appropriate but severe uterine cramps may occur for approximately six hours following treatment and strong oral analgesics should be provided for discharge.

Further studies are underway using other techniques which avoid the problems of fluid absorption. One such endometrial ablation system uses a balloon catheter which conforms to the shape of the endometrial cavity. The catheter is linked to a thermistor to maintain the saline in the balloon at up to 92°C.

Distending medium

Distension of the uterine cavity under pressure is necessary for procedures under direct vision. The medium should provide optical clarity and where electrodiathermy is utilised, it must be non-conductive. Disadvantages of uterine liquid distension include the potential need for a greater cervical diameter to allow for circulation of fluid within the cavity, plus the inconvenience of external leakage. Various distending media have been used including carbon dioxide, dextrose 5%, 32% dextran 70 in dextrose 5%, saline, glycine 1.5%, sorbitol 5%, and mannitol 5%.

Carbon dioxide was the first medium used to distend the uterus. Air, nitrous oxide (N_2O), and oxygen (O_2) have all been used but they are all unsuitable.[59] Carbon dioxide has the same refractive index as air and provides optimal clarity. Successful use depends on a secure seal between the hysteroscope and the cervix. A constant-volume, variable-pressure gas source should be used to achieve optimal distension of the uterine cavity and prevent carbon dioxide embolism with a maximal gas flow of 100 ml/min and an intrauterine pressure less than 13.3 kPa. Carbon dioxide cannot be used with operative hysteroscopy as it could pass into the circulation via open vessels, leading to a carbon dioxide gas embolus (see below).

Dextrose 5% is not suitable, as hyperglycaemia and dilutional hyponatraemia are potential problems. Dextran 70 in dextrose 5% is electrolyte free, non-conductive, and optically clear with a high refractive index and provides excellent visualisation. Adverse reactions include volume overload, pulmonary oedema, coagulopathy, and dextran-induced anaphylactoid/anaphylactic reaction (incidence one in 10 000).

More recently normal saline has been used for diagnostic hysteroscopy. It avoids the problems of gas embolus and hyponatraemia. There is evidence that compared, to carbon dioxide in outpatient hysteroscopy, it has comparable visualisation, with reduced procedure time and patient discomfort.

Electrodiathermy requires the use of solutions which do not conduct electricity. Glycine 1.5%, sorbitol 5%, mannitol 5%, and dextran 70 32% are all potentially suitable. However, sorbitol 5% is isotonic with a short half-life of 35 minutes. It is seldom used as it causes toffee-like deposits on the electrode, making resection technically difficult. Mannitol 5% is isotonic and has a long half-life but it is rarely used because it may cause visual distortion and crystallisation on instruments.[62]

Glycine

As with transurethral resection of the prostate (TURP), glycine 1.5% is the most commonly used solution for operative hysteroscopy. Glycine is an amino acid which is rapidly distributed throughout the extracellular space, with an intravascular half-life of 85 minutes. About 10% is excreted in the urine, leading to a brisk diuresis. Oxidative deamination occurs in the liver resulting in ammonia, oxalate, proline, aminobutyrate and alanine.[59]

Excessive amounts of irrigation fluid may be absorbed during surgery through blood vessels opened up by resection and later from the fluid which can enter the peritoneal cavity via patent Fallopian tubes during the procedure. This can result in a clinical condition similar to the TURP syndrome, where hypotonic irrigation fluid is absorbed from the exposed prostatic bed.[63] The amount of fluid absorbed depends on the infusion pressure of the irrigation fluid, vascularity of the uterus, the number and size of uterine venous sinuses opened, duration of the surgery, and surgical technique.[59,63] Absorption through endometrial veins may occur more readily than during a TURP as it is easier to generate higher pressures in the less compliant uterus.

Although images of the uterine cavity are possible at 5.3 kPa, the pressure must be increased to 13.3–14.7 kPa to identify the tubal orifices. It is usually performed during the midproliferative phase when the endometrium is relatively avascular or following pretreatment with danazol, progesterone or GnRH analogues which makes the endometrium atrophic.

The absorption of large amounts of electrolyte-free irrigation solution is potentially dangerous as it may result in increased intravascular volume, haemodilution, and hyponatraemia.[59,62] These may then lead to the development of left heart failure, pulmonary oedema, and cerebral oedema.

Hyponatraemia may develop rapidly and can produce:[64]

1 headaches
2 nausea and vomiting
3 weakness
4 confusion and restlessness
5 hallucinations
6 faecal and urinary incontinence
7 hypoventilation
8 manifestations of increased intracranial pressure such as:
   • seizures
   • coma

- bradycardia
- dilated pupils
- respiratory arrest

9 electrocardiographic changes:
  - widening of the QRS complex
  - loss of the P wave
  - bradycardia and T wave inversion
  - ventricular tachycardia and standstill

Treatment is usually with 0.9% saline although in more severe cases hypertonic sodium chloride is required. The aim is to increase the serum sodium concentration to above 130 mmol/l but limiting the size of the correction to no more than 25 mmol/l during the initial 24–48 hours. The required correction of the serum sodium (in mmol/l) should be the same as the number of hours over which the serum sodium is corrected. Frusemide and intubation may be necessary, especially if there is evidence of respiratory compromise. These patients should be managed in an intensive care unit. Formulae have been described to act as a guide in the management of the electrolyte disturbance.[64]

Formula 1
$$N1 = [130 - \text{serum sodium}] \times TBW$$

where   N1 = correction of sodium deficit in mmol
        TBW = total body water in litres (equal to half body weight in kg)

Formula 2
$$N2 = N1 \times 1000 \times 1/514$$

where   N2 = volume in ml of hypertonic sodium chloride (514 mmol/l)

Formula 3
$$N3 = N2 \times 1/T$$

where   N3 = infusion rate in ml/h of hypertonic sodium chloride
        T = number of hours to correct serum sodium deficit

Limiting operating time to one hour or less has been recommended to minimise the development of TURP syndrome. However, the syndrome can occur much earlier. McSwiney *et al.* studied plasma sodium levels in 21 patients undergoing endometrial ablation using the diathermy resection.[63] The mean duration of the procedure was 26.4 min (range 15–35, SD 5.3). In five patients the decrease in plasma sodium was greater than 10 mmol/l. The greatest rate of decrease occurred in the first 15 minutes. The decrease in sodium concentration correlated with the irrigation deficit. Consequently, it is important to monitor irrigation deficit continuously to provide an early warning of excessive absorption. It is recommended that surgery be stopped as soon as possible when the deficit is 1000–2000 ml and immediately when the deficit exceeds 2000 ml. Ananthanarayan *et al.* recommended checking plasma sodium concentration once a deficit of 500 ml was noted and the administration of frusemide 20 mg IV if a deficit of 1000 ml occurred.[59] Endometrial rollerball coagulation carries the least risk of the various methods as there is no cutting of blood vessels or tissue and therefore less fluid absorption and haemorrhage.

A method of monitoring irrigation fluid absorption using ethanol has been described. The irrigation fluid was tagged with ethanol and expired breath ethanol measured using an alcohol analyser. Nomograms have been developed for transurethral prostatic resections relating ethanol concentrations in expired gas to the volumes of irrigant fluid absorbed and the serum sodium concentration but a nomogram has not been developed for use with endometrial ablation.[62]

There have been reports of gas embolism with loop diathermy and Nd-YAG laser ablation. The Nd-YAG laser requires the use of carbon dioxide gas flowing between the outer sheath and the inner fibre as a coolant. If this system is used care must be taken to ensure that the outer sheath does not inadvertently extend close to the laser tip and into the hysteroscope, conducting carbon dioxide into the uterine cavity and resulting in carbon dioxide embolism. Other problems have been attributed to the use of glycine, including nausea and transient blindness secondary to ammonia toxicity.

Laparoscopic surgery

Before the mid–1980s, the laparoscope was predominantly used for diagnostic and sterilisation procedures. Since then, more complex procedures have been undertaken. There are a number of potential problems with the procedure related to the surgical technique and patient position, including:

1 trauma from the introduction of trocars and other instruments into the peritoneal cavity;
2 gas insufflation;
3 effects of tension pneumoperitoneum;
4 hypercarbia;
5 patient positioning;
6 miscellaneous problems.

Trauma from instruments introduced into the peritoneal cavity

Accidental injuries of intra-abdominal structures such as bowel, stomach, liver, uterus, and the liver have been reported. Major haemorrhage can occur if large vessels such as the aorta, iliac vessels or epigastric artery are injured.

Gas insufflation

Carbon dioxide is the insufflation gas of choice as it does not support combustion, is highly soluble in blood and tissues, decreasing the risk of gas embolism, and is inexpensive. Nitrous oxide is still used in some centres but is combustible. Arrhythmias such as AV dissociation, nodal rhythm, sinus bradycardia, and asystole probably result from a vagally mediated reflex initiated by stretching of the peritoneum. Management of significant bradycardia consists of communication with the surgeon to release the intra-abdominal pressure, the administration of atropine, and waiting for a response before reinflating. Subcutaneous emphysema, pneumomediastinum, pneumopericardium, and pneumothorax most commonly occur because of a misplaced Verres needle but also through existing defects in the diaphragm or along surgically traumatised tissue planes.[65]

Venous gas embolism is a rare complication of laparoscopy. It can occur at any time during a laparoscopy. During the initial phase of the procedure there may be inadvertent puncture of intra-abdominal vessels or direct transuterine gas injection. Subsequently it may result from the presence of an open venous channel where there is a pressure gradient between the abdominal cavity and the venous system. The clinical manifestations are determined by the volume and the rate of entry into the venous circulation. Small volumes may pass through the heart, causing pulmonary hypertension and right heart failure. Larger volumes cause a "gas lock" in the right atrium, obstructing the pulmonary outflow tract, decreasing left atrial filling pressure, and causing a fall in cardiac output.

In the AIMS analysis of the first 2000 incidents, capnography was the most successful first detector of an air embolus with a sudden decrease in carbon dioxide. Tachycardia, ST depression, oxygen desaturation, decreased/loss of cardiac output, and a "mill-wheel" murmur on chest auscultation are other clinical manifestations. Should this occur the following management is advised.

1 Cessation of gas insufflation and release of the pneumoperitoneum.
2 Head down tilt.
3 Manual ventilation with 100% oxygen.
4 Support of the circulation with adrenaline, intravenous fluids and, if required, external cardiac massage.
5 Aspiration of gas from the right heart via a central venous catheter.
6 If available, early hyperbaric oxygen treatment should be considered to prevent the endothelial sequelae to cerebral arterial gas embolus.[66]

Effects of tension pneumoperitoneum

The changes to the cardiovascular system during laparoscopic surgery are complex and are influenced by the cardiopulmonary status of the patient, the surgical position, the intra-abdominal pressure, the length of surgery, the carbon dioxide absorption, the ventilatory technique, and the anaesthetic agents used.[67] These changes were originally described by Kelman et al. using central venous lines and injection of indocyanine green dye for cardiac output measurement.[68] They found that the heart rate, mean arterial pressure, effective cardiac filling pressure (central venous pressure – intrathoracic pressure), and cardiac output all increased as the intra-abdominal pressure increased by 2 kPa. However, as the intra-abdominal pressure increased to around 4 kPa these parameters all fell in association with a fall in blood pressure and tachycardia. It was considered that the increase in intra-abdominal pressure decreases venous return from the legs. Other studies have found an increase in systemic vascular resistance resulting from increased venous resistance, compression of the aorta, and humoral effects such as increased catecholamines, antidiuretic hormone, and renin-angiotensin activity. These changes may be even more pronounced in the elderly.

Airway pressure increases and compliance decreases during laparoscopic surgery. Hirvonen et al. found that during laparoscopic hysterectomy the head down position decreased compliance by 20% and that this fell by a further 30% as intra-abdominal pressure increased.[69] Diaphragmatic movements are reduced. Consequently, the work of breathing is increased in a spontaneously breathing patient. Venous oxygen admixture may increase due to the pneumoperitoneum-induced reduction in functional residual capacity. However, the increased airway pressure adds a degree of intrinsic positive end-expiratory pressure, reversing this trend.

Renal blood flow and glomerular filtration rate can be depressed, especially with intra-abdominal pressures above 2.7 kPa due to the resultant increase in renal vascular resistance and decrease in cardiac output. Antidiuretic hormone (ADH) has been reported to increase with rises in intra-abdominal, intrathoracic and transmural right atrial pressure. ADH is a potent vasoconstrictor and may also act on the heart to decrease cardiac output and heart rate.

Hypercarbia

Hypercarbia occurs as a result of peritoneal absorption of CO_2, plus the adverse ventilatory effects of the tension pneumoperitoneum and surgical position causing an increase in alveolar dead space. The amount of CO_2 absorbed is determined by the intra-abdominal pressure and the duration of the pneumoperitoneum. Haemodynamic changes from hypercarbia occur via its direct cardiovascular effects and its indirect effects via sympatho-adrenal stimulation. These include tachycardia, arrhythmias, high cardiac output, and low systemic vascular resistance. Increased myocardial oxygen consumption can cause ischaemia. Monitoring of end-tidal CO_2, tidal volumes, and airway pressures is essential when adjusting ventilation to maximise cardiorespiratory performance.

329

Patient positioning (see p 317)

Miscellaneous problems

There are numerous other factors which may complicate these procedures. Crowding of the theatre with additional surgical equipment is hazardous. The placement of video monitors may interfere with access to the patient and anaesthetic equipment. The surgeon may request that the theatre lights be dimmed. In these circumstances it is imperative that the anaesthetist has adequate visualisation of the patient. Laser and electrocautery may cause electrical and equipment hazards and hypothermia may occur due to insufflation of dry room temperature gas.

Most of the documented information on the surgical complication rate is limited to case histories and retrospective case series. Consequently, the incidence of complications may be underestimated. A prospective nationwide multicentre study of gynaecological laparoscopies in The Netherlands was published in 1994.[47] Of the 25 764 procedures, there were 145 complications (rate 5.7 per 1000) and two deaths. Both of these were ultimately from multiorgan failure, with the precipitants being major haemorrhage from epigastric vein trauma in one case and following an unrecognised gastrointestinal injury in the other. In 68 cases the complication was caused by insertion of the trocar. Haemorrhage of the epigastric vein and intestinal injury were the most common complications with 76 laparotomies being performed because of bowel injury.

Oncology surgery

Patients with gynaecological malignancies may present the anaesthetist with a range of complex issues. There are problems related to the malignancy and the patient may be elderly with concomitant medical conditions. However, there are exceptions to this as trophoblastic disease occurs in the reproductive years and cervical carcinoma has an incidence which rises rapidly in the 25–40-year age group, reaches a plateau, and declines in the sixth and seventh decades of life.[70]

The optimal surgical approach to malignancy is resection of the tumour with wide surgical margins. In 70% of patients with ovarian tumours this is not attainable because of early metastases. However, several studies have shown increased survival in some patients following cytoreductive or debulking surgery.

Ovarian carcinoma

Ovarian carcinoma causes more deaths than any other gynaecological tumour. It may present late and provides the greatest number of problems for the anaesthetist. The problems include the following.

Intraperitoneal spread

Extensive involvement of serosal surfaces can cause segmental paralytic ileus and ascites.[70] Bowel involvement and ascites increase the risk of regurgitation at induction. The increased intra-abdominal pressure associated with ascites impedes movement of the diaphragm in inspiration, decreases functional residual capacity, and increases the work of breathing. Drainage of ascites preoperatively to relieve symptoms, or at the time of surgery, can lead to hypovolaemia and hypoalbuminaemia as ascitic fluid continues to be formed. Ascites also decreases renal perfusion (see below).

Liver metastases and pleural effusions

These occur in stage IV disease. Preoperative drainage of a pleural effusion is required if symptomatic or large. Thoracocentesis improves lung expansion and enhances ventilation but rapid drainage of a large effusion has on occasion caused acute pulmonary oedema. Patients with large unilateral pleural effusions should not be placed on their side as the sudden shift of fluid may distort the mediastinum and impede venous return and ventilation.[71]

Poor nutritional status

This arises because of the hypercatabolic nature of the disease, intraperitoneal spread, and liver metastases. Anaemia may require correction preoperatively, depending upon its level, speed of onset, and the patient's age and symptoms. A central venous line for total parenteral nutrition may be needed preoperatively and may be useful for pressure monitoring to assist in fluid management.

Chemotherapeutic effects

Drug therapy may cause myelosuppression. Renal toxicity is associated with cis-platinum, which is often used in ovarian and cervical carcinoma. Bleomycin, which may be used to treat ovarian carcinoma, may result in pulmonary toxicity in the form of interstitial fibrosis. This is dose related, increasing significantly when the total dose exceeds 450 mg, although idiosyncratic reactions have occurred at lower doses. The pulmonary toxicity may be increased by hyperoxia, advanced age, especially greater than 70 years, smoking, previous chest irradiation, additional chemotherapeutic agents, especially cyclophosphamide, and overhydration. Baseline arterial blood gas analysis and chest X-ray are recommended in patients who have received bleomycin. Pulmonary function tests may be helpful in determining the extent of damage in known pulmonary fibrosis but are not predictive of subclinical disease. Where the patient has received bleomycin, a target PaO_2 should be chosen and serial arterial blood gas analysis performed with the FiO_2 at the lowest level required to maintain the target PaO_2.[72]

331

Cardiotoxicity is associated with adriamycin. Adriamycin therapy is usually followed with careful monitoring of left ventricular function monitoring by means of ejection fraction studies. Symptoms of cardiac decompensation should be sought and recent cardiac investigations reviewed.

Renal dysfunction

This can result from ascites, hyperosmotic radiocontrast media used in preoperative staging investigations, and cis-platinum. Patients may receive an osmotic cathartic agent to prepare the bowel, causing preoperative dehydration. Attention to hydration and electrolyte balance is therefore important in perioperative care to prevent compromise of renal function. Patients should have a urinary catheter, hourly urine measurement, and consideration of central venous pressure monitoring.

Complicated surgery

Procedures often require prolonged surgical times and extensive pelvic dissection. The patient's temperature should be monitored, intravenous fluids warmed and a convection warming blanket applied to the upper body, head, and arms to prevent hypothermia. Blood transfusion is often required perioperatively and crossmatched blood should be available.

Postoperative analgesia

This may be provided either epidurally, with opioid boluses or an infusion of a mixture of an opioid and a weak local anaesthetic mixture, or via a patient-controlled pump delivering intravenous opioid. As midline incisions are usually necessary, lumbar epidurals are not as effective as mid to lower thoracic epidurals when mixtures of low-dose local anaesthetic and opioid are used for postoperative epidural analgesia.

Thromboembolism (see below)

Operative laparoscopy is used increasingly in some centres. Laparoscopic transperitoneal lymphadenopathy was first reported in 1991 for staging. It has also revived radical vaginal hysterectomy for patients with early cervical cancer. McConnell et al. reported the development of a tension hydrothorax during a laparoscopy for drainage of ascites and placement of an intraperitoneal Infuse-a-Port in a woman with ovarian carcinoma.[73] Following drainage of some of the ascites and establishment of the pneumoperitoneum, the patient developed a tension hydrothorax which resolved once an emergency chest drain was inserted and 1.5 litres of pleural fluid drained under pressure. The authors considered that the acute increase in intraperitoneal pressure during the pneumoperitoneum caused the mass movement of fluid across the diaphragm, presumably through a small defect, and into the pleural space. Anaesthetists should recognise tension hydrothorax as a potential complication of laparoscopy in the presence of ascites.

Hydatidiform moles

These present other problems. They are usually detected between eight and 24 weeks gestation with a peak around 14 weeks and present with vaginal bleeding which may lead to anaemia. The problems include:[74]

1 life-threatening haemorrhage, especially at the time of suction curettage;
2 pre-eclampsia;
3 hyperemesis;
4 hyperthyroidism. High human chorionic gonadotropin (HCG) levels are thyrotropic in bioassays and may cause a biochemical increased thyroid function. Clinical thyrotoxicosis is uncommon;
5 progression to choriocarcinoma which can metastasise to almost any part of the body. The lungs are the commonest site.

Other rare potential complications include uterine perforation, pelvic sepsis, disseminated intravascular coagulopathy, and trophoblastic pulmonary embolisation.

Because of the association with hyperemesis, increased fundal height, and risk of perioperative bleeding, securing the airway with an endotracheal tube is advisable for evacuation of a hydatidiform mole. An oxytocic infusion should be commenced and ergometrine may be required if bleeding is severe. Hysterectomy at that time should be avoided because of the intense vascularity and risk of uncontrollable haemorrhage.[74]

Infertility

Infertility affects at least one in six couples. The first *in vitro* fertilisation (IVF) baby was born in 1978 as a result of an oocyte collected during a natural cycle. Pharmacological stimulation of ovaries to produce numerous oocytes greatly enhances the success rate as ovulatory failure is responsible for 21% of infertility.[75]

Various regimens are used to stimulate ovulation. The simplest uses cyclical oral antioestrogens such as clomiphene. Acylofenil or tamoxifen may also be used. The more complicated approaches use injectable gonadotrophins such as follicle-stimulating hormone (FSH) and a combination of FSH and luteinising hormone (LH) to stimulate ovarian development. Once the follicle has reached a certain size, HCG is given to stimulate the LH surge and stimulate the final maturation and induce ovulation.[75]

There are several methods of gamete and embryo transfer.

1 In IVF, fertilisation takes place outside the body and the embryos are transferred through the cervix into the uterus where transplantation may occur. Surplus frozen embryos can be preserved for future use.

2 In gamete intrafallopian tube transfer (GIFT), oocytes and spermatozoa are laparoscopically inserted into the end of the fallopian tube.

3 In zygote intrafallopian tube (ZIFT), fertilisation occurs outside the body and the embryos are inserted laparoscopically into the end of the fallopian tube. The embryo then travels down the tube to implant within the uterus.

Requirements for anaesthesia with these procedures depend on the specific technique. Transvaginal ultrasound-guided oocyte retrieval is as effective as laparoscopy in terms of conception rates. It is simpler, less expensive and does not require general anaesthesia. It is most commonly used with sedation. Paracervical block has been found to produce less pain for vaginal puncture but not for the remainder of the oocyte retrieval process when compared with a placebo injection. Alfentanil has been compared with patient-controlled sedation with either midazolam (22 patients) or propofol (25 patients) in conjunction with infiltration of the vaginal vault with 20 ml 1% lignocaine. Oversedation occurred in only one patient in the midazolam group. All patients were dressed and ready to leave within one hour. Alsalili *et al.* studied the effect of propofol on *in vitro* oocyte maturation and cleavage in mice. The fertilisation and embryo cleavage rates were not significantly different when compared with controls.[76]

GIFT and ZIFT procedures require general anaesthesia because manipulation of the fallopian tubes is generally too uncomfortable under sedation.[75] The use of propofol in any of these reproductive procedures is acceptable.

Ovarian hyperstimulation syndrome

There are a number of potentially serious problems associated with induction of ovulation including:

1 an increased incidence of multiple births;
2 an increased miscarriage rate;
3 adnexal torsion;
4 ectopic pregnancy;
5 the possibility of ovarian hyperstimulation syndrome (OHSS).

OHSS is of interest to anaesthetists as the severe form is potentially life threatening and requires intensive care admission. There is wide variation in its reported incidence. The United States *in vitro* Fertilization Registry in 1990 reported that 0.2–0.3% of 25 744 stimulation cycles in 180 IVF centres were complicated by OHSS requiring hospitalisation.[77] It is more common in those with polycystic ovarian syndrome, younger patients, and in cycles where conception is successful.

The pathophysiology of OHSS is not entirely clear. It appears that HCG stimulation of the ovaries causes the release of vasoactive substances leading to increased capillary permeability. Increased prostaglandin synthesis, cytokines including the interleukins, tumour necrosis factor-α, endothelin-1 and vascular endothelial growth factor, and factors belonging to the renin-angiotensin system are thought to be involved.[78]

Presentation is usually 3–8 days after the administration of HCG. Features then persist throughout the luteal phase and start to resolve as menstruation approaches.[75] It is characterised by marked ovarian enlargement, due to multiple ovarian cysts, and increased capillary permeability leading to fluid shifting out of the intravascular space and into serous spaces. This may cause ascites, pleural and pericardial effusions. OHSS may also produce depletion of the intravascular space leading to hypovolaemic shock and multiple organ failure. Thromboembolism and cerebrovascular accident may also occur.

In its mildest form the condition is often self-limiting. More severe forms require intravenous fluids to restore blood volume, increase renal perfusion, and prevent venous thrombosis. The most severe presentations require intensive care admission.[75,78] There may be a need for invasive monitoring and extensive supportive management, including drainage of effusions. Consideration should also be given to prophylactic compression stockings and heparin therapy. There is haemoconcentration and haemostatic activation, as evidenced by a shortened activated partial thromboplastin time.

Oral contraceptive pill and surgery

The combined oral contraceptive pill (OCP) has in many studies been associated with a small increase in thromboembolic events. Since its introduction in the 1960s modifications have occurred in attempt to decrease risk. In the 1970s second-generation drugs, containing a lower dose of ethinyloestradiol, were introduced and more recently, third-generation drugs that contain gonane progesterones (desogetrel, gestodone, and norgestimate). A recent study showed a fourfold increase in the relative risk of spontaneous deep vein thrombosis (DVT) in women taking the OCP and that the rate was 1.5 times higher for third-generation when compared with second-generation OCPs. Changes in the haemostatic system are responsible for this small increase. Increased levels of factor VII and X activity, dependent upon the dose of oestrogen and the type of progesterone, occur with most of the combined OCP preparations. Platelet responsiveness also appears to be increased, possibly due to an increased platelet production of thromboxane A_2. However, fibrinolysis is increased, most likely due to increased plasminogen and decreased plasminogen activator inhibitor-I. The progesterone-only preparations, however, are not associated with an increased thromboembolic risk.[79]

Several studies in the 1970s and early 1980s suggested an increased risk of thromboembolic events after surgery in women taking the combined

OCP. Many of these postoperative studies were carried out when the high-dose oestrogen pills were in use. They often relied upon clinical diagnosis of DVT, which is unreliable, and lacked analysis or information of inter-dependent variables. The Oxford Family Planning Association Study analysed the data on 34 cases of postoperative thromboembolism. They found an incidence of 0.96% (12/1244) in those using oral contraceptives during the month before surgery which was twice as high as in the group not doing so (22/4359), but this was not significant.[80] This is considerably lower than the 25% incidence detected by iodine–125 fibrinogen scans in patients undergoing general surgical operations.

An editorial in the *BMJ* in 1985 and subsequent advice in the *British National Formulary* recommended stopping the pill four weeks before surgery.[81] However, this advice exposed women to the risk of unwanted pregnancy, the effects of the surgery and anaesthesia on the pregnancy and possibly a subsequent termination of pregnancy with its associated physical and psychological risks. The RCOG Working Party on Prophylaxis Against Thromboembolism in Gynaecology and Obstetrics and the Thromboembolic Risk Factors (THRIFT) Consensus Group both concluded that there was insufficient evidence to support a policy of routinely stopping the combined OCP before major surgery and that additional risk factors and contraceptive difficulties should be considered before surgery. They also concluded that there was insufficient evidence to support routine heparin prophylaxis in these women without additional risk factors. If other risk factors are present then thromboprophylaxis may be warranted. The risk of a thromboembolic event is greatly increased with emergency surgery and thromboprophylaxis should be employed in such women taking the combined OCP.[79,82]

Thromboprophylaxis

Deep vein thrombosis (DVT) and pulmonary thromboembolism (PTE) are serious complications of gynaecological surgery. PTE is a major cause of death in hospital patients in the developed world. In the United Kingdom, the 1994–95 Report of the National Confidential Enquiry into Perioperative Deaths found that PTE was responsible for 19% of the deaths following gynaecological surgery.[83] DVT also causes long-term morbidity as chronic venous insufficiency may develop.

Relying upon clinical history and physical examination clearly underestimates the incidence of DVT. Less than 20% of patients with proven PTE have clinical features compatible with venous thrombosis in the legs. Most studies on the incidence of postoperative DVTs have used objective techniques such as radiolabelled fibrinogen or venograms. Different procedures have a greater risk. Following meta-analysis of English-language controlled trials, Clagett *et al.* found that without antithrombotic measures, 24–26%

of patients developed venous thrombosis after major general surgery and 47–55% after total hip replacement.[84] The incidence from North American trials following major general surgery was about half that of European trials. The incidence of DVT following gynaecological surgery appears comparable with that associated with general abdominal surgery. Clarke-Pearson *et al.*, studying major gynaecological surgical patients with radiolabelled iodine, found a rate of 6% in those with benign conditions and 18% with malignant tumour and 39% with recurrent tumour.[85] Using meta-analysis of four earlier studies from the 1970s, the incidence of DVTs following major gynaecological surgery for benign disease was 14%.[86]

Macklon and Greer reviewed 745 999 "new" inpatient episodes in gynaecology in Scotland.[87] There were 574 recorded admissions with venous thromboembolism (VTE), an incidence of 0.076%, of which 45% were PTE, a surprisingly low rate. All gynaecological inpatient episodes, however, were included, the vast majority of which were likely to have been young fit women having relatively minor procedures. DVTs may have gone unrecognised and patients may have been readmitted to other services. Some of these patients would have also received thromboprophylaxis.

The risk of VTE depends upon not only the surgical procedure but also patient factors, such as increasing age, obesity, concurrent illness, previous DVTs, and thrombophilia. Table 9.1, which is a modification of previous tables,[79,82] classifies these risks for gynaecological patients into low, moderate and high according to the risk of proximal venous thrombosis and fatal pulmonary embolus. This can be used to establish a protocol for thromboprophylaxis as recommended by the Thromboembolic Risk Factors (THRIFT) Consensus Group.

Mechanical methods of thromboprophylaxis

Mechanical methods have the advantage that they are not associated with any haemorrhagic risk. Graduated elastic stockings exert a pressure gradient which is maximal at the ankle and decreases up the leg. It is thought that they act by preventing passive venous dilation which occurs during surgery, decreasing endothelial damage and exposure of the prothrombotic subendothelial collagen.[87] They reduce the incidence of DVTs (Table 9.2) but studies have been too small to assess their effect on PTE.[86] They can also be combined with other techniques such as low-dose or low molecular weight heparin for high-risk patients. They have the disadvantage that in some patients, large thigh diameter may render them hazardous, as they act as a tourniquet at the knee or midthigh, increasing the risk. They should be worn until the patient is fully mobile. This is usually greater than four days but some patients find them uncomfortable and are non-compliant. Patient education preoperatively, preferably in a preadmission or gynaecological clinic, is important in minimising this problem.

Table 9.1   Risk assessment for thromboprophylaxis in gynaecology

Low risk	(*Proximal vein thrombosis 0.4%, fatal PTE <0.2%*) • Major surgery (<30 minutes), age <40 years • Minor surgery (>30 minutes), no other risk factor (other than age)
Management	**Early mobilisation and hydration**
Medium risk	(*Proximal vein thrombosis 2–4%, fatal PTE 0.2%*) • Major gynaecological surgery and >40 years or one other risk factor • Minor surgery with previous DVT, PTE or thrombophilia • Extended laparoscopic surgery • Major acute medical illness such as myocardial infarction, heart failure, chest infection, cancer or inflammatory bowel disease • Gross varicose veins • Obesity
Management	1. **Early mobilisation and hydration** 2. **Low molecular weight heparin, e.g. enoxaparin 20 mg daily (or unfractionated heparin 5000 units b.d.)** 3. **If heparin contraindicated, compression elastic stockings and intermittent pneumatic leg compression**

High risk	(*Proximal vein thrombosis 10–20%, fatal PTE 1–5%*)
	• Three or more moderate risk factors
	• Major pelvic or abdominal surgery for gynaecological surgery
	• Major surgery (>30 minutes) in patients with:
	  • previous DVT, PTE or thrombophilia
	  • paralysis or immobilisation of the lower limbs

Management	1. **Early mobilisation and hydration** 2. **Low molecular weight heparin, e.g. enoxaparin 20 mg daily (or unfractionated heparin 5000 units b.d.)** 3. **Graduated compression elastic stockings or intermittent pneumatic leg compression**

Modified from Thromboprophylaxis Risk Factor Consensus Group (1992) and RCOG Working Party on Thromboprophylaxis in Obstetrics and Gynaecology (1995)

Table 9.2   Effectiveness of graduated elastic stockings, intermittent pneumatic compression, low-dose subcutaneous heparin and aspirin in the prevention of DVTs in non-orthopaedic randomised controlled trials (fibrinogen uptake or phlephography)

	Control groups		Treatment groups			
	No. of patients	DVT (%)	No. of patients	DVT (%)	Relative risk	95% CI
Graduated compression stockings	457	118 (26)	473	51 (11)	0.41	0.31–0.50
Intermittent pneumatic compression	855	211 (25)	799	61 (7.7)	0.32	0.24–0.42
Low-dose subcutaneous heparin	3339	864 (26)	3512	302 (8.6)	0.33	0.29–0.37
Aspirin	1459	1459 (27)	1434	278 (19)	0.77	0.62–0.82

Intermittent pneumatic compression (IPC) is also effective in the reduction of DVTs (Table 9.2) but it is unknown whether it significantly reduces the incidence of PTE.[86] As it is understood that DVTs begin to develop intraoperatively and in the first 48 hours, it would appear that this time period should be the minimal time for IPC use. In most of the studies into the effectiveness of IPC, their use is continued well into the postoperative period, usually for 4–5 days. Clarke-Pearson *et al.* demonstrated that in patients with gynaecological malignancies intermittent compression of the calf used intraoperatively and for 24 hours postoperatively did not prevent DVTs. The same group then compared low-dose heparin (5000 units eight-hourly) for at least seven days with IPC of the calf for at least five days. Both regimens showed a similar reduction in DVTs.[88] There are insufficient data to critically assess their efficacy when used only intraoperatively.

Pharmacological methods of thromboprophylaxis

Low-dose subcutaneous heparin is perhaps the most widely studied means of prophylaxis. It enhances antithrombin III (ATIII) activity and effectively neutralises a number of activated coagulation factors – IX, X, XI, XII, and II (thrombin). It is usually prescribed as 5000 units eight- or 12-hourly. No laboratory monitoring is required unless heparin is used for greater than five days when a platelet count should be performed to detect heparin-induced thrombocytopenia. It prevents about 66% of both DVTs (Table 9.2) and PTE. There is an associated risk of bruising at injection sites and a risk of wound haematoma, particularly with Pfannenstiel incisions. This can be minimised by avoiding injection close to the wound and choosing a lateral injection site well above the iliac crest. A site on the lateral aspect of the upper thigh is an alternative.[87] Contraindications include uncorrected bleeding problems, haemorrhagic traits (for example, von Willebrand's disease), impaired hepatic or renal function, hypersensitivity to heparin or heparin-induced thrombocytopenia. This occurs with an incidence of less than 0.5%.

Unfractionated heparin has a molecular weight of 12 000–14 000. A variety of low molecular weight heparins (LMWHs) are now in clinical practice with a molecular weight of 4000–5000. Bleeding complications are less likely as the shorter polysaccharide chain of LMWHs is only able to bind to ATIII, which results in inhibition of factor Xa, but not to thrombin. Consequently, it has very little anticoagulant activity (anti-IIa) but good antithrombotic activity, whereas unfractionated heparin has equal levels of activity. The various LMWHs have different molecular weight distribution profiles, specific activities (anti-Xa to anti-IIa activities), and rates of plasma clearance. They should not be interchanged without due consideration. LMWHs are well absorbed after subcutaneous injection and have a bioavailability of 85% compared to 10% with unfractionated heparin, partly because of their lower binding to plasma matrix proteins. LMWHs do not bind to endothelial cells and their clearance is dose dependent. The half-life following a subcutaneous injection is 3–4 hours, 2–4 times that of unfractionated heparin. The dose-response relationship is more predictable. Approximately 50% of peak anti-Xa activity is present 12 hours after injection. It does not prolong the activated partial thromboplastin time and a specific anti-factor Xa assay is used if measurement of the antithrombotic effect is required. The usual prophylactic dose of enoxaparin is 20 mg daily. This may be increased in patients at high risk. The meta-analysis of studies comparing LMWHs with unfractionated heparin indicated that LMWHs were at least as effective and possibly more so.[86]

LMWHs have the advantage of once-daily dosage, with greater patient acceptance, less effect on platelets, and possibly greater efficacy. Their use requires less nursing time, there is less risk of osteoporosis with long-term use and reduced bleeding is expected. They are, however, more expensive.

Spinal and epidural anaesthesia may reduce the incidence of VTEs.[84] It is believed that this may be due to peripheral vasodilation, reduced activation of clotting factors or decreased platelet adhesion, aggregation and release. All the studies have been done on orthopaedic patients undergoing hip surgery and the numbers of patients have been relatively small.

Every hospital anaesthetic department should develop a protocol for the management of thromboprophylaxis when spinal and epidural blocks are performed. In December 1997, the United States FDA Public Health Advisory issued a warning on the concurrent use of LMWH and spinal/epidural anaesthesia or spinal puncture following 30 reports of patients developing epidural or spinal haematomas in such circumstances. As of April 1998, there had been over 50 cases reported to the FDA. Approximately 75% of these patients were women. The median age was about 75 years and the majority were undergoing orthopaedic surgery. At that time in the USA, most LMWH prophylactic regimes for hip or knee replacement used enoxaparin 30 mg twice daily or dalteparin 5000 U daily, large doses in this elderly population. Concurrent use of NSAIDs and the continued use of an indwelling epidural catheter postoperatively were also implicated as increasing the risk. The FDA has stressed the need when performing spinals and epidurals in patients on LMWH or heparinoids to consider the timing of anticoagulation administration. Horlocker et al., in a review of LMWH prophylaxis and regional anaesthesia, recommended waiting 10–12 hours following a dose of LMWH and waiting at least two hours after needle placement for further administration.[90] They also recommended removing the epidural the following day, a conservative approach. Postoperatively, either mixtures of low-dose local anaesthetic/opioid or opioid alone should be used so that neurological assessment can occur to exclude the possibility of an epidural haematoma. The earlier advice of Vandermeulan et al. that catheter removal should be delayed 10–12 hours after a dose of LMWH and subsequent dosing should not occur for at least two hours after catheter removal appears to be far more reasonable.[91]

Dextran has the risks of fluid overload and anaphylactoid reactions. It is best avoided in patients with a history of allergy, hypersensitivity reactions, and asthma. It is believed that fibrin formed in the presence of dextran is not crosslinked. Dextran also affects platelet function by reducing adhesiveness and aggregation. It may be possible to increase the risk of bleeding in the epidural space following regional block. It can also affect crossmatching. Although a compilation of a number of studies showed that it was effective in reducing the number of PTEs, its effect on DVT incidence is relatively small.[86] Consequently it is rarely indicated.

Aspirin has limited efficacy in reducing the incidence of DVTs. Minidose warfarin has been used with effective results in gynaecological patients. Full-dose warfarin has also been used but the increased risk of bleeding and need for blood tests has excluded its use in all but the very high-risk patient.[87]

Risk assessment of patients should occur following a hospital protocol (Table 9.1). Preferably this should be done at a preanaesthetic clinic. Treatment options can then be discussed with the patient before admission. If a neuroaxial block is planned, instructions as to the timing of heparin or alternative treatment should be clearly communicated in the patient's notes and to the gynaecological and nursing staff. All patients should be encouraged to mobilise early if possible and dehydration should be avoided. As it has a number of advantages, LMWH (dose of enoxaparin 20 mg/day, dalteparin 2500 U/day or equivalent) should probably be preferred to unfractionated heparin in patients at moderate risk. An alternative regime would be graduated elastic compression stockings and intermittent pneumatic compression. In high-risk patients the dose of LMWH should be doubled and one of the mechanical methods added. In moderate and high-risk patients the thromboprophylaxis should start before surgery and preferably continue until discharge. It may need to continue following discharge in some patients at particularly high risk.

References

1 Raeder JC. Propofol anaesthesia versus paracervical blockade with alfentanil and midazolam sedation for outpatient abortion. *Acta Anaesthesiol Scand* 1992;**36**:31–7.
2 Jakobsson J, Oddby E, Rane K. Patient evaluation of four different combinations of intravenous anaesthetics for short outpatient procedures. *Anaesthesia* 1993;**48**:1005–7.
3 Cade L, Ross AW. Is fentanyl effective for postoperative analgesia in day-surgery? *Anaesth Intens Care* 1992;**20**:38–40.
4 Alexander GD, Noe FE, Brown EM. Anesthesia for pelvic laparoscopy. *Anesth Analg* 1969;**48**:14–18.
5 Swann DG, Spens H, Edwards SA, *et al.* Anaesthesia for gynaecological laparoscopy – a comparison between the laryngeal mask airway and tracheal intubation. *Anaesthesia* 1993;**48**:431–4.
6 Brimacombe JR, Brain AIJ, Berry AM, eds. *The laryngeal mask airway: a review and practical guide.* London: WB Saunders, 1997.

341

7 Griffin RM, Hatcher IS. Aspiration pneumonia and the laryngeal mask airway. *Anaesthesia* 1990;**45**:1039–40.

8 Valentine J, Stakes AF, Bellamy MC. Reflux during positive pressure ventilation through the laryngeal mask. *Br J Anaesth* 1994;**73**:543–4.

9 Zarmakoupis PN, Duvivier R, Schulman H. Office tubal sterilisation. *J Am Assoc Gynecol Laparosc* 1994;**1** (suppl):S40.

10 Green CR, Pandit SK, Levy L, et al. Intraoperative ketorolac has an opioid-sparing effect in women after diagnostic laparoscopy but not after laparoscopic tubal ligation. *Anesth Analg* 1996;**82**:732–7.

11 Tool AL, Kammerer-Doak DN, Ngyuen CM, et al. Postoperative pain relief following laparoscopic sterilization with silastic bands. *Obstet Gynecol* 1997;**90**:731–4.

12 Watcha MF, White PF. New antiemetic drugs. *Int Anesthesiol Clin* 1995;**33**:1–20.

13 Watcha MF, White PF. Postoperative nausea and vomiting. Its etiology, treatment and prevention. *Anesthesiology* 1992;**77**:162–84.

14 Raftery S, Sherry E. Total intravenous anaesthesia with propofol and alfentanil protects against postoperative nausea and vomiting. *Can J Anaesth* 1992;**39**:37–40.

15 Zelcer J, Wells DG. Anaesthetic related recovery room complications. *Anaesth Intens Care* 1987;**15**:168–74.

16 Cohen MM, Cameron CB, Duncan PG. Paediatric anaesthetic morbidity and mortality in the perioperative period. *Anesth Analg* 1990;**70**:160–7.

17 Kamath B, Curran J, Hawkey C, et al. Anaesthesia, movement, and emesis. *Br J Anaesth* 1990;**64**:728–30.

18 Honkavaara P, Lehtinen A, Hovorka J, et al. Nausea and vomiting after gynaecological laparoscopy depends on the phase of the menstrual cycle. *Can J Anaesth* 1991;**38**:876–9.

19 Eriksson H, Haasio J, Korttila K. Recovery from sevoflurane and isoflurane anaesthesia after outpatient gynaecological laparoscopy. *Acta Anaesthesiol Scand* 1995;**39**:377–80.

20 Raeder J, Gupta A, Pederson FM. Recovery characteristics of sevoflurane- or propofol-based anaesthesia for day-care surgery. *Acta Anaesthesiol Scand* 1997;**41**:988–94.

21 Divatia JV, Vaidya JS, Badwe RA, et al. Omission of nitrous oxide during anesthesia reduces the incidence of postoperative nausea and vomiting: a meta-analysis. *Anesthesiology* 1996;**85**:1055–62.

22 Edwards ND, Barclay K, Catling SJ, et al. Day case laparoscopy: a survey of postoperative pain and an assessment of the value of diclofenac. *Anaesthesia* 1991;**46**:1077–80.

23 Rowbotham DJ. Current management of postoperative nausea and vomiting. *Br J Anaesth* 1992;**69** (suppl):S46–S49.

24 Rothenberg DM, Parnass SM, Litwack K, et al. Efficacy of ephedrine in the prevention of postoperative nausea and vomiting. *Anesth Analg* 1991;**72**:58–61.

25 Haigh CG, Kaplan LA, Durham JM, et al. Nausea and vomiting after gynaecological surgery: a meta-analysis of factors affecting their incidence. *Br J Anaesth* 1993;**71**:517–22.

26 Tramer MR, Moore RA, Reynolds DJM, et al. A quantitative systematic review of ondansetron in treatment of established postoperative nausea and vomiting. *BMJ* 1997;**314**:1088–92.

27 Malins AF, Field JM, Nesling PM, et al. Nausea and vomiting after gynaecological laparoscopy: comparison of premedication with oral ondansetron, metoclopramide and placebo. *Br J Anaesth* 1993;**72**:231–3.

28 Sniadach MS, Alberts MS. A comparison of the prophylactic antiemetic effect of ondansetron and droperidol on patients undergoing gynecologic laparoscopy. *Anesth Analg* 1997;**85**:797–800.

29 Tang J, Watcha MF, Mehernoor F, et al. A comparison of costs and efficacy of ondansetron and droperidol as prophylactic antiemetic therapy for elective outpatient gynecologic procedures. *Anesth Analg* 1996;**83**:304–13.

30 Capouet V, de Pauw C, Vernet B, et al. Single dose i.v. tropisetron in the prevention of postoperative nausea and vomiting after gynaecological surgery. *Br J Anaesth* 1996;**76**:54–60.

31 Purhonen S, Kauko M, Koski EMJ, et al. Comparison of tropisetron, droperidol, and saline in the prevention of postoperative nausea and vomiting after gynecologic surgery. *Anesth Analg* 1997;**84**:662–7.

32 Fujii Y, Tanaka H, Toyooka H. The effects of dexamethasone on antiemetics in female patients undergoing gynecologic surgery. *Anesth Analg* 1997;**85**:913–17.

33 Stanley G, Appadu B, Mead M, *et al*. Dose requirements, efficacy and side-effects of morphine and pethidine delivered by patient-controlled analgesia after gynaecological surgery. *Br J Anaesth* 1996;**76**:484–6.

34 Macintyre PE, Jarvis DA. Age is the best predictor of postoperative morphine. *Pain* 1996;**64**:357–64.

35 Mansfield MD, James KS, Kinsella J. Influence of dose and timing of administration of morphine on postoperative pain and analgesic requirements. *Br J Anaesth* 1996;**76**:358–61.

36 Scott RM, Jennings PN. Rectal diclofenac analgesia after abdominal hysterectomy. *Aust NZ J Obstet Gynaecol* 1997;**37**:112–14.

37 Balestrieri P, Simmons G, Hill D, *et al*. The effect of intravenous ketorolac given intraoperatively versus postoperatively on outcome from gynecologic abdominal surgery. *J Clin Anesth* 1997;**9**:358–64.

38 Montgomery JE, Sutherland CJ, Kestin IG, *et al*. Morphine consumption in patients receiving rectal paracetamol and diclofenac alone and in combination. *Br J Anaesth* 1996;**77**:445–7.

39 Dakin MJ, Osinubi OY, Carli F. Preoperative spinal bupivacaine does not reduce postoperative morphine requirement in women undergoing total abdominal hysterectomy. *Reg Anesth* 1996;**21**:99–102.

40 Espinet A, Henderson DJ, Faccenda KA, *et al*. Does pre-incisional thoracic extradural block combined with diclofenac reduce postoperative pain after abdominal hysterectomy? *Br J Anaesth* 1996;**76**:209–13.

41 Eriksson-Mjoberg M, Svensson JO, Almkvist O, *et al*. Extradural morphine gives better pain relief than patient-controlled i.v. morphine after hysterectomy. *Br J Anaesth* 1997;**78**:10–16.

42 Ding Y, Fredman, B, White PF. Use of ketorolac and fentanyl during outpatient gynecologic surgery. *Anesth Analg* 1993;**77**:205–10.

43 White PF, Joshi GP, Carpenter RL, *et al*. A comparison of ketorolac and hydrocodone-acetominophen for analgesia after ambulatory surgery: arthroscopy versus laparoscopic tubal ligation. *Anesth Analg* 1997;**85**:37–43.

44 Gillberg LE, Harsten AS, Stahl LB. Preoperative diclofenac sodium reduces post-laparoscopy pain. *Can J Anaesth* 1993;**40**:406–8.

45 Pollard RC, Cooper GM. The laryngeal mask in day surgery: a survey of current practices and usage. *Ambulatory Surg* 1995;**3**:37–42.

46 Carron Brown JA, Chamberlain GVP, Jordon JA, *et al*. *Gynaecological laparoscopy*. Report of the Working Party of the Confidential Enquiry into Gynaecological Laparoscopy. London: Royal College of Obstetricians and Gynaecologists, 1978.

47 Jansen FW, Kapiteyen K, Trimbos-Kemper T, *et al*. Complications of laparoscopy: a prospective multicentre observational study. *Br J Obstet Gynaecol* 1997;**104**:595–600.

48 Joshi GP, Inagaki Y, White PF, *et al*. Use of the laryngeal mask airway as an alternative to the tracheal tube during ambulatory anesthesia. *Anesth Analg* 1997;**85**:573–7.

49 Brimacombe JR, Berry A. The incidence of aspiration associated with the laryngeal mask airway: a meta-analysis of published literature. *J Clin Anesth* 1995;**7**:297–305.

50 Blackshear R, Gravenstein N. Positioning the surgical patient. In: Kirby RR, Gravenstein N, eds. *Clinical anaesthetic practice*. Philadelphia: WB Saunders, 1994.

51 Warner MA, Martin JT, Schroeder DR, *et al*. Lower-extremity motor neuropathy associated with surgery performed on patients in a lithotomy position. *Anesthesiology* 1994;**81**:6–12.

52 Strunin L. How long should patients fast before surgery? Time for new guidelines. *Br J Anaesth* 1993;**70**:1–3.

53 Maltby JR, Lewis P, Martin A, Sutherland LR. Gastric fluid volume and pH in elective patients following unrestricted oral fluid until three hours before surgery. *Can J Anaesth* 1991;**38**:425–9.

54 Phillips S, Hutchinson S, Davidson T. Preoperative drinking does not affect gastric contents. *Br J Anaesth* 1993;**70**:6–9.

55 Whitehead EM, Smith M, Dean Y, *et al*. An evaluation of gastric emptying times in pregnancy and the puerperium. *Anaesthesia* 1993;**48**:53–7.

56 Lam KK, So HY, Gin T. Gastric pH and volume after oral fluids in the postpartum patient. *Can J Anaesth* 1993;**40**:218–21.

343

57 Yogendran S, Asokumar B, Cheng DCH, *et al.* A prospective randomized double-blinded study of the effect of intravenous fluid therapy on adverse outcomes on outpatient surgery. *Anesth Analg* 1995;**80**:682–6.

58 Rudkin GE, Bacon AK, Burrow B, *et al.* Review of efficiencies and patient satisfaction in Australian and New Zealand day surgery units: a pilot study. *Anaesth Intens Care* 1996;**24**:74–8.

59 Ananthanarayan C, Paek W, Dhanidina K. Hysteroscopy and anaesthesia. *Can J Anaesth* 1996;**43**:56–64.

60 Garry R. Endometrial ablation and resection; validation of a new surgical concept. *Br J Obstet Gynaecol* 1997;**104**:1329–31.

61 Lewis BW. Radiofrequency induced endometrial ablation. *Baillière's Clin Obstet Gynaecol* 1995;**9**:347–55.

62 Williamson KM, Mushambai MC. Complications of hysteroscopic treatments of menorrhagia (editorial). *Br J Anaesth* 1996;**77**:305–7.

63 McSwiney M, Myatt J, Hargraves M. Transcervical resection syndrome. *Anaesthesia* 1995;**50**:254–8.

64 Ariel AI. Management of hyponatraemia. *BMJ* 1993;**307**:305–8.

65 Chui PT, Gin T, Oh TE. Anaesthesia for laparoscopic general surgery. *Anaesth Intens Care* 1993;**21**:163–71.

66 Williamson JA, Webb RK, Russell WJ, *et al.* Air embolism – an analysis of 2000 incident reports. *Anaesth Intens Care* 1993;**21**:638–41.

67 Sharma KC, Brandstetter RD, Brensilver JM, *et al.* Cardiopulmonary physiology and pathophysiology as a consequence of laparoscopic surgery. *Chest* 1996;**110**:810–15.

68 Kelman GR, Swapp GH, Smith I, *et al.* Cardiac output and arterial blood-gas tension during laparoscopy. *Br J Anaesth* 1972;**44**:1155–62.

69 Hirvonen EA, Nuutinten LS, Kauko M. Ventilatory effects, blood gas changes, and oxygen consumption during laparoscopic hysterectomy. *Anesth Analg* 1995;**80**:961–6.

70 Day R. Epidemiology in gynaecological oncology. In: Shaw R, Soutter P, Stanton S, eds. *Gynaecology*. London: Churchill Livingstone, 1992.

71 Mahoney PF, Hassen A, Conacher ID. Pleural effusions and anaesthesia. *Anaesthesia* 1994;**49**(7):650.

72 Waid-Jones MI, Coursin DB. Perioperative considerations for patients treated with bleomycin. *Chest* 1991;**99**:993–9.

73 McConnell MS, Finn JC, Feeley TW. Tension hydrothorax during laparoscopy in a patient with ascites. *Anesthesiology* 1994;**80**:1390–3.

74 Rustin GJS. Trophoblastic disease. In: Shaw R, Soutter P, Stanton S, eds. *Gynaecology*. London: Churchill Livingstone, 1992.

75 Williamson K, Mushambai MC. Ovarian hyperstimulation syndrome (editorial). *Br J Anaesth* 1994;**73**:731–3.

76 Alsalili M, Thornton S, Fleming S. The effect of the anaesthetic, propofol on in-vitro oocyte maturation, fertilization and cleavage in mice. *Human Reprod* 1997;**12**:1271–4.

77 Medical Research International, Society for Assisted Reproductive Technology. the American Fertility Society. Embryo transfer (IVF-ET) in the United States: 1990 results from the IVF-ET Registry. *Fertil Steril* 1992;**57**:15–24.

78 Brinsden PR, Wada I, Tan SL, Balen A, Jacobs HS. Diagnosis, prevention and management of ovarian hyperstimulation syndrome. *Br J Obstet Gynaecol* 1995;**102**:767–72.

79 Shaw RW, Bonnar J, Greer IA, *et al. Report of RCOG working party on thromboprophylaxis in obstetrics and gynaecology*. London: Chameleon, 1995.

80 Vessey MP, Mant D, Smith A, *et al.* Oral contraceptives and venous thromboembolism: findings in a large prospective study. *BMJ* 1986;**292**:526.

81 Guillebebaud J. Surgery and the pill. *BMJ* 1985;**291**:498–9.

82 Thromboembolic Risk Factors (THRIFT) Consensus Group. Risk of and prophylaxis for thromboembolism in hospital patients. *BMJ* 1992;**305**:567–74.

83 Gallimore SC, Hoile RW, Ingram GS, *et al. The report of the national confidential enquiry into perioperative deaths 1994/1995*. London: National CEPOD, 1997.

84 Clagett GP, Anderson FA, Heit J, *et al.* Prevention of venous thromboembolism. *Chest* 1995;**108**:312S–328S.

85 Clarke-Pearson, Delong ER, Synan IS, *et al.* Variables associated with postoperative deep

venous thrombosis: a prospective study of 411 gynaecological patients and creation of a prognostic model. *Obstet Gynecol* 1987;**69**:146–50.

86 Consensus Statement. Prevention of venous thromboembolism. *Int Angiogr* 1997;**16**:3–38.

87 Greer IA. Epidemiology, risk factors and prophylaxis of venous thrombo-embolism in obstetrics and gynaecology. *Baillère's Clin Obstet Gynaecol* 1997;**11**:403–30.

88 Clarke-Pearson DL, Synan IS, Dodge R, *et al.* A randomised trial of low-dose heparin and intermittent pneumatic calf compression for the prevention of deep venous thrombosis after gynaecological oncology surgery. *Am J Obstet Gynecol* 1993;**168**:1146–54.

89 FDA Public Health Advisory. Reports of epidural or spinal hematomas with the concurrent use of low molecular weight heparin and spinal/epidural anaesthesia or spinal puncture. Washington DC: US Department of Health and Human Services, 1997.

90 Horlocker TT, Heit JA. Low molecular weight heparin: biochemical, pharmacology, perioperative prophylaxis regimens and guidelines for regional anaesthetic management. *Anesth Analg* 1997;**85**:874–85.

91 Vandermeulan EP, van Aken H, Vermylan J. Anticoagulants and spinal-epidural anesthesia. *Anesth Analg* 1994;**79**:1165–77.

Index